Respiratory Medicine

Series Editor:
Sharon I.S. Rounds

More information about this series at http://www.springer.com/series/7665

Janet S. Lee • Michael P. Donahoe
Editors

Hematologic Abnormalities and Acute Lung Syndromes

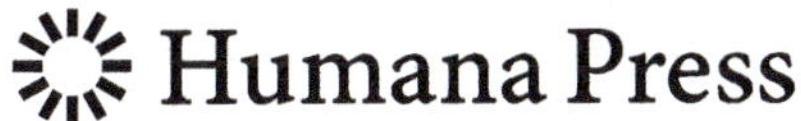

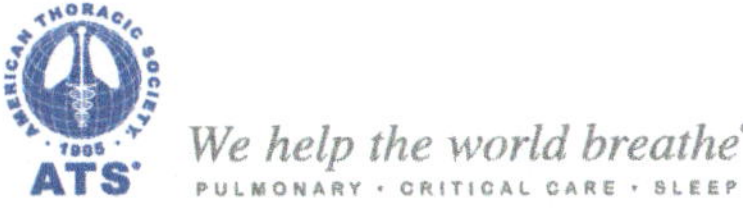

Editors
Janet S. Lee, MD
Professor of Medicine
Division of Pulmonary, Allergy, and Critical Care Medicine
Department of Medicine
University of Pittsburgh School of Medicine
Pittsburgh, PA, USA

Michael P. Donahoe, MD
Professor of Medicine
Division of Pulmonary, Allergy, and Critical Care Medicine
Department of Medicine
University of Pittsburgh School of Medicine
Pittsburgh, PA, USA

ISSN 2197-7372 ISSN 2197-7380 (electronic)
Respiratory Medicine
ISBN 978-3-319-41910-7 ISBN 978-3-319-41912-1 (eBook)
DOI 10.1007/978-3-319-41912-1

Library of Congress Control Number: 2016951643

Printed on acid-free paper

This Humana Press imprint is published by Springer Nature
The registered company is Springer International Publishing AG Switzerland

Preface

Standard textbooks in Respiratory Medicine do not typically organize their contents to specifically address hematologic abnormalities in acute lung syndromes. However, the main function of the lung is gas exchange at the interface between the external environment and blood. Thus, by definition, blood and its components are an integral part of the lungs and, given the large surface area of the pulmonary vascular beds, the lungs harbor a significant fraction of the circulating blood volume at any one time. While red cells are the vehicles for gas transfer, platelets provide hemostasis, and leukocytes vital for lung homeostasis and immunity, components of the hematopoietic system, can also serve as agents of injury to the lungs in disease states. So, it is not surprising that primary hematologic disorders or disorders secondary to immunopathology can lead to acute lung dysfunction. The purpose of this book is to provide a unique framework for acute lung syndromes that arise from hematologic disorders or is defined by a hematologic abnormality as a key feature. These acute lung processes can present as life-threatening conditions, and as such, the pulmonary physician or critical care physician is often directly involved in their care or called upon to provide expertise.

The book emphasizes the pathogenesis and current understanding of mechanisms and is organized into three parts. It begins with an overview containing the central theme of the lungs as the direct interface between the external environment and blood and a description of individual components of the hematopoietic system, their function, and relevance to the lungs. The overview also discusses the concept of the lungs as an organ site of leukocyte sequestration and a target organ of injury and how cells of hematopoietic origin can serve as agents of injury. The second part of the book focuses upon primary hematologic disorders that can lead to acute pulmonary manifestations. This section is organized by benign and malignant hematologic disorders and the specific clinical entities affecting the lungs associated with these disorders. The third part of the book focuses upon transfusion-related complications occurring in the ICU setting.

These chapters provide a unique framework for discussing unusual clinical entities encountered largely in the acute hospital setting. These acute pulmonary syndromes are typically not organized in such a way for easy reference. However, recent advances in medicine have allowed for patients with severe comorbidities such as sickle cell anemia, hemophilia, hematologic malignancies, or immunopathologies to survive, and thus many of the syndromes discussed have not had full representation in respiratory medicine textbooks historically. Thus, the book encompasses disease entities that specialists will encounter. The book is written in detail, emphasizing primary literature and pathophysiology, and catered to clinicians who take care of these patients.

Pittsburgh, PA, USA Janet S. Lee, MD
Pittsburgh, PA, USA Michael P. Donahoe, MD

Contents

Contributors

Afua Darkwah Abrahams, MBChB, FWACP Department of Pathology, University of Ghana Medical School and Korle Bu Teaching Hospital, University of Ghana, Accra, Ghana

Olufolake Adetoro Adisa, MD Department of Pediatrics, Emory University, Atlanta, GA, USA

Margaret F. Bennewitz, PhD Division of Pulmonary, Allergy and Critical Care Medicine, Pittsburgh Heart, Lung, and Blood Vascular Medicine Institute, University of Pittsburgh School of Medicine, Pittsburgh, PA, USA

Guang-Shing Cheng, MD Fred Hutchinson Cancer Research Center, University of Washington School of Medicine, Seattle, WA, USA

Michael P. Donahoe, MD Division of Pulmonary, Allergy, and Critical Care Medicine, Department of Medicine, University of Pittsburgh School of Medicine, Pittsburgh, PA, USA

Andra Fee-Mulhearn, DO, MPH Division of Pulmonary, Allergy, Critical Care and Sleep Medicine, The Ohio State University, Columbus, OH, USA

Stefanie Forest, MD, PhD Department of Pathology and Cell Biology at Columbia University Medical Center, New York Presbyterian Hospital, New York, NY, USA

Mario V. Fusaro, MD Division of Telehealth, Division of Pulmonary and Critical Care Medicine, Westchester Medical Center, Valhalla, NY, USA

Division of Pulmonary and Critical Care Medicine, Department of Medicine, and Department of Epidemiology and Public Health, University of Maryland School of Medicine, Baltimore, MD, USA

Samit Ghosh, PhD Division of Hematology/Oncology, Department of Medicine, University of Pittsburgh School of Medicine, Pittsburgh, PA, USA

Shani Gunning-Carter, MD Division of Hematology/Oncology, Department of Medicine, Monongahela Valley Hospital, Monongahela, PA, USA

Eldad A. Hod, MD Department of Pathology and Cell Biology at Columbia University Medical Center, New York Presbyterian Hospital, New York, NY, USA

Nicole P. Juffermans, MD, PhD Laboratory of Experimental Intensive Care and Anesthesiology, Department of Intensive Care Medicine, Academic Medical Center, Amsterdam, The Netherlands

Gregory J. Kato, MD Division of Hematology-Oncology, Department of Medicine, Monongahela Valley Hospital, Monongahela, PA, USA

Division of Hematology/Oncology, Pittsburgh Heart, Lung, and Blood Vascular Medicine Institute, Department of Medicine, University of Pittsburgh School of Medicine, Pittsburgh, PA, USA

Janet S. Lee, MD Division of Pulmonary, Allergy, and Critical Care Medicine, Pittsburgh Heart, Lung, and Blood Vascular Medicine Institute, Department of Medicine, University of Pittsburgh School of Medicine, Pittsburgh, PA, USA

Roberto Machado, MD Division of Pulmonary, Critical Care, Sleep and Allergy, Department of Medicine, University of Illinois College of Medicine at Chicago, Chicago, IL, USA

Department of Pharmacology, University of Illinois at Chicago, Chicago, IL, USA

David K. Madtes, MD Fred Hutchinson Cancer Research Center, University of Washington School of Medicine, Seattle, WA, USA

Hannah C. Mannem, MD Division of Pulmonary, Allergy, and Critical Care Medicine, Department of Medicine, University of Pittsburgh School of Medicine, Pittsburgh, PA, USA

Patrick Nana-Sinkam, MD Division of Pulmonary, Allergy, Critical Care and Sleep Medicine, The Ohio State University, Columbus, OH, USA

Division of Medical Oncology, The Ohio State University, Columbus, OH, USA

James Thoracic Oncology Center, The Ohio State University, Columbus, OH, USA

Faculty Advancement, Mentorship and Engagement, Center for FAME, The Ohio State University, Columbus, OH, USA

Giora Netzer, MD, MSCE Division of Pulmonary and Critical Care Medicine, Department of Medicine, and Department of Epidemiology and Public Health, University of Maryland School of Medicine, Baltimore, MD, USA

Solomon Fiifi Ofori-Acquah, PhD Department of Pathology, University of Ghana Medical School and Korle Bu Teaching Hospital University of Ghana, Accra, Ghana

Center for Translational and International Hematology, Pittsburgh Heart, Lung, and Blood Vascular Medicine Institute, University of Pittsburgh, Pittsburgh, PA, USA

Amma Owusu-Ansah, MD, MBBS Division of Hematology/Oncology, Department of Medicine, University of Pittsburgh School of Medicine, Pittsburgh, PA, USA

Margaret V. Ragni, MD Division of Hematology/Oncology, Department of Medicine, University of Pittsburgh School of Medicine, Pittsburgh, PA, USA

Francesca Rapido, MD Department of Pathology and Cell Biology at Columbia University Medical Center, New York Presbyterian Hospital, New York, NY, USA

Department of Medical Surgical Pathophysiology and Organ Transplantation, Universita' degli Studi di Milano, Milan, Italy

Belinda Rivera-Lebron, MD, MS Division of Pulmonary, Allergy, and Critical Care Medicine, Department of Medicine, University of Pittsburgh School of Medicine, Pittsburgh, PA, USA

Craig D. Seaman, MD Division of Hematology/Oncology, Department of Medicine, University of Pittsburgh School of Medicine, Pittsburgh, PA, USA

Prithu Sundd, PhD Division of Pulmonary, Allergy and Critical Care Medicine, Pittsburgh Heart, Lung, and Blood Vascular Medicine Institute, University of Pittsburgh School of Medicine, Pittsburgh, PA, USA

Justin R. Sysol, BS Division of Pulmonary, Critical Care, Sleep and Allergy, Department of Medicine, University of Illinois College of Medicine at Chicago, Chicago, IL, USA

Department of Pharmacology, University of Illinois at Chicago, Chicago, IL, USA

Eleftherios C. Vamvakas, MD, PhD, MPH Formerly, Rita and Taft Schreiber Chair in Transfusion Medicine, Cedars-Sinai Medical Center, Los Angeles, CA, USA

Alexander P. Vlaar, MD, PhD Laboratory of Experimental Intensive Care and Anesthesiology, Department of Intensive Care Medicine, Academic Medical Center, Amsterdam, The Netherlands

Peng Zhang, MD Division of Pulmonary, Allergy, and Critical Care Medicine, Pittsburgh Heart, Lung, and Blood Vascular Medicine Institute, Department of Medicine, University of Pittsburgh School of Medicine, Pittsburgh, PA, USA

Part I
Overview

Chapter 1
The Lung–Blood Interface

Peng Zhang and Janet S. Lee

Introduction

The central function of the lung is to perform gas exchange, that is, to deliver oxygen from the air to the blood, and to remove carbon dioxide from the blood back to the external environment. The unique organizational features of the lung, such as branching airways that enable the creation of a large surface area for gas exchange, and the ultrastructure of the alveolar membrane to facilitate diffusion, support this central function. As the lungs are in direct contact with the external environment, the lungs are exposed to inhaled particulate matter, antigens, noxious gases, and microbial pathogens. Thus, it is no wonder that the lungs are characterized by a sophisticated host defense mechanism comprised of the mucociliary clearance system, the epithelial barrier, alveolar macrophages that survey the airspaces, and secretion of molecules that facilitate recognition of danger signals and removal of foreign particles, damaged cells, cellular debris, and pathogens.

In addition, the large surface area of the pulmonary vascular beds allows for the lungs to harbor a significant fraction of the circulating blood volume at any one time. However, the unique features of the lung architecture that define its core function of gas exchange may also predispose the lungs to injury. While red cells are the vehicles for gas transfer, platelets provide hemostasis, and macrophages vital for lung homeostasis and immunity, abnormalities of the hematopoietic system can serve to incite or propagate injury to the lungs in disease states. So, it is not surprising that primary hematologic disorders or disorders secondary to immunopathology can lead to acute lung dysfunction or worsen existing conditions. This chapter

P. Zhang, MD • J.S. Lee, MD (✉)
Division of Pulmonary, Allergy, and Critical Care Medicine, Pittsburgh Heart, Lung, and Blood Vascular Medicine Institute, Department of Medicine, University of Pittsburgh School of Medicine, Pittsburgh, PA, USA
e-mail: leejs3@upmc.edu

J.S. Lee, M.P. Donahoe (eds.), *Hematologic Abnormalities and Acute Lung Syndromes*, Respiratory Medicine, DOI 10.1007/978-3-319-41912-1_1

discusses the central theme of the lungs as the direct interface between the external environment and blood. Thus, the focus is to introduce the readers to the physiologic principles that govern lung structure–function relationships, but is in no way intended to be comprehensive. For a more in-depth understanding, we refer the readers to some excellent reviews [1–4].

Airway Structure

The airway of the human lungs, similar to other mammalian lungs, is a dichotomous branching system. For human lungs, there are on average 23 generations of branching airways, as shown by the airway diagram in Fig. 1.1 [5]. However, due to inter-individual variations in the shape of the thoracic cavity, the actual number of branched airways in the human lung is between 18 and 30 generations [5]. The terminology of the branching airways has changed little since the original description by ER Weibel and depicted in Fig. 1.1. The first few generations of airways are termed bronchi, and are characterized by the presence of cartilage. The next few generations of branching airways are termed bronchioles, and they are defined histologically by the absence of cartilage. The last generation of conducting airways is terminal bronchioles that begin roughly at generation fourteen. The generation of airway branching that follows the terminal bronchioles is referred as the transitional bronchiole. The airway diameter relative to the airway generation is presumed to be different above and below the transitional bronchiole [6].

Alveoli begin to appear within the walls of the transitional bronchiole, and gradually increase in number in the next several generations of airway branching, i.e., respiratory bronchioles, before alveolar ducts appear and terminate into alveolar sacs. The boundary between respiratory bronchioles and alveolar ducts is somewhat arbitrary, as it relies on the relative degree of "alveolarization." An airway is considered an alveolar duct when alveoli completely cover the airway [7]. The last eight generations of airways are together referred to as the acinus. In the human lungs, there are approximately 30,000 acini, with an average volume of 187 mm^3 (SD: ± 79 mm^3) [8]. These acini comprise a total of approximately eight million end branches, also known as alveolar sacs, and these alveolar sacs finally connect to approximately 300 million alveoli. Contrary to the common model of "parallel alveoli," where all the alveoli are arranged at the end of alveolar sacs, alveoli actually start to appear in the last six to nine generations of airways [9, 10].

When comparing airway structures between different species, the most noticeable difference lies in the number of terminal bronchioles, which is the result of differences in generations of airway branching. This is largely determined by the size and shape of the thoracic cavity [1]. Another difference is the presence or absence of respiratory bronchioles [7]. In humans, there are approximately 1–3 generations of respiratory bronchioles before the appearance of alveolar ducts. However, rats and mice, which represent common animal model systems, possess only either one generation of respiratory bronchioles or are absent [7]. When these animals are

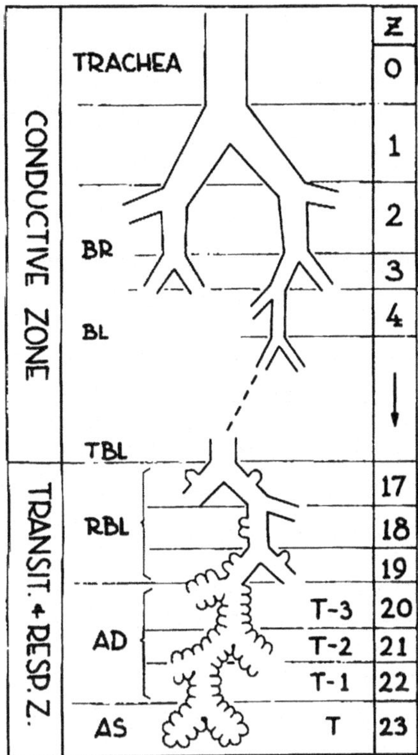

Fig. 1.1 Diagram of the human airway system. There are 23 generations of branching airways on average, beginning with larger airways in the conducting zone, consisting of the trachea, bronchi (BR), bronchioles (BL), and finally terminal bronchioles and transitional bronchioles (TBL). The acinar airways begin to appear following the TBL, with respiratory bronchioles (RBL), alveolar ducts (AD) that terminate into alveolar sacs (AS). (Used with permission from Weibel ER: Morphometry of the Human Lung. Heidelberg: Springer-Verlag; 1963)

used to study human diseases such as cigarette smoke-induced emphysema, which are presumed to originate in the respiratory bronchioles [11], one needs to consider anatomical differences of the model system.

Effective gas exchange depends on the large surface area of the alveolar membrane. This is made possible by arranging alveoli closely along the alveolar ducts, allowing for a large number of alveoli within the relatively confined space of the thoracic cavity. Another advantage of having this arrangement is to minimize the distance for oxygen molecules to diffuse before coming into contact with the alveolar membrane. In fact, the average longitudinal distance from transitional bronchiole to the alveolar sacs, is approximately 8.3 mm (SD: ±1.4 mm) [8, 10].

Features of the Blood Vessel Tree

As the airway tree branches, so does the vascular tree. The pulmonary artery follows the airway tree closely, although the arterial vascular tree branches more frequently than the airway [3]. Compared with an average of 23 airway generations, there are approximately 28 generations of the pulmonary arterial branching within the human lung [3]. The pulmonary artery begins as a single trunk, branches into 70 million pre-capillary arterioles, and terminates into approximately 280 billion capillary segments [12]. At any given moment, there are approximately 200 ml of capillary blood volume bathing the entire alveolar surface [12].

As the artery branches, the accessory structures of the vessel wall also change. The walls of the major pulmonary arteries consist of a large number of collagen and elastic lamina, so they can sustain the pressure generated by the cardiac output from the right ventricle [13]. Vessels surrounded by smooth muscle fibers begin to appear when the vascular diameter falls below 1 mm [13]. The smooth muscle fibers enable these small arteries to regulate blood flow via constriction and dilation [13]. As the pulmonary artery continues to branch, the muscular wall gradually tapers until there is only one layer of smooth muscle, marking the appearance of arterioles [14]. Eventually, the muscular wall becomes incomplete, and this defines the pre-capillary region [14]. In general, the amount of smooth muscle along the pulmonary arterial wall is less compared with systemic arteries, which contributes to the low resistance of the pulmonary artery tree [1]. In the more peripheral region of the human lung, the pulmonary vein travels closely with the artery and airway within the bronchovascular bundle [13]. In the more central region of the lung, the veins travel separately to the hilum from the artery and airway [13]. For cow, pig, and sheep lung, the pulmonary veins travel along with the airway and artery within the bronchovascular bundle. For smaller mammals such as rabbit, guinea pig, and rat, the pulmonary veins course independently from the airway–artery bundle [15, 16]. Compared with the capillary networks of other organ systems, the structure of the pulmonary capillary network is quite unique. Rather than an individual capillary unit interacting with a discrete alveolar unit, pulmonary capillaries are spread across the alveolar surface of multiple alveolar units [12]. This structure of the pulmonary capillary network maximizes the contact surface area between alveolar membrane and the capillary blood for oxygenation, and minimizes the extent of shunting [10].

Bronchial Artery System

The bronchial artery system normally accounts for ~1 % of cardiac output, and mainly functions to deliver nutritive support to the large airway and vessels under basal conditions [17]. At the level of alveoli and respiratory bronchioles, bronchial arteries form connections with the pulmonary arteries via microvascular anastomoses, and create physiological shunts in the lung, as bronchial arteries do not participate in gas exchange [18]. The bronchial artery system is also a high-pressure system compared with the pulmonary arterial system [17]. Thus, when pathological changes occur in the pulmonary artery, increased bronchopulmonary collaterals and collateral blood flow may form, diverting more blood from the cardiac output through bronchopulmonary shunts, and, if significant, compromise blood oxygenation [19]. Some conditions that are associated with bronchial artery dilatation include bronchiectasis, primary pulmonary hypertension, lung cancer, Takayasu's arteritis, and chronic thromboembolic disease [1, 18]. In some extreme disease states such as in chronic thromboembolic disease, the percentage of cardiac output circulating through bronchopulmonary collaterals may increase by 18–30 % [20, 21].

Convection–Diffusion in Airway Conductance

Oxygen transport through the large airways occurs by convective, or bulk, flow [3]. As airway branches, the diameter of the airway decreases, but the degree of airway narrowing is not uniform [3]. The degree of airway narrowing in successive generations (i.e., the more peripheral regions of the lung) is less than that of the airway located in the central regions of the lung. As previously mentioned, the transition point where this occurs is at the level of the transitional bronchiole. In fact, the airway diameters of respiratory bronchioles and alveolar ducts change very little. Given that the number of airways doubles after each generation, the total cross-sectional area of the respiratory bronchioles and alveolar ducts rapidly increases. With a given volume of gas, the oxygen bulk flow will therefore decrease, to a point where it is slower than the rate of simple diffusion [22]. After this point, diffusion becomes the predominant process. This structure–function relationship is ideal, because the airway terminates into blind ends, and the only way oxygen is delivered to the peripheral lung is by diffusion [1]. In human lungs, at rest, the convection–diffusion transition point occurs at approximately the 14–16th generation of airway branching, which corresponds roughly to the transitional bronchiole or the first generation of respiratory bronchioles [3]. The diffusion-dominant zone in human lung at rest starts at approximately generation 16 [3]. During exercise, the point of convection–diffusion transition will move more peripherally, as the initial bulk flow (convection) velocity can increase by tenfold [1, 9, 10, 23].

Interdependence of Alveolar pO_2, and Independence of Arterial pO_2

In addition to the large contact surface area between the alveolar membrane and capillary blood, another important determinant of gas exchange is the pressure gradient of oxygen between alveolar (P_AO_2) and the capillary blood (P_aO_2) [1]. This pressure gradient is maintained by effective ventilation-diffusion in the airway to ensure high alveolar oxygen pressure, and sufficient capillary perfusion to supply deoxygenated blood that provides a lower capillary oxygen partial pressure [1, 4].

The acinar capillaries are arranged in parallel, so for each capillary unit, its oxygen partial pressure will be the same, and is independent of other capillary units [3]. On the contrary, alveoli first appear within the walls of the respiratory bronchiole, and are arranged in series along the acinar airway [3]. Given the finite amount of oxygen in each breath, the alveoli that are close to the entrance of the acinar airway will be ventilated first. As the oxygen diffuses across the blood-gas membrane of these proximal alveoli, the amount of oxygen that is left decreases, and therefore the alveolar oxygen partial pressure decreases as it moves towards more peripheral alveoli [23]. In other words, the P_AO_2 is interdependent between the proximal and distal alveoli [23]. About half the surface area of the gas-exchange membrane of an acinar airway is located in the last generation. If the gas-exchange membrane is too permeable to oxygen, then by the time oxygen reaches the last generation of airway, the P_AO_2 will be so low that little oxygen can diffuse across the membrane, and the peripheral gas-exchange surface is underutilized, or "screened," for diffusion [23]. If oxygen permeability of the alveolar membrane is too low, oxygen will require a much larger total surface area for gas-exchange to sustain metabolic activity of the organism, and this will require a larger thoracic cavity size [23]. With the convection–diffusion transition point moving more distally during exercise, less alveolar surface area is screened for diffusion, compared with the area being screened when the subject is at rest [23]. By mathematical modeling, others have shown that in human lungs, the relationship between oxygen permeability across the gas-exchange membrane and oxygen diffusion capacity in the distal airways provides functional reserve for oxygenation while avoiding strong diffusion screening at rest [9, 10, 23].

Oxygen Diffusion Capacity

The capacity of oxygen molecules to travel from alveolar air to red blood cells is called the oxygen diffusion capacity. It is comprised of two serial events, the first of which is the oxygen transfer across the blood-gas membrane by passive diffusion. The second event is the binding of oxygen to hemoglobin [1]. The surface area available for gas exchange, the extreme thinness of the membrane structure, and the oxygen partial pressure gradient across the alveolar and capillary compartment enhances diffusion capacity [24]. The binding of oxygen molecules to hemoglobin is determined by the biochemical properties of the hemoglobin, as well as the content of total hemoglobin that is available for oxygenation. Clinically, the oxygen diffusing capacity is reflected by the diffusing capacity of the lungs for carbon monoxide (DLCO) [25]. Carbon monoxide is chosen as the testing agent because of its high affinity to hemoglobin, and therefore the test result will not be sensitively affected by changes in cardiac output [25]. DLCO is the product of two measurements, the first measurement of which is the rate constant (K_{CO}), reflecting the rate of CO uptake from alveolar gas, and the second is the alveolar volume (V_A). K_{CO} is, by definition, a direct characterization of the diffusion capacity through the gas-exchange membrane and the binding of hemoglobin [25]. K_{CO} is reduced when there is pulmonary capillary destruction (i.e., pulmonary vasculitis), remodeling, and dilatation (i.e., pulmonary arteriovenous malformation), or alveolar destruction (such as emphysema), and increased when there is increased pulmonary blood volume (as seen in alveolar hemorrhage, congestive heart failure, left-to-right intracardiac shunts), or with reduced alveolar expansion (such as respiratory muscle weakness or pneumonectomy) [26]. The passage for CO_2 is similar but in reverse direction. Because CO_2 is more readily capable of diffusing across the blood-gas membrane than O_2, the exchange of CO_2 will not be impaired as long as there is enough ventilation [1].

Red Blood Cell as Vehicles of Gas Exchange

The principle carrier of oxygen in the blood is hemoglobin, which transports approximately 20 mL of oxygen per 100 mL of blood [4]. A small portion of oxygen (0.3 mL/100 mL) is directly dissolved in blood [4]. As the fraction of inspired oxygen (FiO_2) increases from 0.21 to 1.0, the oxygen partial pressure increases accordingly, and more oxygen is directly dissolved in the blood. When breathing in FiO_2 of 1.0, the directly dissolved oxygen reaches 2 mL/100 mL, and constitutes a more significant portion of the total oxygen carrying capacity of blood [4]. Hemoglobin A, the most prevalent hemoglobin in humans, is comprised of four globin proteins, two alpha and two beta globin subunits ($\alpha 2\beta 2$), noncovalently bound to each other to form a tetramer [27, 28]. A pocket is created within each globin subunit that contains heme, an iron-containing porphyrin, that binds molecular oxygen when iron is in the ferrous state [4]. The relationship between oxyhemoglobin, or the total % hemoglobin saturated with oxygen, and the partial pressure of oxygen follows a nonlinear sigmoidal-shaped curve [4]. This oxyhemoglobin disassociation curve reflects cooperative interaction between the four oxygen-binding sites resulting from conformational change of the hemoglobin structure upon binding the initial oxygen molecule that increases the affinity of hemoglobin for subsequent oxygen molecules until all four binding sites are saturated [28, 29]. The oxyhemoglobin disassociation curve encapsulates the essential function of red blood cells, that is, oxygen binding and ability to unload as a function of the partial pressure of oxygen. Hemoglobinopathies such as sickle cell anemia are single-gene mutations that lead to abnormal hemoglobin structure and can show altered oxyhemoglobin dissociation curve [30]. In sickle cell disease, sickling occurs under conditions of hypoxic stress [30]. As discussed in subsequent chapters, vaso-occlusive crisis due to the sickling of red blood cells within the pulmonary microvasculature contributes to the acute chest syndrome in sickle cell disease (see Chap. 3).

Ultrastructure of the Alveolus

There are several distinguishable cell populations comprising the alveolus, including type I alveolar epithelial (AE1), type II alveolar epithelial (AE2), and lung fibroblasts [5]. AE1 is flat and elongated, and is the main structural barrier for gas exchange together with the endothelial cell. AE2 cells are smaller and cuboidal in morphology, serve as the alveolar stem cell, and actively carry out metabolic and secretory functions, as well as immune defense, the latter function also modulated and executed by resident mononuclear phagocytes [31]. Finally, lung fibroblasts help maintain the alveolar structure by secreting extracellular matrix proteins [1, 32].

Type I Alveolar Epithelial Cells

The three determinants of effective gas exchange are (1) the large surface area of contact, (2) oxygen partial-pressure gradient across the alveolar and capillary blood, and (3) permeability of the airway-blood barrier [1]. As previously mentioned, the mammalian lung achieves the large surface area of gas exchange by generations of branching airways that end in alveoli [5]. A strategically located convection–diffusion transition point maintains an oxygen pressure gradient, as do ample amounts of deoxygenated blood coursing through the pulmonary vascular beds [23].

The gas-exchange membrane is comprised of the AE1 cells, capillary endothelial cell, and a fused basement membrane [5, 12], as shown by the electron microscopy image in Fig. 1.2. The blood-gas barrier is notable for its extreme thinness (~0.3 μm in total thickness in mammalian lung [33]), in part, due to the highly specialized morphology of the AE1 cells. AE1 cells only comprise 8 % of the total cells in the normal adult human lung, but covers 95 % of the alveolar surface [32]. If we divide the total alveolar surface area by the number of AE1 nuclei, the surface area covered by one

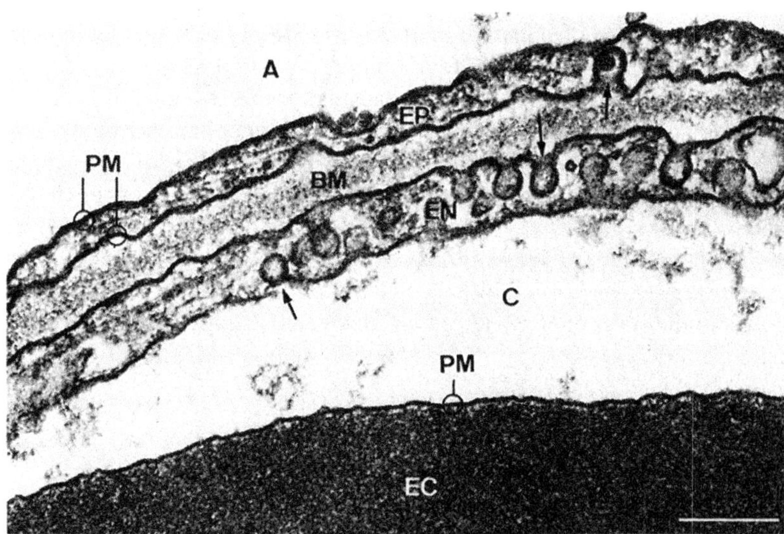

Fig. 1.2 Ultrastructure of the alveolar-capillary membrane by electron microscopy. Note the very thin epithelium (EP) with minimal cytoplasm, and the equally thin endothelium (EN) in close contact, separated only by the fused basement membrane (BM). *A* alveolar space, *C* capillary space, *PM* plasma membrane, *EC* erythrocyte. Scale marker: 0.2 μm (Used with permission from Weibel ER: The pathway for oxygen: structure and function in the mammalian respiratory system. Massachusetts: Harvard University Press; 1984)

type I epithelial cell is approximately 4000–5000 μm^2, which is larger than what is observed under the microscope of any single AE1 cell surface [34]. This is because the Type I alveolar epithelial cell is not a simple squamous cell, but branched cells with multiple apical faces, and its cell body is spread out over several vast surfaces with minimal cytoplasm in between, except in regions near the nuclei [34]. These regions correspond respectively to the observed thin portions of the gas-exchange membrane, comprising approximately 50 % of the total surface area. In the thick portions of the blood-gas barrier, elastic fibers, collagen fibrils, and fibroblasts can be observed [1, 4]. The research on AE1 has been challenging, due to its "flatness" in morphology, and the difficulty in separating intact AE1 cells from the rest of the lung tissue.

Type II Alveolar Epithelial Cells

Apart from being the progenitor cell of the alveolar epithelium, the AE2 cell actively participates in multiple functions including maintenance of homeostasis, surfactant production, alveolar fluid balance, and host defense [35]. AE2 cells are usually located in the corners of alveoli, or near the inter-alveolar pores of Kohn. Following alveolar injury, AE2 cells can form clusters during proliferation [1]. In contrast to AE1 cells, AE2 cells comprise approximately 60 % of alveolar epithelial cells, and approximately 15 % of all lung parenchymal cells, but they only cover approximately 5 % of alveolar membrane surface [36].

As previously discussed, AE1 cells are crucial for gas exchange function. However, AE1 cells are fragile and easily damaged, and they are replenished from AE2 cells [35]. The cell turnover time for alveolar epithelium, defined as the time required to renew all cells in a given population, is approximately 4–5 weeks in adult mammals [37]. This is much slower than the bronchial epithelium where cell turnover time is approximately 2–10 days [37]. However, it is suspected that the cell turnover time is faster following injury [38], where AE2 cells begin to proliferate, and cell turnover takes 2–5 days in experimental mouse models [39]. The initially formed cells express markers of both AE1 and AE2 cells, and morphologically form a thick cuboidal lining, also known as "cuboidal metaplasia." This lining may be effective as a barrier to prevent alveolar fluid collection, but it does not provide enough oxygen permeability for efficient gas exchange. It may take weeks for the lining to mature and transform into the thin gas-exchange lining of AE1 cells. This may explain why patients with acute respiratory distress syndrome (ARDS) remain hypoxic while pulmonary edema is resolving [4]. Apart from AE2 cells as progenitor cells for the alveolar epithelium, recent studies also shed light into the possible existence of a different progenitor cell generating both AE1 cells and AE2 cells [40, 41]. Potential progenitor cell population includes the bronchioalveolar stem cell, distal airway stem cell, and/or mesenchymal stem cell in both mouse models and human tissue samples [40–42].

Maintaining the Alveolar Lining

A thin, continuous layer of surfactants covers the alveolar surface [43]. Four types of surfactants have been identified: SP-A, -B, -C, and -D. They are synthesized, secreted, and recycled by AE2 cells [38]. In fact, AE2 cells are the only cell type in the lung that can synthesize all components of the surfactant, and SP-C is considered synthesized only by AE2 cells [38]. Apart from regulating the surface tension and preventing alveolar collapse, surfactants also help regulate alveolar fluid balance [44]. SP-A and SP-D are structurally related to collectins, or collagen containing C-type lectins, and participate in host defense [38, 45]. Between the surfactant lining and the actual alveolar epithelium, a thin layer of fluid, or hypophase, exists [38]. This hypophase is functionally important, as it serves as the immediate extracellular environment for the intra-alveolar surface [46]. In addition, it is the reaction milieu for extracellular biochemical processes. It is not surprising that the chemical properties of the hypophase are closely regulated. Studies have shown that AE2 cells possess membrane-bound water channels and ion pumps, and evidence supports the notion that AE2 cells are crucial regulators of the hypophase through regulation of, for example, pH and calcium concentrations [38, 47].

Capillary Endothelium

Compared with AE1 cells, the endothelial cell is notable for the simpler architecture of a typical flat cell. Endothelial cells cover a smaller surface area per cell of approximately 1000 μm^2, which is approximately 1/4 the surface area of a typical AE1 cell [3]. Endothelial cells form leaky occluding junctions compared with the tight occluding junctions formed between AE1 cells [3]. Thus, the exchange of solutes, water, and some small molecular-weight macromolecules between blood and the interstitial space is less restrained in contrast to the tightly regulated barrier provided by the AE1 cells [1]. In contrast to the endothelium of the pulmonary arteries and veins, the capillary endothelium is less metabolically active, and Weibel–Palade bodies, storage organelles specific to endothelial cells that contain and involved in regulated secretion of von Willebrand factor [48], are not commonly observed [1]. The thin portion of the gas exchange membrane is characterized by approximately 0.2 μm of tissue separating the capillary endothelium from the alveolar epithelial surface [33]. Given the scant protection surrounding the pulmonary capillary endothelium, it implies a considerable fragility. This fragility is made evident when normal lungs undergo extreme conditions such as the athlete during severe exercise, and the damage can present as hemoptysis [33].

Alveolar Fluid Balance

Gas exchange is compromised when the air inside the alveolar space is replaced by blood, purulence, or edema fluid. The pathophysiology of pulmonary edema formation has been the focus of intense research. Cardiogenic pulmonary edema is the result of elevated vascular pressure, while noncardiogenic pulmonary edema, i.e. acute respiratory distress syndrome (ARDS), is secondary to increased permeability of both the lung vasculature and epithelium [49, 50]. The resolution process of pulmonary edema has been a less understood process until recently. Experimental evidence indicates that alveolar edema resolution depends upon active ion transport across the alveolar epithelium resulting in the generation of an osmotic gradient for absorption of water from the alveolar space [4, 51]. In healthy alveolar epithelium, both AE1 cells and AE2 cells are involved in maintaining alveolar fluid balance, through epithelial sodium channels and aquaporins, and the rate of alveolar fluid clearance can be regulated by factors including dopamine, thyroid hormone, or corticosteroids [49]. In injured alveolar epithelium, the epithelial barrier is more "leaky," thus the passive barrier function is compromised. Due to the loss of functional AE1 and AE2 cells, the rate of active fluid clearance is also reduced [49].

Hose Defense Mechanisms of the Lung

In larger airways, the mucociliary clearance system plays an important role in host defense. The process of mucus being transported to the pharynx from the lower respiratory tract by the rhythmic movement of cilia is termed mucociliary clearance [52]. This clearance system is comprised of mucus, secreted from submuosal glands and goblet cells, and the layer of bronchial epithelial cells with their apical cilia [52]. In healthy individuals, there is only modest amount of mucus, and inhaled particulate matter and substances are asymptomatically removed [52]. Dysfunctional mucociliary clearance can be the result of disturbance in the quantity of mucus, such as in chronic bronchitis with marked mucus hypersecretion, or in the quality of the mucus, as observed in cystic fibrosis where the mucus is dehydrated due to the cystic fibrosis transmembrane conductance regulator *(CFTR)* gene mutation, or due to disruption of ciliary function, either primary from genetic disorders of ciliary dyskinesia or secondary from insults like tobacco smoke [4, 53].

Cell populations involved in lung immune defense include recruited neutrophils and monocytes, resident mononuclear phagocytes such as macrophages and dendritic cells (DCs), in addition to B cells and T cells [4]. Because of the small caliber of pulmonary capillaries, neutrophils migrate slowly and form a functional lung capillary neutrophil reservoir that can be quickly activated, and recruited into the airspace [4, 54]. This "marginated pool" of neutrophils and proposed mechanisms of neutrophil migration into the lungs are extensively discussed in the subsequent chapter (see Chap. 2). Macrophages are located in different compartments of the lung and include bronchial macrophages, alveolar surface macrophages, and interstitial macrophages [55]. There is also evidence for the presence of intravascular macrophages in humans, monkeys, but not in rodents; these macrophages reside on the inner surface of capillary lumen, and may constitute a line of defense against hematogenous pathogens [55, 56].

The roles of macrophages include clearance of alveolar surfactant [57], phagocytosis of inhaled pathogens or particles and modulation of the local immune response [58]. Based on in vivo murine models and human lung tissues, lung-resident DCs are also comprised of several subpopulations with distinct cellular origins and functions. These include conventional DCs, plasmacytoid DCs, and monocyte-derived DCs [55, 59]. They are important in the initiation of the immune response to foreign material and pathogens by constantly sampling and presenting antigens to lymphocytes, and the establishment of immune tolerance to harmless antigens [55].

Bronchial-associated lymphoid tissues (BALT), an ectopic lymphoid organ containing T cells, B cells, and a germinal center, do not exist in normal lungs, but can be observed in autoimmune disorder related interstitial lung diseases such as in Sjogren's disease, or in chronic inflammatory states such as in chronic obstructive pulmonary disease (COPD) [60]. It remains to be seen whether BALT tissues are the consequence of or contribute to the pathogenesis of these diseases. Recent studies imply that the appearance of BALT may be influenced by the presence of neutrophil inflammation, and regulated by T cells [61].

Conclusion

The lung's major function of performing gas exchange is supported by its unique anatomical structure. Given this primary function, the lungs rely upon an exquisitely thin barrier membrane, and enormous cross-sectional area consisting of an intricate pulmonary capillary network for effective gas transport and delivery. This ultrastructure renders the lungs susceptible to perturbations from the vascular space and hematologic system, resulting in small or large vessel occlusion, remodeling of pulmonary vascular beds, alveolar hemorrhage, or the development of pulmonary edema. These perturbations can lead to lung injury, such as in the form of vaso-occlusive crisis of sickle cell disease, pulmonary thromboembolism from inherited or acquired thrombophilias, idiopathic pneumonia syndrome following bone marrow transplantation, or ARDS following intense neutrophilic inflammation during severe pneumonia. In the following chapters, we will examine closely disorders resulting from pathologic interactions between the lung and the hematologic system.

Acknowledgements The authors are supported by research funding from the National Heart, Lung and Blood Institute (Award Number: HL086884) and the National Institute for Allergy and Infectious Diseases (Award Number: AI119042).

References

1. Grippi MA. Fishman's pulmonary diseases and disorders, vol. 5. New York: McGraw-Hill Education; 2015. p. 20–103.
2. West JB. Respiratory physiology—the essentials. 4th ed. Baltimore: Williams and Wilkins; 1990. p. 1–122.
3. Weibel ER. The pathway for oxygen: structure and function in the mammalian respiratory system. Cambridge, MA: Harvard University Press; 1984. p. 138–376.
4. Murray JF, Mason RJ. Murray and Nadel's textbook of respiratory medicine. 5th ed. Philadelphia, PA: Saunders/Elsevier; 2010. p. 1–132.
5. Weibel ER. Morphometry of the human lung. Berlin: Springer; 1963. p. 51–126.
6. Zeman KL, Scheuch G, Sommerer K, Brown JS, Bennett WD. In vivo characterization of the transitional bronchioles by aerosol-derived airway morphometry. J Appl Physiol. 1999;87(3):920–7.
7. Parent RA. Comparative biology of the normal lung. 2nd ed. Boston, MA: Elsevier; 2015. p. 21–49.
8. Haefeli-Bleuer B, Weibel ER. Morphometry of the human pulmonary acinus. Anat Rec. 1988;220(4):401–14.
9. Sapoval B, Filoche M, Weibel ER. Smaller is better—but not too small: a physical scale for the design of the mammalian pulmonary acinus. Proc Natl Acad Sci U S A. 2002;99(16):10411–6.
10. Weibel ER, Sapoval B, Filoche M. Design of peripheral airways for efficient gas exchange. Respir Physiol Neurobiol. 2005;148(1–2):3–21.
11. Flenley DC, Downing I, Greening AP. The pathogenesis of emphysema. Bull Eur Physiopathol Respir. 1986;22(1):245s–52. Review.
12. Weibel ER. Morphological basis of alveolar-capillary gas exchange. Physiol Rev. 1973;53(2):419–95. Review.
13. Townsley MI. Structure and composition of pulmonary arteries, capillaries, and veins. Compr Physiol. 2012;2(1):675–709.
14. Reid L. Structural and functional reappraisal of the pulmonary artery system. Sci Basis Med Annu Rev. 1968:289–307.
15. McLaughlin RF, Tyler WS, Canada RO. A study of the subgross pulmonary anatomy in various mammals. Am J Anatomy. 1961;108(2):149–65.
16. McLaughlin RFJ, Tyler WS, Canada RO. Subgross pulmonary anatomy of the rabbit, rat, and guinea pig, with additional notes on the human lung. Am Rev Respir Dis. 1966;94(3):380–7.
17. Widdicombe J. Physiologic control Anatomy and physiology of the airway circulation. Am Rev Respir Dis. 1992;146(5 Pt 2):S3–7. Review.
18. Walker CM, Rosado-de-Christenson ML, Martinez-Jimenez S, Kunin JR, Wible BC. Bronchial arteries: anatomy, function, hypertrophy, and anomalies. Radiographics. 2015;35(1):32–49.
19. Wagenvoort CA, Wagenvoort N. Arterial anastomoses, bronchopulmonary arteries, and pulmobronchial arteries in perinatal lungs. Lab Invest. 1967;16(1):13–24.
20. Endrys J, Hayat N, Cherian G. Comparison of bronchopulmonary collaterals and collateral blood flow in patients with chronic thromboembolic and primary pulmonary hypertension. Heart. 1997;78(2):171–6.
21. Ley S, Kreitner KF, Morgenstern I, Thelen M, Kauczor HU. Bronchopulmonary shunts in patients with chronic thromboembolic pulmonary hypertension: evaluation with helical CT and MR imaging. Am J Roentgenol. 2002;179(5):1209–15.
22. Yeh HC, Schum GM. Models of human lung airways and their application to inhaled particle deposition. Bull Math Biol. 1980;42(3):461–80.
23. Felici M, Filoche M, Sapoval B. Diffusional screening in the human pulmonary acinus. J Appl Physiol. 2003;94(5):2010–6.
24. Gehr P, Bachofen M, Weibel ER. The normal human lung: ultrastructure and morphometric estimation of diffusion capacity. Respir Physiol. 1978;32(2):121–40.

25. Cotes JE. Lung function : assessment and application in medicine, Chapter 9. 1st ed. Oxford: Blackwell Scientific; 1965. p. 209–28.
26. Hughes JMB, Pride NB. Examination of the carbon monoxide diffusing capacity (DL(CO)) in relation to its KCO and VA components. Am J Respir Crit Care Med. 2012;186(2):132–9. Review.
27. Berg JM, Tymoczko JL, Stryer L. Biochemistry. 7th ed. New York: W.H. Freeman; 2012.
28. Chanutin A, Curnish RR. Effect of organic and inorganic phosphates on the oxygen equilibrium of human erythrocytes. Arch Biochem Biophys. 1967;121(1):96–102.
29. Mills FC, Johnson ML, Ackers GK. Oxygenation-linked subunit interactions in human hemoglobin: experimental studies on the concentration dependence of oxygenation curves. Biochemistry. 1976;15(24):5350–62.
30. Bunn HF. Pathogenesis and treatment of sickle cell disease. N Engl J Med. 1997;337(11):762–9. Review.
31. Reid L, Meyrick B, Antony VB, Chang LY, Crapo JD, Reynolds HY. The mysterious pulmonary brush cell: a cell in search of a function. Am J Respir Crit Care Med. 2005;172(1):136–9.
32. Herzog EL, Brody AR, Colby TV, Mason R, Williams MC. Knowns and unknowns of the alveolus. Proc Am Thorac Soc. 2008;5(7):778–82.
33. West JB. Fragility of pulmonary capillaries. J Appl Physiol. 2013;115(1):1–15.
34. Weibel ER. The mystery of "non-nucleated plates" in the alveolar epithelium of the lung explained. Acta Anat. 1971;78(3):425–43.
35. Mason RJ, Williams MC. Type II alveolar cell. Defender of the alveolus. Am Rev Respir Dis. 1977;115(6 Pt 2):81–91.
36. Crapo JD, Barry BE, Gehr P, Bachofen M, Weibel ER. Cell number and cell characteristics of the normal human lung. Am Rev Respir Dis. 1982;126(2):332–7.
37. Bowden DH. Cell turnover in the lung. Am Rev Respir Dis. 1983;128(2 Pt 2):S46–8.
38. Fehrenbach H. Alveolar epithelial type II cell: defender of the alveolus revisited. Respir Res. 2001;2(1):33–46.
39. Adamson IY, Bowden DH. The type 2 cell as progenitor of alveolar epithelial regeneration. A cytodynamic study in mice after exposure to oxygen. Lab Invest. 1974;30(1):35–42.
40. Kim CF, Jackson EL, Woolfenden AE, Lawrence S, Babar I, Vogel S, et al. Identification of bronchioalveolar stem cells in normal lung and lung cancer. Cell. 2005;121(6):823–35.
41. Moodley Y. Evidence for human lung stem cells. N Engl J Med. 2011;365(5):464. author reply 5–6.
42. Guillot L, Nathan N, Tabary O, Thouvenin G, Le Rouzic P, Corvol H, et al. Alveolar epithelial cells: master regulators of lung homeostasis. Int J Biochem Cell Biol. 2013;45(11):2568–73.
43. Ochs M, Nenadic I, Fehrenbach A, Albes JM, Wahlers T, Richter J, et al. Ultrastructural alterations in intraalveolar surfactant subtypes after experimental ischemia and reperfusion. Am J Respir Crit Care Med. 1999;160(2):718–24.
44. Clements JA. Pulmonary edema and permeability of alveolar membranes. Arch Environ Health. 1961;2:280–3.
45. Hills BA. An alternative view of the role(s) of surfactant and the alveolar model. J Appl Physiol. 1999;87(5):1567–83.
46. Stephens RH, Benjamin AR, Walters DV. Volume and protein concentration of epithelial lining liquid in perfused in situ postnatal sheep lungs. J Appl Physiol. 1996;80(6):1911–20.
47. Eckenhoff RG, Somlyo AP. Rat lung type II cell and lamellar body: elemental composition in situ. Am J Physiol. 1988;254(5 Pt 1):C614–20.
48. Ewenstein BM, Warhol MJ, Handin RI, Pober JS. Composition of the von Willebrand factor storage organelle (Weibel-Palade body) isolated from cultured human umbilical vein endothelial cells. J Cell Biol. 1987;104(5):1423–33.
49. Matthay MA. Resolution of pulmonary edema. Thirty years of progress. Am J Respir Crit Care Med. 2014;189(11):1301–8.

50. Wiedemann HP, Wheeler AP, Bernard GR, Thompson BT, Hayden D, deBoisblanc B, et al. Comparison of two fluid-management strategies in acute lung injury. N Engl J Med. 2006;354(24):2564–75.
51. Matthay MA, Folkesson HG, Clerici C. Lung epithelial fluid transport and the resolution of pulmonary edema. Physiol Rev. 2002;82(3):569–600.
52. Burns MW. Fertility, immotile cilia and chronic respiratory infections. Med J Aust. 1979;2(6):287–8.
53. Afzelius BA. A human syndrome caused by immotile cilia. Science. 1976;193(4250):317–9.
54. Kolaczkowska E, Kubes P. Neutrophil recruitment and function in health and inflammation. Nat Rev Immunol. 2013;13(3):159–75.
55. Kopf M, Schneider C, Nobs SP. The development and function of lung-resident macrophages and dendritic cells. Nat Immunol. 2015;16(1):36–44.
56. Balhara J, Gounni AS. The alveolar macrophages in asthma: a double-edged sword. Mucosal Immunol. 2012;5(6):605–9.
57. Trapnell BC, Whitsett JA, Nakata K. Pulmonary alveolar proteinosis. N Engl J Med. 2003;349(26):2527–39.
58. Westphalen K, Gusarova GA, Islam MN, Subramanian M, Cohen TS, Prince AS, et al. Sessile alveolar macrophages communicate with alveolar epithelium to modulate immunity. Nature. 2014;506(7489):503–6.
59. Demedts IK, Brusselle GG, Vermaelen KY, Pauwels RA. Identification and characterization of human pulmonary dendritic cells. Am J Respir Cell Mol Biol. 2005;32(3):177–84.
60. Moyron-Quiroz JE, Rangel-Moreno J, Kusser K, Hartson L, Sprague F, Goodrich S, et al. Role of inducible bronchus associated lymphoid tissue (iBALT) in respiratory immunity. Nat Med. 2004;10(9):927–34.
61. Foo SY, Zhang V, Lalwani A, Lynch JP, Zhuang A, Lam CE, et al. Regulatory T cells prevent inducible BALT formation by dampening neutrophilic inflammation. J Immunol. 2015;194(9):4567–76.

Chapter 2
Leukocyte Kinetics and Migration in the Lungs

Prithu Sundd and Margaret F. Bennewitz

Introduction

The primary function of the lungs is to enable the oxygenation of venous blood [1]. The blood–air barrier in the lungs (described in Chap. 1), which is continuously exposed to inhaled microbes and inflammatory stimuli, also serves as a site of host defense [2]. Leukocyte trafficking to sites of inflammation is central to the maintenance of homeostasis in the lung [3, 4]; however, unregulated profuse recruitment of leukocytes can promote lung injury and respiratory failure [5]. Neutrophils are the most abundant leukocytes in human blood and the first subset of leukocytes to reach a site of inflammation [3, 6]. More than 60 % of the lung microcirculation is made up of pulmonary capillaries, which are mostly smaller in diameter than neutrophils [7, 8]. As a result, neutrophils are required to deform into an elongated shape when entering the pulmonary capillaries, which slows down their transit, leading to their concentration in the noninflamed lung [9]. Thus, the anatomy of the lung microcirculation serves to promote homeostasis in the noninflamed lung by concentrating neutrophils within the pulmonary capillaries in the form of a "marginated pool," which can be readily recruited in response to an inflammatory stimulus [10]. Following an inflammatory insult, neutrophils sequester primarily within the pulmonary capillaries in large numbers [11] and infiltrate into the alveolar air spaces, which contributes to the disruption of the blood-air barrier and progression of lung injury [5]. Unlike the well-characterized sequential steps of rolling, activation, arrest, crawling, and transmigration that drive neutrophil recruitment in the systemic venules [6], neutrophils do not roll in the pulmonary capillaries but rather undergo a series of overlapping steps of cell stiffening and sequestration followed

P. Sundd, PhD (✉) • M.F. Bennewitz, PhD
Division of Pulmonary, Allergy and Critical Care Medicine, Pittsburgh Heart, Lung and Blood Vascular Medicine Institute, University of Pittsburgh School of Medicine, Pittsburgh, PA, USA
e-mail: prs51@pitt.edu

J.S. Lee, M.P. Donahoe (eds.), *Hematologic Abnormalities and Acute Lung Syndromes*, Respiratory Medicine, DOI 10.1007/978-3-319-41912-1_2

by trans-endothelial, trans-interstitial, and trans-epithelial migration [2]. The major adhesion molecules such as selectins and β_2-integrins that enable neutrophil rolling and arrest, respectively in the systemic microcirculation seem to be dispensable for neutrophil sequestration in the pulmonary capillaries [4].

Intravital microscopy (IVM) in mice has been used extensively to study neutrophil recruitment to different vascular beds during inflammation [12–15]. Such studies of the cremaster microcirculation in mice have been instrumental in establishing the multistep adhesion paradigm of neutrophil recruitment in the systemic venules [14]. However, the high-resolution IVM observations in the lungs of mice have been limited by the invasiveness of the surgical procedure required to access the pulmonary vascular bed as well as the motion artifacts caused by the breathing pattern and beating of the heart. Recently, fluorescence IVM approaches [13, 16–20] that allow studying leukocyte kinetics at high temporal and spatial resolution in the mouse lung have been introduced. These IVM studies in mice have confirmed the findings made previously in dogs [9, 11], rats [17], humans [7] and rabbits [21].

This chapter will provide an overview of the molecular and biophysical mechanisms that regulate neutrophil trafficking in the lung during homeostasis and inflammation. The first section "Intravital microscopy of the lung microcirculation in mice" will introduce the readers to IVM of the lung in mice and the advantage of using it to study leukocyte trafficking. The second section "The blood–air barrier in the lung" will describe the structure of the lung microcirculation. The third section "Leukocyte kinetics in the noninflamed lung" will highlight the mechanisms that dictate the transit and margination of neutrophils in the noninflamed lung. Lastly, the fourth section "Leukocyte kinetics in the inflamed lung" will highlight the cascade of adhesive events and molecular pathways that drive neutrophil recruitment into the alveolar air spaces during lung inflammation. The chapter will conclude with a discussion on future studies required for further improvement in our understanding of the leukocyte kinetics in the lung.

Intravital Microscopy of the Lung Microcirculation in Mice

The mouse is the most widely used vertebrate to study the molecular mechanism of acute lung syndromes [22]. The choice of the mouse as a vertebrate model has been promulgated by the availability and ease of creating transgenic/knock-in mutant or fluorescent reporter strains. Although leukocyte trafficking in the lung microcirculation has been studied previously using IVM in vertebrates like dogs [9, 11], rabbits [21] and rats [17], the need to identify the molecular mechanisms using genetically deficient mouse strains warrants that such imaging studies be performed in mice. The small size of mice, fragility of the lung tissue and large scale movements (on the order of millimeters) of the lung vasculature caused by the breathing and cardiac cycle [13, 19, 23] makes IVM a challenge. Furthermore, visualizing cellular trafficking in real-time within the pulmonary microcirculation necessitates the use of multiphoton-excitation (MPE) fluorescence microscopy, due to its high resolution in the z-direction, reduced photobleaching, less phototoxicity, and deeper tissue penetration [24]. Neutrophil trafficking within the lung microcirculation can be visualized using knockin/transgenic mice that express fluorescence exclusively in neutrophils. *Lyz2-EGFP* mice have enhanced green fluorescent protein (GFP) knocked into the murine lysozyme M locus, resulting in green fluorescence within neutrophils and a small subset of monocytes [25]. Recently, the "Catchup" mouse was introduced, which has tdTomato knocked into the Ly-6G locus [26]. The Catchup mouse expresses red fluorescence specifically localized to neutrophils and would thus be useful for in vivo MPE-IVM studies of neutrophil trafficking in the lung [26]. Alternatively, neutrophils can be labeled in vivo in mice through intravascular administration of fluorescent antibodies (<20 μg per mouse) against the neutrophil surface marker Ly-6G [27]. The microcirculation in mice can be visualized through the intravascular administration of dyes such as fluorescent dextrans, quantum dots, and Evans blue [13, 16, 28].

Recently, Looney et al. [13] introduced an IVM approach that relies on stabilization of a small region of the mouse lung through the application of a gentle vacuum. This approach enabled real-time visualization of neutrophil trafficking within the pulmonary microcirculation of live mice. Using a relatively similar approach, Kreisel et al. [28] showed that a resident pool of neutrophils resides in the pulmonary microcirculation of mice under baseline conditions. Inspired by Looney et al. [13], our lab introduced a modified MPE-IVM fluorescence methodology and used it to visualize neutrophil trafficking through the pulmonary microcirculation of mechanically ventilated mice [16]. This approach allowed us to visualize the pulmonary microcirculation, assess the kinetics of neutrophil trafficking through the mouse lung and also reproduce the findings made in previous studies using other vertebrate models [7, 9, 11, 17, 21]. We found that neutrophil transit through the lung microcirculation is several folds slower than that of red blood cells (RBCs), a marginated pool of neutrophils exists in the pulmonary capillary bed of noninflamed lungs, a majority of these marginated neutrophils are elongated and they entirely fill the lumen of the capillaries.

The Blood–Air Barrier in the Lung

The blood-air interface has been described in detail in Chap. 1. The human lung is composed of two subunits, the central airways and the peripheral parenchyma. The central airways consist of the trachea, bronchi, and terminal bronchioles, while the peripheral parenchyma includes the respiratory bronchioles, alveolar ducts, and alveoli [1, 2]. Alveolar ducts terminate into alveolar sacs, which are air spaces enclosed within numerous polygonal structures known as "alveoli." An adult human lung has 300 million alveoli, each ~0.25 mm in diameter, resulting in a total alveolar surface area of ~100 m^2 [1, 2, 10, 29], which is covered by type-I and type-II pneumocytes. Transmission electron microscopic studies of the fixed sections of peripheral canine lung [29] have revealed that the alveolar wall is thin (<200 nm) on one

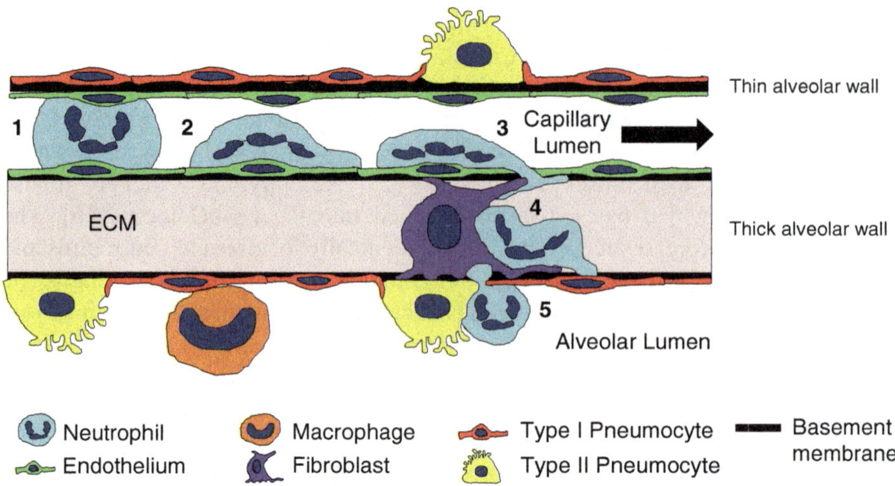

Fig. 2.1 Neutrophil emigration into the alveolar air space. The thick alveolar wall is the preferred site for neutrophil emigration. (1) Initial mechanical sequestration followed by prolonged retention of a neutrophil within the lumen of a pulmonary capillary. (2) Trans-luminal crawling of a neutrophil towards the junction of endothelial cells. (3) Paracellular trans-endothelial migration of a neutrophil. (4) Neutrophils migrate through the holes in the endothelial basement membrane (*thick black line*) followed by migration through the ECM along the interstitial fibroblast and finally into the basal-lateral space beneath the type-II pneumocyte through the holes in the epithelial basement membrane (*thick black line*). (5) Neutrophils enter the alveolar lumen preferentially at the junction of type I and type II pneumocytes

side and thick (~2.5 μm) [1] on the other side. The thin wall contains the capillary endothelium and the alveolar epithelium separated by a common basement membrane rich in fibronectin and collagen (Fig. 2.1). The thick wall (Fig. 2.1) consists of endothelium and epithelium separated by an interstitial matrix, which consists of separate endothelial and epithelial basement membranes, fibroblasts, mast cells, pericytes, and an extracellular matrix (ECM) rich in collagen, elastin, and proteoglycans [2, 29]. Using transmission electron microscopy and serial section reconstruction of the rabbit lung, Walker et al. [2, 30] revealed that the junction of the thick and thin alveolar wall is the primary site for neutrophil emigration in the inflamed lung.

The structure of the pulmonary microcirculation has been described elegantly in the recent review by Townsley et al. [31]. A single alveolus is surrounded by ~1000 inter-connected short tubular capillary segments arranged in a spheroidal mesh. The alveolar wall separating adjacent alveoli has a single network of capillaries which is exposed to the alveolar air on both sides [1, 32]. The average length and diameter of pulmonary capillary segments in the human lung is 15 and 7.5 μm, respectively, and the entire pulmonary capillary network is connected to 300 million arterial and venular end branches [2, 10, 29]. The lumen of the pulmonary capillaries is lined with pulmonary endothelial cells and a single endothelial cell is estimated to cover the walls of three adjacent capillary segments [33]. Figure 2.2 shows an MPE-IVM

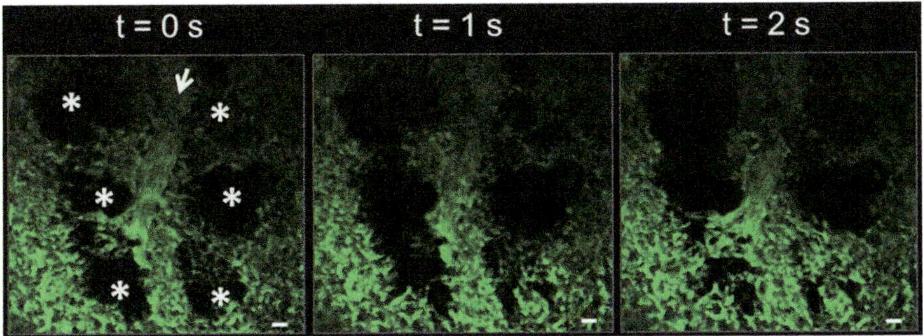

Fig. 2.2 Structure of the pulmonary microcirculation in mice. MPE-IVM fluorescence image of the pulmonary microcirculation in a WT C57BL/6 mouse following IV infusion of FITC-dextran (*green*). The pulmonary capillaries surrounding the alveoli (*) can be seen moving in and out of the imaging plane in the *z*-direction due to the dynamic expansion and contraction of the alveoli (*) with mechanical ventilation. Movement of the alveoli starts from the bottom of the image at $t=0$ s and moves up to the top with increasing time. Alveoli are marked by asterisks. Intravascular FITC dextran highlights the pulmonary capillaries and a feeding arteriole in green. The open arrow denotes the direction of blood flow within the feeding arteriole. The times displayed are relative to the frame at $t=0$ s. Scale bars are 20 μm. The feeding arteriole has a diameter of 33 μm, while the capillaries have an average diameter of 6 ± 2 μm. Figure adapted from Ref. [16]

fluorescence microscopy image of the lung microcirculation in a wild type (WT) C57BL/6 mouse following intravascular infusion of FITC-dextran (green). As shown in Fig. 2.2, the terminal pulmonary arteriole branches out into networks of inter-connected short capillary segments, which surround alveoli (visible as dark polygons) and drain into the pulmonary venule (not visible in Fig. 2.2). These terminal arterioles and venules have a diameter in the range of 20–30 μm [13, 16, 19]. Also the physiological pressure difference across the whole pulmonary capillary network (between a pulmonary arteriole and venule) is ~6 mmHg, while that across a single pulmonary capillary segment is 0.15–0.6 mmHg [34, 35]. Thus, the pressure across a single pulmonary capillary segment is 10 times smaller than that across the whole pulmonary capillary network.

Leukocyte Kinetics in the Noninflamed Lung

As described in the section “The blood–air barrier in the lung,” the average diameter of a pulmonary capillary segment in the human lung is ~7.5 μm, which is smaller than the average diameter of a human neutrophil ~ 8 μm [2, 4, 7, 36]. Therefore, neutrophils are required to deform in order to transit through the pulmonary capillary network (capillary network between a pulmonary arteriole and a venule). Based on in vivo studies performed in canine or rabbit lungs [7, 8, 21, 37], a neutrophil is estimated to pass through 40–100 capillary segments during a single transit from an arteriole to a venule and 30–60 % of these segments require the

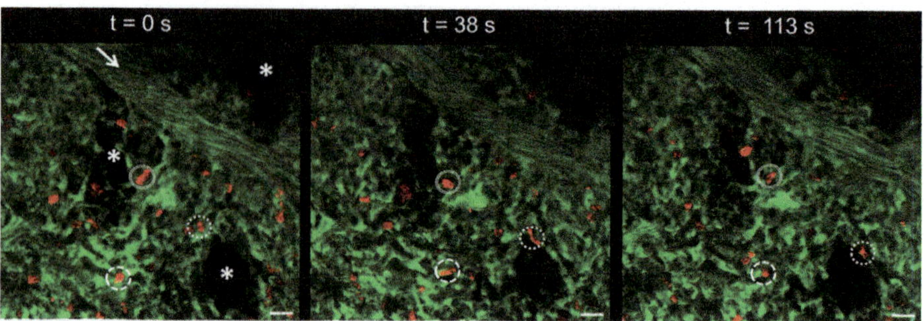

Fig. 2.3 Neutrophil kinetics in the noninflamed lung. MPE-IVM fluorescence image of the pulmonary microcirculation in a WT C57BL/6 mouse. Intravascular FITC dextran (*green*) highlights the pulmonary capillaries and a feeding arteriole. The arrow denotes the direction of blood flow within the feeding arteriole. Neutrophils shown in red were stained by IV infusion of Alexa Fluor 546 Gr-1 mAb (*red*). The marginated pool of neutrophils is visible as elliptical cells (*red*) within the pulmonary capillary segments (*green*). The solid and dotted circles denote three elliptical neutrophils slowly transiting through the pulmonary capillaries over a 2 min observation period. The times displayed are relative to the frame at $t = 0$ s. The pulmonary arteriole has a diameter of 30 μm. Alveoli are marked by asterisks. The scale bars are 20 μm

neutrophil to deform. Studies using scanning electron microscopy of fixed human lung tissue [7] and in vivo video microscopy of canine lungs [11] have revealed that neutrophils which are spherical in the pulmonary arterioles appear to be elliptical in shape inside the pulmonary capillaries. Recently, these findings were confirmed by high-resolution MPE-IVM studies performed in mice [13, 16], which revealed ellipsoid neutrophils slowly transiting through the capillary segments in the mouse lung (Fig. 2.3).

Deformation of neutrophils from a spherical to an elliptical shape is not instantaneous [38, 39]. Neutrophils are known to pause for a while at the entrance, as well as at the capillary junctions to deform, and the pause time is referred to as the "entrance time" [4, 7]. Computational models of the pulmonary capillary network, which were inspired by in vivo video microscopic images of rabbit and canine lungs, reveal that the pressure drop across a single pulmonary capillary segment needs to exceed a critical value to allow the cell to enter a capillary segment [34, 35]. This critical pressure is determined by the ratio of the capillary to neutrophil diameter [34, 38] and the cortical tension of the neutrophil ~35 pN/μm [39], which is the surface tension that enables the cell to maintain a spherical shape [40]. The cortical tension is dictated by the presence of a layer of actin cytoskeleton known as the "cortex" beneath the plasma membrane [39, 41]. Using in vitro pulmonary capillary sized microfluidic channels, Gabriele et al. [42] have shown that the entrance and transit time of passive leukocytes through 4 μm capillaries is determined by the degree of actin polymerization and therefore, stiffer cells take more time to enter into a capillary segment. In vivo, the pressure drop across a capillary segment can be smaller than the critical pressure; however, the blockage of the capillary entrance by a neutrophil can result in a 100–300 % increase in the pressure drop, which eventually pushes the neutrophil through the capillary [35].

Once inside a capillary segment, neutrophils also stop in the straight segments between junctions and these straight segment pauses are four to five times more frequent than in the junctions [11, 16]. The hemodynamic force acting on a stationary neutrophil that completely fills the lumen of the capillary segment can be estimated $F \approx \Delta P \pi R_p^2$, where ΔP is the pressure difference (~0.15–0.6 mmHg) and R_p is the radius of the capillary segment [36, 43, 44]. Based on IVM studies done in canine lungs, Lien et al. [9] showed that the RBCs being highly deformable, easily transit through a single pulmonary capillary network with a transit time of 1.4–4.2 s, while neutrophils being less deformable have a mean transit time of 6.1 min. The pauses responsible for the increased transit time of neutrophils result in at least a 50-fold higher concentration of neutrophils in the pulmonary than the systemic circulation and this resident pool of neutrophils is referred to as the "marginated pool" [4, 7, 21, 45]. The prolonged transit time and margination of neutrophils in the lung microcirculation also serves to promote host defense by allowing these cells to respond promptly to an inflammatory stimulus [10]. At the same time, the interconnected architecture of the pulmonary capillary network ensures that there are enough alternative routes for RBC transit around those capillary segments which are plugged with neutrophils [4].

Recent data from our lab (Fig. 2.3) and others [13, 28] using MPE-IVM of the lung in WT C57BL/6 mice revealed that the neutrophils are present in large numbers in the noninflamed lung, completely fill the lumen of the capillaries and therefore, appear ellipsoidal as they transit through the pulmonary capillaries [16]. Similar to previous reports [4, 11, 13, 28, 46], our analysis of neutrophil track lengths and speed revealed that the neutrophil transit through the pulmonary capillaries is indeed a combination of "hopping (stop and go)" and slow continuous motion. As shown in Figure 2.3, we found that some capillaries even in the noninflamed lung are effectively occluded temporarily as neutrophils transit slowly through them, which can take longer than 5 min as shown previously [35]. Although the ratio of neutrophil to capillary diameter and the forces of deformation are believed to dictate the transit time and margination of neutrophils within the noninflamed pulmonary capillary network, a role for neutrophil–endothelial adhesion cannot be entirely ruled out.

Neutrophil–endothelial adhesion plays a pivotal role in neutrophil margination within the systemic microcirculation. The neutrophil adhesion to the systemic venular endothelium starts with rolling, which is mediated by P-selectin on the endothelium binding to P-selectin-glycoprotein-ligand-1 (PSGL-1) on neutrophils [6]. Interleukin-8 (IL-8/CXCL-8) on human endothelium or KC (CXCL-1) on mouse endothelium binds to CXCR1 and CXCR2 on rolling neutrophils to activate β_2-integrins CD11b/CD18 (Mac-1) and CD11a/CD18 (LFA-1) expressed on neutrophils, which then bind to intercellular-adhesion-molecule-1 (ICAM-1) on the endothelium to enable arrest [6]. Although endothelial P-selectin is central to leukocyte rolling in venules and arterioles [47], its role in leukocyte margination within the pulmonary capillaries is debatable [4]. To test the role of P-selectin (if present on the capillary wall) in mediating leukocyte margination in the lungs, undifferentiated HL-60 promyelocytic leukemia cells (diameter 13.5 μm) were allowed to flow in 7.5 μm diameter glass capillaries coated with recombinant human P-selectin or bovine serum albumin (BSA) under physiological conditions [43]. HL-60 cells were observed to deform into an elliptical shape and flow freely with minimal arrest in BSA coated capillaries but paused for long durations in P-selectin coated capillaries [43]. Although this may imply that P-selectin if present on the capillary endothelium can mediate neutrophil sequestration in pulmonary capillaries, there is conflicting evidence to support that such a scenario may exist in pulmonary capillaries in vivo [4]. P-selectin is expressed on the pulmonary arteriolar and venular endothelium [11, 48–50] and supports leukocyte rolling in these vessels in vivo [11, 47, 51]. However, the immunohistochemistry performed on noninflamed canine lung sections revealed that P-selectin is absent from the pulmonary capillary endothelium [11]. Alternatively, it has been proposed that the P-selectin expression on the pulmonary capillary endothelium can be low enough to be detected by the immunohistochemical techniques [2].

L-selectin is constitutively expressed on passive neutrophils and is known to mediate neutrophil margination in the systemic venules [52]; however, the requirement of L-selectin in neutrophil margination within the noninflamed lung is unclear. Using IVM of the rabbit lung under baseline conditions, Kuebler et al. [51] found that the intravenous infusion of fucoidin, which inhibits both P-selectin and L-selectin, led to the reduced rolling of leukocytes in both pulmonary venules and arterioles and also a reduction in the neutrophil transit time through the pulmonary capillary bed, suggesting a role for P- or L-selectin in leukocyte margination in the lung. A role for L-selectin was further supported by Gebb et al. [11], which used IVM to show that L-selectin mediates neutrophil rolling in the pulmonary arterioles and venules of noninflamed canine lungs. In contrast, Doyle et al. [53] revealed that the margination of neutrophils in pulmonary capillaries as well as venules and arterioles was normal in L-selectin deficient mice, suggesting that L-selectin may not be necessary for neutrophil margination in the noninflamed pulmonary capillaries.

Although β_2-integrin-ICAM-1-mediated firm arrest is critical to neutrophil margination in the systemic microcirculation [6], both β_2-integrin and ICAM-1 seem to be not required for neutrophil margination in the noninflamed lung. Aoki et al. [46] used IVM of the ex vivo perfused rat lung to show that ICAM-1 is constitutively expressed on both the pulmonary venular and capillary endothelium, suggesting that ICAM-1 may mediate neutrophil margination in the pulmonary capillaries. CD18 (β_2-) integrins on circulating neutrophils are maintained in the bent passive state in the absence of inflammation and the binding of β_2-integrins to ICAM-1 requires their activation to an extended high-affinity state, suggesting no role for β_2-integrins in the noninflamed lung [54]. Anderson et al. [55] demonstrated that the neutrophil deformation followed by migration through a 3 μm polycarbonate filter resulted in the upregulation of CD18 expression on neutrophils, which led to their enhanced adhesion to the immobilized recombinant ICAM-1. Similar to this observation, other in vitro studies have shown that neutrophils activate following aspiration into glass capillaries smaller than 5 μm in diameter [43, 44]. Whether such deformation induced activation and upregulation of CD18 expression occurs in pulmonary capillaries in vivo is debatable [56] but the role of CD18 in neutrophil margination can be tested by inhibiting CD18 function. Animals injected with functional blocking antibodies (Abs) against CD18 showed no increase in circulating neutrophil count, suggesting that CD18 is not required for the margination of neutrophils in the non-inflamed lung [4]. Finally, mice deficient in both P-selectin and ICAM-1 do not show a defect in neutrophil margination in the noninflamed lung and surprisingly, the size of the marginated pool in these double deficient mice was significantly larger than the WT mice suggesting that both endothelial P-selectin and ICAM-1 are not necessary for neutrophil margination in the lung [50].

Although chemokine-GPCR (G-protein-coupled receptor) signaling is known to mediate integrin activation and cytoskeletal remodeling of neutrophils during inflammation [52], a role of GPCRs in neutrophil margination within the noninflamed lung is unclear. Recently, Devi et al. [57] provided evidence to support a role for chemokine signaling in neutrophil margination in the noninflamed lung. Using both mice and primates, Devi et al. [57] demonstrated that neutrophils marginated within the lung show a relatively higher expression of the chemokine receptor CXCR4, which facilitates neutrophil margination in the healthy lung by binding to its ligand CXCL-12 (SDF-1) expressed on the pulmonary capillary endothelium. Taken together, these studies suggest that the role of adhesion in neutrophil margination in the healthy lung cannot be excluded but it seems to be less important than the role of neutrophil resistance to deformation and the presence of the large number of capillary segments with diameters smaller than the neutrophil.

Leukocyte Kinetics in the Inflamed Lung

Neutrophil recruitment to a site of systemic inflammation takes place primarily in the post-capillary venules through sequential steps of rolling, activation, arrest, trans-luminal crawling, trans-endothelial migration, and migration across the ECM into the inflammatory foci [6]. PSGL-1 on neutrophils binds to members of the selectin family (P-, E-selectin on the endothelium, and L-selectin on neutrophils) to mediate rolling, while β_2-integrins (LFA-1 and Mac-1) on neutrophils bind to ICAM-1 on the inflamed endothelium or ECM components to mediate arrest and subsequent steps of migration, respectively [6, 58]. Unlike the systemic microcirculation, neutrophil recruitment to the inflamed lungs occurs predominantly (>90 %) in the pulmonary capillary network with minimal contribution (<10 %) from the pulmonary arterioles and venules [2, 4, 45, 46].

In vivo studies performed in dogs, mice, rabbits, and other rodents using diverse pulmonary or systemic stimuli have been instrumental in establishing the current paradigm of neutrophil recruitment in the inflamed lung. Intratracheal (IT) [13, 59, 60], intraperitoneal (IP) [61] and intravascular (IV) administration [62, 63] of gram-negative bacterial endotoxin, lipopolysaccharide (LPS), has been shown to induce neutrophil sequestration in the pulmonary capillaries of mice. Neutrophils have also been shown to sequester in the pulmonary capillaries of the canine [45], mouse [53] and rabbit [64] lung following IV infusion of complement fragments. In addition to these studies, hyper-mechanical ventilation [65], IV IL-6 [66], IV cobra venom factor

(CVF) [50, 67], IV activated plasma [68], IT IgG immune complex [67, 69], IT IL-1β [70], IT phorbol-12-myristate-13-acetate (PMA) [56] and IT hydrochloric acid (HCl) [71] have been used to induce pulmonary inflammation in animal models. Also IT instillation of pneumonia inducing microbes such as *Escherichia coli* (*E. coli*) [53, 72, 73], *Streptococcus pneumoniae* (*S. pneumoniae*) [49, 53, 56, 72], *Pseudomonas aeruginosa* (*P. aeruginosa*) [74, 75] and *Staphylococcus aureus* (*S. aureus*) [73] have been widely used in animal models to elucidate the molecular and biophysical mechanism of neutrophil recruitment in the inflamed lung.

The release of pathogen or danger associated molecular patterns (PAMPs or DAMPs) by microbial pathogens or necrotic host cells, respectively, is central to the progression of inflammation [76]. The recognition of PAMPs and DAMPs by the pattern recognition receptors (PPRs) on alveolar macrophages, pulmonary endothelial cells, alveolar epithelial cells, and interstitial mast cells results in the release of pro-inflammatory mediators such as IL-1β, TNF, IL-6, G-CSF, and chemokines such as IL-8 (CXCL8; human), KC (CXCL1; mice), MIP2α (CXCL2; mice), and MCP-1 (CCL2) [5, 76]. These mediators cause activation of the neutrophils and endothelial cells by binding to their cognate receptors expressed on these cell types. Activated neutrophils sequester within the pulmonary microcirculation and migrate across the endothelial-epithelial barrier into the alveolar air space. Emigrated neutrophils may release chemokines to further amplify neutrophil recruitment and undergo degranulation, oxidative burst, and NETosis [5]. NETosis involves the release of neutrophil extracellular traps (NETs), which are composed of strands of decondensed chromatin decorated with histones and granule proteins such as neutrophil elastase (NE) or myeloperoxidase (MPO). NETosis has been described in detail elsewhere [12, 77]. These effector functions of neutrophils which are critical to the clearance of bacteria and the resolution of inflammation are tightly regulated; otherwise, the release of neutrophil derived oxidants and proteases can contribute to the disruption of the endothelial–epithelial barrier [76, 78, 79]. Eventually, apoptotic neutrophils are cleared away from the alveolar air space by alveolar macrophages through the process of "efferocytosis" [5, 80, 81].

Neutrophil recruitment into the air spaces of the inflamed lung can be roughly classified into five sequential steps (Fig. 2.1): capillary sequestration and retention, trans-luminal crawling, trans-endothelial migration, trans-interstitial migration, and trans-epithelial migration [2, 4, 5, 59, 76, 82]. In the following text, capillary sequestration and retention is described as a single step, while trans-luminal crawling, trans-endothelial migration, trans-interstitial migration, and trans-epithelial migration are discussed collectively under "Neutrophil emigration into the alveolar air space."

Neutrophil Sequestration and Retention in the Pulmonary Capillaries

In response to a systemic or pulmonary inflammatory insult, neutrophils sequester within the pulmonary capillaries in large numbers which exceed the baseline marginated pool by several folds [4]. In fact, acute neutrophil sequestration in the inflamed lung is known to be associated with transient peripheral blood neutropenia

[45, 64, 72]. Entrapment in the pulmonary capillaries (step 1 in Fig. 2.1) is one of the primary steps in the recruitment of neutrophils to the alveolar air spaces during pulmonary inflammation [2, 4]. Unlike the well-characterized multistep adhesion cascade that mediates neutrophil-endothelium interaction in the inflamed venules [58]; the molecular and biophysical mechanism that enables neutrophil entrapment in the inflamed pulmonary capillaries is incompletely understood [2, 76].

As described in the section "Leukocyte kinetics in the noninflamed lung," neutrophils pause in both the straight segments and junctions of the pulmonary capillaries in the noninflamed lung. Neutrophils are much smaller in diameter than most of the pulmonary capillaries and have to deform into an elliptical shape prior to entering a pulmonary capillary segment. Once inside the capillary, the forces of deformation push the neutrophil membrane against the capillary wall, resulting in a large surface area of contact with the capillary endothelium [7, 43]. Neutrophils constitutively express PSGL-1 [83, 84], L-selectin, inactivated β_2-integrins, and other glycoprotein ligands for E-selectin [52]. ICAM-1 is known to be constitutively expressed on the lung capillary endothelium and the expression increases following pulmonary inflammation [46, 85]. Based on the quintessential role of these adhesion molecules in the systemic microcirculation and the large contact area that exists between an elliptical neutrophil and the pulmonary capillary endothelium, it would be plausible to expect a role for adhesion molecules in neutrophil sequestration in the inflamed pulmonary capillaries.

The role for selectins in mediating neutrophil capillary sequestration during pulmonary inflammation was supported by early studies. Selectin-IgG chimeras were used to show that P- and L-selectin mediate IV cobra venom factor (CVF)-induced lung injury in rats, while L-selectin and E-selectin mediate IT IgG-immune complex induced lung injury in rats [86] and a P-selectin like epitope is upregulated on the lung capillary endothelium of rats following CVF infusion [87]. Also Mulligan et al. [67] demonstrated that the treatment of rats with an L-selectin blocking Ab inhibited neutrophil recruitment in the lungs following IV infusion of CVF or IT instillation of an IgG-immune complex. However, Bullard et al. [49] raised skepticism about the role of both P-selectin and ICAM-1 by showing that neutrophil recruitment during *S. pneumoniae* induced pneumonia was unchanged in the lungs of P-selectin/ICAM-1 double mutant mice compared to wild type mice, suggesting no role for P-selectin or ICAM-1.

The discrepancy in these early reports was explained by Doerschuk et al. [50] using a mouse model of CVF-induced lung injury. In this study [50], Abs against P-selectin and ICAM-1 inhibited neutrophil sequestration in the pulmonary capillaries supporting a role for endothelial P-selectin and ICAM-1 [50]; however, mutant mice lacking P-selectin, ICAM-1 or both had no defect in CVF induced neutrophil sequestration, suggesting that neither P-selectin nor ICAM-1 is required [50]. Similarly, functional blocking Abs against ICAM-1 and β_2-integrins, LFA-1, and Mac-1, were shown to partially inhibit the acute neutrophil recruitment in the lungs of mice challenged with IT endotoxin [88] or *P. aeruginosa* [75]; however, the recruitment was completely normal in ICAM-1 deficient mice challenged with either stimuli [75, 88]. As an attempt to explain the difference in the role for adhesion molecules based on functional blocking vs. genetic deletion, it has been suggested that the immune system in mutant animals may have evolved at the embryonic stage to substitute the roles of these molecules with some other molecules or the Abs may inhibit neutrophil adhesion by other mechanisms in addition to functional blocking [4, 49, 50].

Understanding the role of adhesion molecules in neutrophil sequestration in the pulmonary capillaries was further refined by later studies aimed at the temporal kinetics of neutrophil dynamics in the inflamed lung. Using IV infusion of complement fragments in L-selectin deficient mice, Doyle et al. [53] revealed that L-selectin is not required for the initial rapid (<1 min) sequestration but is necessary for the prolonged retention (>5 min) of the sequestered neutrophils within the pulmonary capillaries. In vivo studies using functional blocking monoclonal Abs revealed that neither β_2-integrins (CD18) nor L- or P-selectin was essential for the initial sequestration of neutrophils in the pulmonary capillaries of rabbits immediately following infusion of complement fragments [64] or activated plasma [68]. However, both β_2-integrins and L-selectin were required to keep the neutrophils arrested within the pulmonary capillaries for greater than 4–7 min [64, 68]. Similarly, Kuebler et al. [63] demonstrated that L-selectin was required for prolonged leukocyte sequestration in the pulmonary capillaries of rabbits following IV infusion of LPS. Also, ICAM-1 was shown to be upregulated on the rat lung capillary endothelium following LPS treatment and mediate prolonged leukocyte sequestration by binding to β_2-integrins expressed on stimulated leukocytes [46, 89].

Further studies explored the hypothesis that neutrophil-endothelium interactions in the inflamed lung can be stimulus dependent. Doyle et al. [53] have shown that L-selectin plays a role in neutrophil sequestration within the pulmonary capillaries during *E. coli* but not *S. pneumoniae* induced pneumonia, suggesting that the requirement for L-selectin could be possibly dictated by the type of stimulus. Similarly, Doerschuk et al. [56] reported an important observation that β_2-integrins are required for prolonged pulmonary capillary sequestration and the recruitment of neutrophils in response to an IT challenge of rabbits with PMA but not *S. pneumoniae* or HCl, suggesting that the requirement of β_2-integrins might also be dependent on the stimuli inducing the pulmonary inflammatory response [56]. This observation was further supported by animal studies performed with diverse inflammatory stimuli. β_2-integrin-ICAM-1 adhesion was shown to mediate neutrophil sequestration in the pulmonary capillaries following IV infusion of CVF [90], intrapulmonary instillation of IgG immune complex [69] in rats and intrabronchial challenge with IL-1α but not complement fragments in rabbits [70]. Using a functional blocking Ab against CD18, neutrophil recruitment in the rabbit lungs was shown to be CD18-dependent following IT administration of *P. aeruginosa* [74] and intrapulmonary *E. coli* [73] but CD18-independent in response to intrapulmonary *S. aureus* [73]. Also, acute neutrophil sequestration in the pulmonary capillaries of rats during HCl induced pneumonia was shown to be independent of β_2-integrin Mac-1 [91]. Using functional blocking Abs and mice deficient in LFA-1 or ICAM-1, LFA-1-ICAM-1 interaction was shown to be responsible for 50 % of neutrophil recruitment in the lung in response to aerosolized LPS [82]. As shown by the previous studies, the remaining 50 % of recruitment was believed to be mediated by CD18-independent mechanisms [82]. Thus, the requirement of both β_2-integrins and L-selectin for prolonged (>1 min) neutrophil sequestration within the inflamed pulmonary capillaries is dictated by the stimulus eliciting the pulmonary inflammatory response [4].

Since adhesion molecules do not seem to be required for the initial (<1 min) sequestration of neutrophils, it is believed that pulmonary inflammation leads to stiffening of neutrophils and a reduction in their deformability, which may result in slower transit and acute mechanical sequestration of neutrophils within the pulmonary capillaries [4]. Cytoskeletal remodeling in neutrophils occurs following the interaction of neutrophil receptors with the inflammatory mediators, cytokines, and danger signals released by tissue macrophages, necrotic host cells, mast cells, and endothelial cells in response to a pulmonary or systemic insult [3, 5, 6, 58]. Several in vitro and in vivo studies support the role of mechanical stiffening in the initial (within <1 min) sequestration of neutrophils within the inflamed pulmonary capillaries. Suwa et al. [66] has shown that the high F-actin content in circulating neutrophils was associated with reduced deformability and an increased retention in the pulmonary capillaries of rabbits. Also, IV infusion of complement fragments in rabbits was shown to cause rapid sequestration of neutrophils in the pulmonary capillaries [92]. Remarkably, the immuno-electron microscopy of the rabbit lung tissue revealed that the sequestered neutrophils were less deformable, round but not elongated in shape and had an actin rich layer under the plasma membrane [92]. Choudhury et al. [65] demonstrated that the initial neutrophil sequestration within the pulmonary capillaries of mice challenged with injurious mechanical ventilation was mediated by stiffening of neutrophils, while the prolonged retention was dependent on L-selectin but not β_2-integrins. Also using a rat model of bacterial pneumonia, Yoshida et al. [72] was able to show that the inflammatory mediators in the blood induced cytoskeletal changes resulting in the formation of an F-actin rim under the plasma membrane of circulating neutrophils. These F-actin-rim containing neutrophils were found to be preferentially sequestering within the lungs, which was independent of the β_2-integrin-mediated adhesion to the vascular wall [72]. These findings suggested that inflammatory mediators induce a reduction in neutrophil deformability that is responsible for their initial (<1 min) sequestration during pulmonary inflammation.

Based upon the collective evidence, the acute neutrophil entrapment in the inflamed pulmonary capillaries is believed to occur in two steps [4]: The first step involves rapid (<1 min) mechanical sequestration of stiff neutrophils within the pulmonary capillaries. Mechanical sequestration is immediately followed by the second step of prolonged retention (>5 min) that is mediated by adhesive interactions between the sequestered neutrophils and the inflamed capillary endothelium. Depending upon the inflammatory stimulus, the neutrophil-endothelium adhesion during prolonged retention can be either mediated by β_2-integrins and L-selectin on neutrophils binding to their cognate ligands on the inflamed endothelium or adhesive pathways that are still elusive.

Although P-selectin is critical for neutrophil rolling along the inflamed systemic venules [93], the role for P-selectin in neutrophil sequestration in the pulmonary capillaries has been treated with skepticism because the immunohistochemistry studies to date were unable to detect P-selectin expression on the lung capillary endothelium [2, 4, 11]. However, Weibel-Palade bodies (which in venules are the vehicles for rapid P-selectin expression on the endothelium) have been shown to be present in the lung endothelium [2, 94]. In a recent study, P-selectin expression was observed on the lung endothelium of mice, which was upregulated 6 h following LPS infusion [95]; however, although 6 h is enough for relocation of P-selectin to the endothelial membrane, the likelihood of P-selectin expressed on platelets adhering to the endothelium was not ruled out [95]. Another study on the role of P-selectin in acid-induced lung injury revealed that intravascular sequestration of neutrophils in the lungs is reduced in mice with no endothelial P-selectin compared to wild type mice, although the lack of P-selectin did not lead to a reduction in lung injury [71]. Asaduzzaman et al. [96, 97] and Roller et al. [47] have also shown that both endothelial and platelet P-selectin contribute to neutrophil sequestration in the lung microcirculation during abdominal sepsis-driven ALI by binding to neutrophil PSGL-1. Recently, a recombinant form of PSGL-1-Ig fusion protein attenuated neutrophil recruitment in the lungs of endotoxin challenged mice, suggesting a role for P-selectin–PSGL-1 interaction in neutrophil sequestration [98]. In addition to P-selectin, E-selectin can also bind to neutrophil PSGL-1 and may mediate neutrophil sequestration; however, E-selectin is not expressed on the noninflamed pulmonary capillary endothelium [4]. Also unlike P-selectin, which is stored preformed in Weibel-Palade bodies of endothelial cells and expressed on the cell surface within minutes in response to an inflammatory stimulus [99], E-selectin requires *de novo* mRNA synthesis which is unlikely to happen during the acute (1–5 min) neutrophil sequestration response following an inflammatory challenge.

Besides L-selectin and β_2-integrins, recent studies have shown that the endothelial surface layer (ESL) and platelets can play a role in neutrophil–endothelium interactions in the inflamed lung. Degradation of the ESL by endothelial heparanase has been suggested to mediate neutrophil sequestration within the pulmonary microcirculation of mice following systemic LPS challenge [20]. Degradation of the ESL was shown to expose ICAM-1 on the pulmonary endothelium, which is normally hidden within the thick ESL and is thus inaccessible to leukocyte β_2-integrins [20]. There is also growing evidence to support a role for platelets in neutrophil sequestration and recruitment within inflamed lungs. Neutrophil sequestration in the pulmonary capillaries of mice has been shown to be mediated by platelet-neutrophil aggregation during HCl [71] or endotoxin [78] induced pneumonia and transfusion [100] or abdominal sepsis [47, 96] induced ALI. This platelet-neutrophil aggregation was shown to be mediated by P-selectin on activated platelets binding to PSGL-1 on neutrophils [71, 78, 100] and the PSGL-1-P-selectin engagement triggered outside-in signaling leading to the upregulation of Mac-1 on neutrophils [96, 100].

Neutrophil Emigration into the Alveolar Air Space

The current understanding of the molecular mechanism of neutrophil emigration across the inflamed endothelial–epithelial barrier is based on IVM studies done in nonpulmonary vascular beds in mice [58, 101, 102], in vitro transmigration assays [103–105], electron microscopy and serial section reconstruction of rabbit pulmonary capillaries, arterioles, and venules [2, 104, 106]. Similar to the step of neutrophil sequestration within the lumen of inflamed pulmonary capillaries, the pathway for neutrophil emigration (trans-luminal, trans-endothelial, trans-interstitial, and trans-epithelial migration) into the alveolar air spaces could be CD18-dependent or independent based on the stimulus eliciting the inflammatory response [4]. Since the adhesion pathways mediating CD18-independent emigration are largely unknown, only the molecular events driving CD18-dependent emigration will be discussed here.

In preparation for emigrating across the pulmonary capillary endothelium, arrested neutrophils are required to crawl towards the junctions of endothelial cells (step 2 in Fig. 2.1). ICAM-1 and ICAM-2 are expressed on the pulmonary capillary endothelium [46, 85, 107] and are known to bind activated β_2-integrins LFA-1 and Mac-1 on neutrophils to mediate trans-luminal crawling in the systemic venules [102, 105]. The process of trans-luminal crawling requires transient and regional changes in the mechanical properties and adhesion molecule distribution of neutrophils and pulmonary endothelial cells [4, 76]. Signaling pathways triggered by CD18-ICAM-1 mediated neutrophil–endothelial adhesion, chemokine–GPCR interaction, and chemokine gradient sensing collectively result in the activation of small GTPases and the actomyosin machinery within the neutrophils [6, 52, 58, 100, 101]. These activation events enable trans-luminal crawling of leukocytes by triggering spatial and temporal changes in the cytoskeletal organization, generation of a protrusive leading edge and a contractile uropod, clustering of PSGL-1 and recycling of CD18 to the leading edge of the leukocytes. Recently, P-selectin-PSGL-1-mediated platelet interactions with adhered neutrophils have also been shown to trigger signaling events that result in neutrophil polarization, redistribution of CD18 and CXCR2 and trans-luminal crawling in the inflamed cremaster venules of mice [100]. Although platelet-neutrophil aggregation is known to occur in the inflamed pulmonary microcirculation [78], it is not known whether these interactions contribute to intra-luminal crawling within the pulmonary capillaries.

The current understanding of the molecular mechanism of leukocyte trans-endothelial migration (TEM; step 3 in Fig. 2.1) across pulmonary capillaries is largely based on in vitro cell culture transmigration studies or IVM studies of the systemic microcirculation in mice. Due to the difference in the primary site of neutrophil recruitment in the lungs (pulmonary capillaries) vs. systemic circulation (post-capillary venules), the molecular mechanism of TEM in the two vascular beds may not be exactly the same. Nevertheless, the current paradigm of TEM serves to explain the kinetics of leukocyte trafficking in the inflamed lungs. Based on in vitro endothelial cell culture studies [103–105] and electron microscopy of the rabbit lung during *S. pneumoniae* induced pneumonia [2, 106], leukocytes crawling in the pulmonary capillaries are believed to undergo TEM in less than 2 min [104]. TEM occurs predominantly (60 %) through a paracellular (between endothelial cells) pathway at the junction of three endothelial cells (tricellular corners) and less frequently (20 %) at the junction of two endothelial cells (bicellular corners) or (20 %) through the cytoplasm (transcellular pathway) of endothelial cells.

The paracellular TEM of an adhered leukocyte is regulated by endothelial cell junction integrity, which is dependent on the two primary junctional structures "adherens junctions" and "tight junctions" located within the endothelial cleft [2, 5, 52, 58, 104, 105, 108–111]. Adherens junctions are formed by homophilic interactions between VE-cadherin molecules on adjacent endothelial cells [112]. The stability of adherens junctions is dependent on the linkage of VE-cadherin to the endothelial cell actin-cytoskeleton by cytoplasmic catenins (α, β, and γ) [58]. Tight junctions consist of homophilic interactions between members of the junctional adhesion molecule (JAM) family (JAM-A, JAM-B, JAM-C, and endothelial cell-selective adhesion molecule (ESAM)) and claudins [112]. Depending on the vascular bed and the inflammatory stimulus, the borders of adjacent endothelial cells can also express PECAM-1, CD99, ICAM-2, and the polio virus receptor (PVR) [58, 108]. Human lung endothelial junctions are known to express JAM-A and C, while mouse lung endothelial junctions express only JAM-A [2]. PECAM-1 and CD99 contribute to the endothelial cell junction integrity by undergoing homophilic interaction [108].

The preference for TEM at the tricellular corners is supported by the presence of higher discontinuity in tight junctions at the tricellular (pore diameter ~27 nm [106]) than bicellular (pore diameter ~3–6 nm) junctions [113, 114]. However, the pore size required for leukocyte TEM is 1–2 μm [109, 110, 115], which is 100-folds larger than the pore size at the tricellular corners, suggesting that additional mechanisms are involved. Based on in vitro fluorescence microscopy of cultured endothelial monolayers and IVM of the systemic microcirculation in mice, the lateral displacement or sliding of cell–cell junctional complexes is believed to enable paracellular leukocyte TEM [58, 105, 109, 116].

The protrusion of an adhered leukocyte into the endothelial cleft triggers signaling events within the endothelial cell leading to sequential disassembly of the junctional complexes [6, 52, 58, 108, 117]. CD18-mediated adhesion of leukocytes to the apical surface of the endothelial cell junction results in clustering of ICAM-1 and ICAM-2 on the endothelial cell border [58, 118], an increase in cytosolic free Ca^{2+} [118, 119], generation of endothelial reactive oxygen species (ROS) [118, 120], phosphorylation of p38-mitogen-activated protein kinase (MAPK) [118], activation of endothelial proline-rich tyrosine kinase-2 (Pyk2) and Src kinase [121], and activation of small GTPase Rho-A, Rho-associated protein kinase (ROCK), and endothelial myosin light-chain kinase [111, 118, 122, 123]. These signaling events lead to local variation in the F-actin polymerization, an increase in the stiffness of endothelial cells and activation of actomyosin machinery [58, 108, 118, 122, 124], which facilitates opening of the endothelial cleft to allow passage of the emigrating leukocyte [58, 108].

As the leukocyte migrates between the junctions of endothelial cells, the tight junctions are dis-assembled and homotypic or heterotypic adhesions are established between members of the tight junctions with receptors on the leukocyte surface [108]. JAM-A and JAM-C on endothelial cells can bind to LFA-1 and Mac-1, respectively, on the emigrating leukocyte. In addition, PECAM-1 and CD99 on the endothelial borders can undergo homotypic adhesion with PECAM-1 and CD99, respectively, expressed on the leukocyte surface [125]. These interactions trigger signaling events that drive reversible endocytosis of VE-cadherin, enabled by tyrosine phosphorylation and dephosphorylation events [126], which lead to the transient disassembly of the VE-cadherin adherens junctions [127]. The coordinated disruption of tight junctions, the generation of actin-myosin tension and the disassembly of VE-cadherin adherens junctions facilitates leukocyte migration through the endothelial cell–cell junction.

Following successful TEM, the emigrated neutrophil is required to cross the interstitial matrix (step 4 in Fig. 2.1) separating the pulmonary endothelium from the alveolar epithelium, before it can enter the inflamed air space. As shown in Fig. 2.1, the interstitial matrix consists of the sub-endothelial basement membrane followed by an ECM maintained by a fibroblast and the sub-epithelial basement membrane. As described in the section "The blood–air barrier in the lung," the ECM is rich in collagen, elastin, and proteoglycans, and may also be populated with mast cells and pericytes [2]. Although neutrophils can release proteases such as elastase and gelatinase to degrade the endothelial basement membrane [128], the in vitro and in vivo studies performed with inhibitors or neutrophils from mice deficient in elastase or gelatinase do not support a necessary role for proteolytic degradation in neutrophil migration across the basement membrane [129–133].

Using transmission electron microscopy and serial section reconstruction of the rabbit lung, Walker and colleagues [2, 30] identified preexisting holes in the sub-endothelial basement membrane, which were occupied by the cytoplasmic extensions of the interstitial fibroblast during steady state (refer to Fig. 2.1). These preexisting holes were found to serve as a point of entry for migrating neutrophils during *S. pneumoniae* induced pulmonary inflammation. At steady state, these holes allowed physical contact between endothelial cells and the fibroblast. These preexisting holes are believed to become available for neutrophil passage as the fibroblast contracts in response to mechanical stress, an inflammatory stimulus or neutrophil–ECM adhesion triggered signaling events [76]. Walker et al. [2, 30] also identified similar preexisting holes in the sub-epithelial basement membrane below the type-II pneumocytes (Fig. 2.1). These preexisting holes were occupied by the cytoplasmic extensions of the type-II pneumocytes and served as a point of physical contact between the interstitial fibroblast and the type-II pneumocyte at steady state. Thus, the interstitial fibroblast was shown to serve as a physical bridge connecting endothelial cells to the type-II pneumocytes through preexisting holes in the two basement membranes [134].

Interstitial fibroblasts were also proposed to serve as a directional as well as an adhesive substrate for neutrophils migrating across the interstitium during *S. pneumoniae* induced pulmonary inflammation in the rabbit [134]. Neutrophils were observed to migrate alongside the interstitial fibroblast with ~70 % of the surface area in close contact with the fibroblast and the ECM [134]. Based on in vitro and in vivo studies [135–137], neutrophil crawling and adhesion along the fibroblast is believed to be partially mediated by β_2-integrin-ICAM-1 and β_1-integrin-VCAM-1 adhesive interactions. During migration along the interstitial fibroblast, neutrophils also undergo adhesive interactions with the components of the ECM. The ECM is rich in fibronectin, fibrinogen, laminin, collagens, entactin, tenascin, thrombospondin, and vitronectin [2]. In vivo studies performed in rats and mice show that neutrophil adhesion and migration across the lung ECM is also mediated by the interaction of β_2- and β_1-integrins on migrating neutrophils with ECM components [138, 139]. Once a neutrophil has migrated along the fibroblast and the ECM, it enters the basal lateral space of the type-II pneumocyte through one of the preexisting holes in the sub-epithelial basement membrane. Following entrance into the basal-lateral space of the type-II pneumocyte, the neutrophil is required to transmigrate across the epithelium (step 5 in Fig. 2.1).

The current understanding of the molecular mechanism of trans-epithelial migration is less profound than that of trans-endothelial migration and it is largely based on in vitro studies performed with cultured monolayers of intestinal epithelial cells, a few studies done with lung epithelial cells and rare in vivo studies [30, 140, 141]. Electron microscopy studies performed in the canine [140] and rabbit lung [30] have been instrumental in establishing that neutrophils enter the alveolar air space preferentially at the tricellular junctions where the borders of two type-I pneumocytes meet one type-II pneumocyte. This observation was supported by the freeze-fracture studies of the rabbit lung conducted by Walker and colleagues, which revealed tight-junction discontinuities at the tricellular junction of two type-I and one type-II pneumocyte [2]. Based on these findings, it is believed that the discontinuity at the epithelial tricellular junctions likely serves as a "migration tunnel" for emigrating neutrophils during pulmonary inflammation and therefore, trans-migration is not dependent on tight-junction disruption by neutrophil oxidants or proteases [2, 117, 141]. During migration through these tunnels, neutrophils are required to adhere and crawl along the borders of epithelial cells by sequentially engaging with epithelial adhesion molecules [117, 141]. Neutrophil adhesion to the alveolar epithelium basal-lateral surface is believed to be mediated by the β_2-integrin Mac-1 on neutrophils binding to JAM-C and fucosylated proteoglycans on epithelial cells [141, 142]. The β_2-integrin-mediated adhesion of neutrophils is believed to trigger phosphorylation of tight junction proteins and the activation of the actomyosin machinery within the epithelial cells, which collectively results in transient opening of the inter-epithelial cleft to allow the migration of the neutrophil [141, 143].

As the migrating neutrophil enters the inter-epithelial cleft, several adhesive interactions are possible with the epithelial membrane [2, 141]. CD47 expressed on both neutrophils and epithelial cell borders can interact with its cognate ligands on either cell type; JAM-L on neutrophils can bind to CAR (coxsackie and adenovirus receptor) expressed on epithelial cells and JAM-A on epithelial cells can bind to both JAM-A and LFA-1 on neutrophils [141]. However, the evidence to support the role of these interactions in alveolar epithelial migration of neutrophils currently does not exist [2, 141]. Following complete migration, neutrophil adhesion to the apical surface of the epithelium is believed to be mediated by β_2-integrins on neutrophils binding to ICAM-1 [144] expressed on epithelial cells. Although β_2-integrins seem to play an important role in neutrophil trans-epithelial migration during pulmonary inflammation [2, 4, 76, 141, 144–147], a role for β_1-integrins [139], CD44 [148] and β_2-integrin-independent pathways [56] cannot be ruled out [2, 4].

Conclusion

In vitro and in vivo studies performed over the last two decades have substantially improved our understanding of the molecular mechanism behind neutrophil recruitment in noninflamed and inflamed lungs. Based on the current understanding, this chapter attempts to describe the molecular adhesive paradigm of neutrophil recruitment to the alveolar air spaces during inflammation. However, there are several steps in the neutrophil recruitment cascade, which are still incompletely understood and warrant future investigations. The adhesion and signaling pathways that mediate stimulus specific CD18/ICAM-1-independent emigration into the air spaces are still unclear [76]. Although pro-inflammatory mediators are believed to trigger neutrophil stiffening and the initial mechanical sequestration within the inflamed pulmonary capillaries, the signaling events that elicit this stiffening response are not well understood. Recently, monocytes were found to regulate neutrophil recruitment in the alveolar air space during pulmonary inflammation [28], suggesting that future studies should be designed to address whether neutrophil recruitment can be controlled by other leukocytes. In the systemic circulation, P-, E-, and L-selectin–PSGL-1 interaction induced outside-in signaling has been shown to play a role in β_2-integrin activation and neutrophil adhesion to the inflamed endothelium [93]. Although the presence of P-selectin on the pulmonary capillary endothelium is debatable, activated platelets express P-selectin which can bind to PSGL-1 on neutrophils. Recently, P-selectin-PSGL-1-mediated platelet–neutrophil interaction was shown to trigger neutrophil trans-luminal crawling within the systemic venules of mice [100]. MPE-IVM studies of the mouse lung should be conducted to identify the role of P-selectin-PSGL-1 signaling and platelet–neutrophil interaction in neutrophil sequestration in the inflamed pulmonary capillaries.

As described in the section "Neutrophil emigration into the alveolar air space," our current understanding of the molecular events that enable neutrophil emigration into the air spaces is primarily based on the lessons learned in nonpulmonary vascular beds. MPE-IVM of the lung should be conducted in mice to elucidate the molecular pathways that drive neutrophil emigration across the blood–air barrier. Rolling neutrophils are known to form long cell-autonomous adhesive structures known as "slings," which enable neutrophils to roll efficiently in the inflamed systemic venules [149, 150]. Although rolling does not happen in the pulmonary capillaries, neutrophils are known to roll in pulmonary arterioles of mice during inflammation [11, 47, 51]. Neutrophils rolling in the pulmonary arterioles can have slings, which may play a role in capillary sequestration following the entrance of these neutrophils into a pulmonary capillary. MPE-IVM fluorescence and scanning electron microscopic studies are needed to identify whether slings are involved in neutrophil sequestration in pulmonary capillaries during inflammation. As authors, we have tried to acknowledge most studies which have contributed to the understanding of neutrophil kinetics in the lungs. Exclusion of a study from the discussion, by no means suggests that the study was not as equally important as the ones acknowledged in this work.

Acknowledgements This study was supported by the 11SDG7340005 from the American Heart Association (P.S.) and the VMI startup funds (P.S.). M.F.B. is supported by the National Heart, Lung, and Blood Institute of the National Institutes of Health under the T32 training grant NHLBI 5T32 HL110849-02.

References

1. Fraser RG, Pare JAP. Structure and function of the lung: with emphasis on roentgenology. Philadelphia: Saunders; 1977. p. 2–4.
2. Burns AR, Smith CW, Walker DC. Unique structural features that influence neutrophil emigration into the lung. Physiol Rev. 2003;83(2):309–36.
3. Nauseef WM, Borregaard N. Neutrophils at work. Nat Immunol. 2014;15(7):602–11.
4. Doerschuk CM. Mechanisms of leukocyte sequestration in inflamed lungs. Microcirculation. 2001;8(2):71–88.
5. Matthay MA, Ware LB, Zimmerman GA. The acute respiratory distress syndrome. J Clin Invest. 2012;122(8):2731–40.
6. Kolaczkowska E, Kubes P. Neutrophil recruitment and function in health and inflammation. Nat Rev Immunol. 2013;13(3):159–75.
7. Doerschuk CM, Beyers N, Coxson HO, Wiggs B, Hogg JC. Comparison of neutrophil and capillary diameters and their relation to neutrophil sequestration in the lung. J Appl Physiol. 1993;74(6):3040–5.
8. Hogg JC, McLean T, Martin BA, Wiggs B. Erythrocyte transit and neutrophil concentration in the dog lung. J Appl Physiol. 1988;65(3):1217–25.
9. Lien DC, Wagner Jr WW, Capen RL, Haslett C, Hanson WL, Hofmeister SE, et al. Physiological neutrophil sequestration in the lung: visual evidence for localization in capillaries. J Appl Physiol. 1987;62(3):1236–43.
10. Hogg JC, Doerschuk CM. Leukocyte traffic in the lung. Annu Rev Physiol. 1995;57:97–114.
11. Gebb SA, Graham JA, Hanger CC, Godbey PS, Capen RL, Doerschuk CM, et al. Sites of leukocyte sequestration in the pulmonary microcirculation. J Appl Physiol. 1995;79(2):493–7.
12. Tanaka K, Koike Y, Shimura T, Okigami M, Ide S, Toiyama Y, et al. In vivo characterization of neutrophil extracellular traps in various organs of a murine sepsis model. PLoS One. 2014;9(11):e111888.
13. Looney MR, Thornton EE, Sen D, Lamm WJ, Glenny RW, Krummel MF. Stabilized imaging of immune surveillance in the mouse lung. Nat Methods. 2011;8(1):91–6.

14. Ley K, Mestas J, Pospieszalska MK, Sundd P, Groisman A, Zarbock A. Chapter 11. Intravital microscopic investigation of leukocyte interactions with the blood vessel wall. Methods Enzymol. 2008;445:255–79.
15. Hickey MJ, Westhorpe CL. Imaging inflammatory leukocyte recruitment in kidney, lung and liver—challenges to the multi-step paradigm. Immunol Cell Biol. 2013;91(4):281–9.
16. Bennewitz MF, Watkins SC, Sundd P. Quantitative intravital two-photon excitation microscopy reveals absence of pulmonary vaso-occlusion in unchallenged Sickle Cell Disease mice. Intra Vital. 2014;3(1):e29748.
17. Presson Jr RG, Brown MB, Fisher AJ, Sandoval RM, Dunn KW, Lorenz KS, et al. Two-photon imaging within the murine thorax without respiratory and cardiac motion artifact. Am J Pathol. 2011;179(1):75–82.
18. Yang Y, Yang G, Schmidt EP. In vivo measurement of the mouse pulmonary endothelial surface layer. J Vis Exp. 2013;72:e50322.
19. Tabuchi A, Mertens M, Kuppe H, Pries AR, Kuebler WM. Intravital microscopy of the murine pulmonary microcirculation. J Appl Physiol. 2008;104(2):338–46.
20. Schmidt EP, Yang Y, Janssen WJ, Gandjeva A, Perez MJ, Barthel L, et al. The pulmonary endothelial glycocalyx regulates neutrophil adhesion and lung injury during experimental sepsis. Nat Med. 2012;18(8):1217–23.
21. Wiggs BR, English D, Quinlan WM, Doyle NA, Hogg JC, Doerschuk CM. Contributions of capillary pathway size and neutrophil deformability to neutrophil transit through rabbit lungs. J Appl Physiol. 1994;77(1):463–70.
22. Matute-Bello G, Frevert CW, Martin TR. Animal models of acute lung injury. Am J Physiol. 2008;295(3):L379–99.
23. Looney MR, Bhattacharya J. Live imaging of the lung. Annu Rev Physiol. 2014;76:431–45.
24. Cella F, Diaspro A. Two-photon excitation microscopy: a superb wizard for fluorescence imaging. In: Diaspro A, editor. Nanoscopy and multidimensional optical fluorescence microscopy. Boca Raton, FL: CRC Press; 2010. 7-1-12.
25. Faust N, Varas F, Kelly LM, Heck S, Graf T. Insertion of enhanced green fluorescent protein into the lysozyme gene creates mice with green fluorescent granulocytes and macrophages. Blood. 2000;96(2):719–26.
26. Hasenberg A, Hasenberg M, Mann L, Neumann F, Borkenstein L, Stecher M, et al. Catchup: a mouse model for imaging-based tracking and modulation of neutrophil granulocytes. Nat Methods. 2015;12(5):445–52.
27. Yipp BG, Kubes P. Antibodies against neutrophil LY6G do not inhibit leukocyte recruitment in mice in vivo. Blood. 2013;121(1):241–2.
28. Kreisel D, Nava RG, Li W, Zinselmeyer BH, Wang B, Lai J, et al. In vivo two-photon imaging reveals monocyte-dependent neutrophil extravasation during pulmonary inflammation. Proc Natl Acad Sci U S A. 2010;107(42):18073–8.
29. Weibel ER. The pathway for oxygen: structure and function in the mammalian respiratory system. Cambridge, MA: Harvard University Press; 1984. 425 p.
30. Walker DC, Behzad AR, Chu F. Neutrophil migration through preexisting holes in the basal laminae of alveolar capillaries and epithelium during streptococcal pneumonia. Microvasc Res. 1995;50(3):397–416.
31. Townsley MI. Structure and composition of pulmonary arteries, capillaries, and veins. Compr Physiol. 2012;2(1):675–709.
32. Guntheroth WG, Luchtel DL, Kawabori I. Pulmonary microcirculation: tubules rather than sheet and post. J Appl Physiol. 1982;53(2):510–5.
33. Hogg JC. Neutrophil kinetics and lung injury. Physiol Rev. 1987;67(4):1249–95.
34. Bathe M, Shirai A, Doerschuk CM, Kamm RD. Neutrophil transit times through pulmonary capillaries: the effects of capillary geometry and fMLP-stimulation. Biophys J. 2002;83(4):1917–33.
35. Huang Y, Doerschuk CM, Kamm RD. Computational modeling of RBC and neutrophil transit through the pulmonary capillaries. J Appl Physiol. 2001;90:545–64.
36. Sundd P. Micropipette cell adhesion assay: a novel in vitro assay to model leukocyte adhesion in the pulmonary capillaries of the lung [Ph.D.]. Athens: Ohio University; 2007.

37. Staub NC, Schultz EL. Pulmonary capillary length in dogs, cat and rabbit. Respir Physiol. 1968;5(3):371–8.
38. Fenton BM, Wilson DW, Cokelet GR. Analysis of the effects of measured white blood cell entrance times on hemodynamics in a computer model of a microvascular bed. Pflugers Arch. 1985;403(4):396–401.
39. Evans E, Yeung A. Apparent viscosity and cortical tension of blood granulocytes determined by micropipet aspiration. Biophys J. 1989;56(1):151–60.
40. Tran-Son-Tay R, Needham D, Yeung A, Hochmuth RM. Time-dependent recovery of passive neutrophils after large deformation. Biophys J. 1991;60(4):856–66.
41. Evans E, Kukan B. Passive material behavior of granulocytes based on large deformation and recovery after deformation tests. Blood. 1984;64(5):1028–35.
42. Gabriele S, Benoliel AM, Bongrand P, Theodoly O. Microfluidic investigation reveals distinct roles for actin cytoskeleton and myosin II activity in capillary leukocyte trafficking. Biophys J. 2009;96(10):4308–18.
43. Sundd P, Zou X, Goetz DJ, Tees DF. Leukocyte adhesion in capillary-sized. P-selectin-coated micropipettes. Microcirculation. 2008;15(2):109–22.
44. Shao JY, Hochmuth RM. The resistance to flow of individual human neutrophils in glass capillary tubes with diameters between 4.65 and 7.75 μm. Microcirculation. 1997;4(1):61–74.
45. Lien DC, Henson PM, Capen RL, Henson JE, Hanson WL, Wagner Jr WW, et al. Neutrophil kinetics in the pulmonary microcirculation during acute inflammation. Lab Invest. 1991;65(2):145–59.
46. Aoki T, Suzuki Y, Nishio K, Suzuki K, Miyata A, Iigou Y, et al. Role of CD18-ICAM-1 in the entrapment of stimulated leukocytes in alveolar capillaries of perfused rat lungs. Am J Physiol Heart Circ Physiol. 1997;273(5):H2361–71.
47. Roller J, Wang Y, Rahman M, Schramm R, Laschke MW, Menger MD, et al. Direct in vivo observations of P-selectin glycoprotein ligand-1-mediated leukocyte-endothelial cell interactions in the pulmonary microvasculature in abdominal sepsis in mice. Inflamm Res. 2013;62(3):275–82.
48. Parthasarathi K, Ichimura H, Monma E, Lindert J, Quadri S, Issekutz A, et al. Connexin 43 mediates spread of Ca2+-dependent proinflammatory responses in lung capillaries. J Clin Invest. 2006;116(8):2193–200.
49. Bullard DC, Qin L, Lorenzo I, Quinlin WM, Doyle NA, Bosse R, et al. P-selectin/ICAM-1 double mutant mice: acute emigration of neutrophils into the peritoneum is completely absent but is normal into pulmonary alveoli. J Clin Invest. 1995;95(4):1782–8.
50. Doerschuk CM, Quinlan WM, Doyle NA, Bullard DC, Vestweber D, Jones ML, et al. The role of P-selectin and ICAM-1 in acute lung injury as determined using blocking antibodies and mutant mice. J Immunol. 1996;157(10):4609–14.
51. Kuebler WM, Kuhnle GE, Groh J, Goetz AE. Contribution of selectins to leucocyte sequestration in pulmonary microvessels by intravital microscopy in rabbits. J Physiol. 1997;501(Pt 2):375–86.
52. Ley K, Laudanna C, Cybulsky MI, Nourshargh S. Getting to the site of inflammation: the leukocyte adhesion cascade updated. Nat Rev Immunol. 2007;7(9):678–89.
53. Doyle NA, Bhagwan SD, Meek BB, Kutkoski GJ, Steeber DA, Tedder TF, et al. Neutrophil margination, sequestration, and emigration in the lungs of L-selectin-deficient mice. J Clin Invest. 1997;99(3):526–33.
54. Luo BH, Carman CV, Springer TA. Structural basis of integrin regulation and signaling. Annu Rev Immunol. 2007;25:619–47.
55. Anderson GJ, Roswit WT, Holtzman MJ, Hogg JC, Van Eeden SF. Effect of mechanical deformation of neutrophils on their CD18/ICAM-1-dependent adhesion. J Appl Physiol. 2001;91(3):1084–90.
56. Doerschuk CM, Winn RK, Coxson HO, Harlan JM. CD18-Dependent and -independent mechanisms of neutrophil emigration in the pulmonary and systemic microcirculation of rabbits. J Immunol. 1990;144(6):2327–33.

57. Devi S, Wang Y, Chew WK, Lima R, A-González N, Mattar CN, et al. Neutrophil mobilization via plerixafor-mediated CXCR4 inhibition arises from lung demargination and blockade of neutrophil homing to the bone marrow. J Exp Med. 2013;210(11):2321–36.
58. Nourshargh S, Alon R. Leukocyte migration into inflamed tissues. Immunity. 2014; 41(5):694–707.
59. Reutershan J, Basit A, Galkina EV, Ley K. Sequential recruitment of neutrophils into lung and bronchoalveolar lavage fluid in LPS-induced acute lung injury. Am J Physiol Lung Cell Mol Physiol. 2005;289(5):L807–15.
60. Rittirsch D, Flierl MA, Day DE, Nadeau BA, McGuire SR, Hoesel LM, et al. Acute lung injury induced by lipopolysaccharide is independent of complement activation. J Immunol. 2008;180(11):7664–72.
61. Andonegui G, Bonder CS, Green F, Mullaly SC, Zbytnuik L, Raharjo E, et al. Endothelium-derived toll-like receptor-4 is the key molecule in LPS-induced neutrophil sequestration into lungs. J Clin Invest. 2003;111(7):1011–20.
62. Andonegui G, Zhou H, Bullard D, Kelly MM, Mullaly SC, McDonald B, et al. Mice that exclusively express TLR4 on endothelial cells can efficiently clear a lethal systemic Gram-negative bacterial infection. J Clin Invest. 2009;119(7):1921–30.
63. Kuebler WM, Borges J, Sckell A, Kuhnle GE, Bergh K, Messmer K, et al. Role of L-selectin in leukocyte sequestration in lung capillaries in a rabbit model of endotoxemia. Am J Respir Crit Care Med. 2000;161(1):36–43.
64. Kubo H, Doyle NA, Graham L, Bhagwan SD, Quinlan WM, Doerschuk CM. L- and P-selectin and CD11/CD18 in intracapillary neutrophil sequestration in rabbit lungs. Am J Respir Crit Care Med. 1999;159(1):267–74.
65. Choudhury S, Wilson MR, Goddard ME, O'Dea KP, Takata M. Mechanisms of early pulmonary neutrophil sequestration in ventilator-induced lung injury in mice. Am J Physiol Lung Cell Mol Physiol. 2004;287(5):L902–10.
66. Suwa T, Hogg JC, Klut ME, Hards J, van Eeden SF. Interleukin-6 changes deformability of neutrophils and induces their sequestration in the lung. Am J Respir Crit Care Med. 2001;163(4):970–6.
67. Mulligan M, Miyasaka M, Tamatani T, Jones M, Ward P. Requirements for L-selectin in neutrophil-mediated lung injury in rats. J Immunol. 1994;152(2):832–40.
68. Doerschuk CM. The role of CD18-mediated adhesion in neutrophil sequestration induced by infusion of activated plasma in rabbits. Am J Respir Cell Mol Biol. 1992;7(2):140–8.
69. Mulligan MS, Wilson GP, Todd RF, Smith CW, Anderson DC, Varani J, et al. Role of beta 1, beta 2 integrins and ICAM-1 in lung injury after deposition of IgG and IgA immune complexes. J Immunol. 1993;150(6):2407–17.
70. Hellewell PG, Young SK, Henson PM, Worthen GS. Disparate role of the beta 2-integrin CD18 in the local accumulation of neutrophils in pulmonary and cutaneous inflammation in the rabbit. Am J Respir Cell Mol Biol. 1994;10(4):391–8.
71. Zarbock A, Singbartl K, Ley K. Complete reversal of acid-induced acute lung injury by blocking of platelet-neutrophil aggregation. J Clin Invest. 2006;116(12):3211–9.
72. Yoshida K, Kondo R, Wang Q, Doerschuk CM. Neutrophil cytoskeletal rearrangements during capillary sequestration in bacterial pneumonia in rats. Am J Respir Crit Care Med. 2006;174(6):689–98.
73. Ramamoorthy C, Sasaki SS, Su DL, Sharar SR, Harlan JM, Winn RK. CD18 adhesion blockade decreases bacterial clearance and neutrophil recruitment after intrapulmonary E. coli, but not after S. aureus. J Leukoc Biol. 1997;61(2):167–72.
74. Kumasaka T, Doyle NA, Quinlan WM, Graham L, Doerschuk CM. Role of CD 11/CD 18 in neutrophil emigration during acute and recurrent Pseudomonas aeruginosa-induced pneumonia in rabbits. Am J Pathol. 1996;148(4):1297–305.
75. Qin L, Quinlan WM, Doyle NA, Graham L, Sligh JE, Takei F, et al. The roles of CD11/CD18 and ICAM-1 in acute Pseudomonas aeruginosa-induced pneumonia in mice. J Immunol. 1996;157(11):5016–21.

76. Williams AE, Chambers RC. The mercurial nature of neutrophils: still an enigma in ARDS? Am J Physiol. 2014;306(3):L217–30.
77. Yipp BG, Kubes P. NETosis: how vital is it? Blood. 2013;122(16):2784–94.
78. Ortiz-Munoz G, Mallavia B, Bins A, Headley M, Krummel MF, Looney MR. Aspirin-triggered 15-epi-lipoxin A4 regulates neutrophil-platelet aggregation and attenuates acute lung injury in mice. Blood. 2014;124(17):2625–34.
79. Caudrillier A, Kessenbrock K, Gilliss BM, Nguyen JX, Marques MB, Monestier M, et al. Platelets induce neutrophil extracellular traps in transfusion-related acute lung injury. J Clin Invest. 2012;122(7):2661–71.
80. Liang J, Jung Y, Tighe RM, Xie T, Liu N, Leonard M, et al. A macrophage subpopulation recruited by CC chemokine ligand-2 clears apoptotic cells in noninfectious lung injury. Am J Physiol. 2012;302(9):L933–40.
81. Bratton DL, Henson PM. Neutrophil clearance: when the party is over, clean-up begins. Trends Immunol. 2011;32(8):350–7.
82. Basit A, Reutershan J, Morris MA, Solga M, Rose Jr CE, Ley K. ICAM-1 and LFA-1 play critical roles in LPS-induced neutrophil recruitment into the alveolar space. Am J Physiol. 2006;291(2):L200–7.
83. Moore KL, Eaton SF, Lyons DE, Lichenstein HS, Cummings RD, McEver RP. The P-selectin glycoprotein ligand form human neutrophils displays sialylated, fucosylated. O-linked poly-N-acetyllactosamine. J Biol Chem. 1994;269(37):23318–27.
84. Moore KL, Patel KD, Bruehl RE, Li F, Johnson DA, Lichenstein HS, et al. P-selectin glycoprotein ligand-1 mediates rolling of human neutrophils on P-selectin. J Cell Biol. 1995;128:661–71.
85. Burns AR, Takei F, Doerschuk CM. Quantitation of ICAM-1 expression in mouse lung during pneumonia. J Immunol. 1994;153(7):3189–98.
86. Mulligan M, Watson S, Fennie C, Ward P. Protective effects of selectin chimeras in neutrophil-mediated lung injury. J Immunol. 1993;151(11):6410–7.
87. Mulligan MS, Polley MJ, Bayer RJ, Nunn MF, Paulson JC, Ward PA. Neutrophil-dependent acute lung injury. Requirement for P-selectin (GMP-140). J Clin Invest. 1992;90(4):1600–7.
88. Kumasaka T, Quinlan WM, Doyle NA, Condon TP, Sligh J, Takei F, et al. Role of the intercellular adhesion molecule-1(ICAM-1) in endotoxin-induced pneumonia evaluated using ICAM-1 antisense oligonucleotides, anti-ICAM-1 monoclonal antibodies, and ICAM-1 mutant mice. J Clin Invest. 1996;97(10):2362–9.
89. Kandasamy K, Sahu G, Parthasarathi K. Real-time imaging reveals endothelium-mediated leukocyte retention in LPS-treated lung microvessels. Microvasc Res. 2012;83(3):323–31.
90. Mulligan MS, Varani J, Warren JS, Till GO, Smith CW, Anderson DC, et al. Roles of beta 2 integrins of rat neutrophils in complement- and oxygen radical-mediated acute inflammatory injury. J Immunol. 1992;148(6):1847–57.
91. Motosugi H, Quinlan WM, Bree M, Doerschuk CM. Role of CD11b in focal acid-induced pneumonia and contralateral lung injury in rats. Am J Respir Crit Care Med. 1998;157(1):192–8.
92. Motosugi H, Graham L, Noblitt TW, Doyle N, Quinlan WM, Li Y, et al. Changes in neutrophil actin and shape during sequestration induced by complement fragments in rabbits. Am J Pathol. 1996;149(5):963–73.
93. McEver RP. Selectins: initiators of leucocyte adhesion and signalling at the vascular wall. Cardiovasc Res. 2015;107(3):331–9.
94. Wang N. Electron microscopy in diagnostic pathology. Nonneoplastic disease. In: Schraufnagel D, editor. Electron microscopy of the lung. Lung biology in health and disease, vol. 48. New York: Dekker; 1990. p. 429–90.
95. Kiefmann R, Heckel K, Schenkat S, Dorger M, Goetz AE. Role of p-selectin in platelet sequestration in pulmonary capillaries during endotoxemia. J Vasc Res. 2006;43(5):473–81.
96. Asaduzzaman M, Lavasani S, Rahman M, Zhang S, Braun OO, Jeppsson B, et al. Platelets support pulmonary recruitment of neutrophils in abdominal sepsis. Crit Care Med. 2009;37(4):1389–96.

97. Asaduzzaman M, Rahman M, Jeppsson B, Thorlacius H. P-selectin glycoprotein-ligand-1 regulates pulmonary recruitment of neutrophils in a platelet-independent manner in abdominal sepsis. Br J Pharmacol. 2009;156(2):307–15.
98. Shao HZ, Qin BY. rPSGL-1-Ig, a recombinant PSGL-1-Ig fusion protein, ameliorates LPS-induced acute lung injury in mice by inhibiting neutrophil migration. Cell Mol Biol. 2015;61(1):1–6.
99. Hattori R, Hamilton K, Fugate R, McEver R, Sims P. Stimulated secretion of endothelial von Willebrand factor is accompanied by rapid redistribution to the cell surface of the intracellular granule membrane protein GMP-140. J Biol Chem. 1989;264(14):7768–71.
100. Sreeramkumar V, Adrover JM, Ballesteros I, Cuartero MI, Rossaint J, Bilbao I, et al. Neutrophils scan for activated platelets to initiate inflammation. Science. 2014;346(6214):1234–8.
101. Hyun YM, Sumagin R, Sarangi PP, Lomakina E, Overstreet MG, Baker CM, et al. Uropod elongation is a common final step in leukocyte extravasation through inflamed vessels. J Exp Med. 2012;209(7):1349–62.
102. Phillipson M, Heit B, Colarusso P, Liu L, Ballantyne CM, Kubes P. Intraluminal crawling of neutrophils to emigration sites: a molecularly distinct process from adhesion in the recruitment cascade. J Exp Med. 2006;203(12):2569–75.
103. Burns A, Bowden R, Abe Y, Walker D, Simon S, Entman M, et al. P-selectin mediates neutrophil adhesion to endothelial cell borders. J Leukoc Biol. 1999;65(3):299–306.
104. Burns AR, Walker DC, Brown ES, Thurmon LT, Bowden RA, Keese CR, et al. Neutrophil transendothelial migration is independent of tight junctions and occurs preferentiallly at tricellular corners. J Immunol. 1997;159:2893–903.
105. Halai K, Whiteford J, Ma B, Nourshargh S, Woodfin A. ICAM-2 facilitates luminal interactions between neutrophils and endothelial cells in vivo. J Cell Sci. 2014;127(Pt 3):620–9.
106. Walker DC, MacKenzie A, Hosford S. The structure of the tricellular region of endothelial tight junctions of pulmonary capillaries analyzed by freeze-fracture. Microvasc Res. 1994;48(3):259–81.
107. Gerwin N, Gonzalo JA, Lloyd C, Coyle AJ, Reiss Y, Banu N, et al. Prolonged eosinophil accumulation in allergic lung interstitium of ICAM-2 deficient mice results in extended hyperresponsiveness. Immunity. 1999;10(1):9–19.
108. Muller WA. The regulation of transendothelial migration: new knowledge and new questions. Cardiovasc Res. 2015;107(3):310–20.
109. Woodfin A, Voisin MB, Beyrau M, Colom B, Caille D, Diapouli FM, et al. The junctional adhesion molecule JAM-C regulates polarized transendothelial migration of neutrophils in vivo. Nat Immunol. 2011;12(8):761–9.
110. Burns AR, Bowden RA, MacDonell SD, Walker DC, Odebunmi TO, Donnachie EM, et al. Analysis of tight junctions during neutrophil transendothelial migration. J Cell Sci. 2000;113(Pt 1):45–57.
111. Carman CV, Springer TA. A transmigratory cup in leukocyte diapedesis both through individual vascular endothelial cells and between them. J Cell Biol. 2004;167(2):377–88.
112. Dejana E. Endothelial cell-cell junctions: happy together. Nat Rev Mol Cell Biol. 2004;5(4):261–70.
113. Simionescu N, Simionescu M, Palade GE. Open junctions in the endothelium of the postcapillary venules of the diaphragm. J Cell Biol. 1978;79(1):27–44.
114. Simionescu N, Simionescu M, Palade GE. Structural basis of permeability in sequential segments of the microvasculature of the diaphragm. I. Bipolar microvascular fields. Microvasc Res. 1978;15(1):1–16.
115. Marchesi VT, Florey HW. Electron micrographic observations on the emigration of leucocytes. Q J Exp Physiol Cogn Med Sci. 1960;45:343–8.
116. Huang MT, Larbi KY, Scheiermann C, Woodfin A, Gerwin N, Haskard DO, et al. ICAM-2 mediates neutrophil transmigration in vivo: evidence for stimulus specificity and a role in PECAM-1-independent transmigration. Blood. 2006;107(12):4721–7.

117. Schmidt EP, Lee WL, Zemans RL, Yamashita C, Downey GP. On, around, and through: neutrophil-endothelial interactions in innate immunity. Physiology. 2011;26(5):334–47.
118. Wang Q, Pfeiffer 2nd GR, Stevens T, Doerschuk CM. Lung microvascular and arterial endothelial cells differ in their responses to intercellular adhesion molecule-1 ligation. Am J Respir Crit Care Med. 2002;166(6):872–7.
119. Huang AJ, Manning JE, Bandak TM, Ratau MC, Hanser KR, Silverstein SC. Endothelial cell cytosolic free calcium regulates neutrophil migration across monolayers of endothelial cells. J Cell Biol. 1993;120(6):1371–80.
120. Martinelli R, Gegg M, Longbottom R, Adamson P, Turowski P, Greenwood J. ICAM-1-mediated endothelial nitric oxide synthase activation via calcium and AMP-activated protein kinase is required for transendothelial lymphocyte migration. Mol Biol Cell. 2009;20(3):995–1005.
121. Allingham MJ, van Buul JD, Burridge K. ICAM-1-mediated, Src- and Pyk2-dependent vascular endothelial cadherin tyrosine phosphorylation is required for leukocyte transendothelial migration. J Immunol. 2007;179(6):4053–64.
122. Kang I, Wang Q, Eppell SJ, Marchant RE, Doerschuk CM. Effect of neutrophil adhesion on the mechanical properties of lung microvascular endothelial cells. Am J Respir Cell Mol Biol. 2010;43(5):591–8.
123. Lessey-Morillon EC, Osborne LD, Monaghan-Benson E, Guilluy C, O'Brien ET, Superfine R, et al. The RhoA guanine nucleotide exchange factor, LARG, mediates ICAM-1-dependent mechanotransduction in endothelial cells to stimulate transendothelial migration. J Immunol. 2014;192(7):3390–8.
124. Tasaka S, Koh H, Yamada W, Shimizu M, Ogawa Y, Hasegawa N, et al. Attenuation of endotoxin-induced acute lung injury by the Rho-associated kinase inhibitor, Y-27632. Am J Respir Cell Mol Biol. 2005;32(6):504–10.
125. Watson RL, Buck J, Levin LR, Winger RC, Wang J, Arase H, et al. Endothelial CD99 signals through soluble adenylyl cyclase and PKA to regulate leukocyte transendothelial migration. J Exp Med. 2015;212(7):1021–41.
126. Wessel F, Winderlich M, Holm M, Frye M, Rivera-Galdos R, Vockel M, et al. Leukocyte extravasation and vascular permeability are each controlled in vivo by different tyrosine residues of VE-cadherin. Nat Immunol. 2014;15(3):223–30.
127. Vestweber D. Relevance of endothelial junctions in leukocyte extravasation and vascular permeability. Ann N Y Acad Sci. 2012;1257:184–92.
128. Kaynar AM, Houghton AM, Lum EH, Pitt BR, Shapiro SD. Neutrophil elastase is needed for neutrophil emigration into lungs in ventilator-induced lung injury. Am J Respir Cell Mol Biol. 2008;39(1):53–60.
129. Mackarel AJ, Cottell DC, Russell KJ, FitzGerald MX, O'Connor CM. Migration of neutrophils across human pulmonary endothelial cells is not blocked by matrix metalloproteinase or serine protease inhibitors. Am J Respir Cell Mol Biol. 1999;20(6):1209–19.
130. Huber AR, Weiss SJ. Disruption of the subendothelial basement membrane during neutrophil diapedesis in an in vitro construct of a blood vessel wall. J Clin Invest. 1989;83(4):1122–36.
131. Belaaouaj A, McCarthy R, Baumann M, Gao Z, Ley TJ, Abraham SN, et al. Mice lacking neutrophil elastase reveal impaired host defense against gram negative bacterial sepsis. Nat Med. 1998;4(5):615–8.
132. Betsuyaku T, Shipley JM, Liu Z, Senior RM. Neutrophil emigration in the lungs, peritoneum, and skin does not require gelatinase B. Am J Respir Cell Mol Biol. 1999;20(6):1303–9.
133. Hirche TO, Atkinson JJ, Bahr S, Belaaouaj A. Deficiency in neutrophil elastase does not impair neutrophil recruitment to inflamed sites. Am J Respir Cell Mol Biol. 2004;30(4):576–84.
134. Behzad AR, Chu F, Walker DC. Fibroblasts are in a position to provide directional information to migrating neutrophils during pneumonia in rabbit lungs. Microvasc Res. 1996;51(3):303–16.

135. Burns AR, Simon SI, Kukielka GL, Rowen JL, Lu H, Mendoza LH, et al. Chemotactic factors stimulate CD18-dependent canine neutrophil adherence and motility on lung fibroblasts. J Immunol. 1996;156(9):3389–401.
136. Shang XZ, Issekutz AC. Beta 2 (CD18) and beta 1 (CD29) integrin mechanisms in migration of human polymorphonuclear leucocytes and monocytes through lung fibroblast barriers: shared and distinct mechanisms. Immunology. 1997;92(4):527–35.
137. Meng H, Marchese MJ, Garlick JA, Jelaska A, Korn JH, Gailit J, et al. Mast cells induce T-cell adhesion to human fibroblasts by regulating intercellular adhesion molecule-1 and vascular cell adhesion molecule-1 expression. J Invest Dermatol. 1995;105(6):789–96.
138. Burns JA, Issekutz TB, Yagita H, Issekutz AC. The alpha 4 beta 1 (very late antigen (VLA)-4, CD49d/CD29) and alpha 5 beta 1 (VLA-5, CD49e/CD29) integrins mediate beta 2 (CD11/CD18) integrin-independent neutrophil recruitment to endotoxin-induced lung inflammation. J Immunol. 2001;166(7):4644–9.
139. Ridger VC, Wagner BE, Wallace WA, Hellewell PG. Differential effects of CD18, CD29, and CD49 integrin subunit inhibition on neutrophil migration in pulmonary inflammation. J Immunol. 2001;166(5):3484–90.
140. Damiano VV, Cohen A, Tsang AL, Batra G, Petersen R. A morphologic study of the influx of neutrophils into dog lung alveoli after lavage with sterile saline. Am J Pathol. 1980;100(2):349–64.
141. Zemans RL, Colgan SP, Downey GP. Transepithelial migration of neutrophils: mechanisms and implications for acute lung injury. Am J Respir Cell Mol Biol. 2009;40(5):519–35.
142. Aurrand-Lions M, Lamagna C, Dangerfield JP, Wang S, Herrera P, Nourshargh S, et al. Junctional adhesion molecule-C regulates the early influx of leukocytes into tissues during inflammation. J Immunol. 2005;174(10):6406–15.
143. Turner JR. "Putting the squeeze" on the tight junction: understanding cytoskeletal regulation. Semin Cell Dev Biol. 2000;11(4):301–8.
144. Jagels MA, Daffern PJ, Zuraw BL, Hugli TE. Mechanisms and regulation of polymorphonuclear leukocyte and eosinophil adherence to human airway epithelial cells. Am J Respir Cell Mol Biol. 1999;21(3):418–27.
145. McDonald RJ, St George JA, Pan LC, Hyde DM. Neutrophil adherence to airway epithelium is reduced by antibodies to the leukocyte CD11/CD18 complex. Inflammation. 1993;17(2):145–51.
146. Celi A, Cianchetti S, Petruzzelli S, Carnevali S, Baliva F, Giuntini C. ICAM-1-independent adhesion of neutrophils to phorbol ester-stimulated human airway epithelial cells. Am J Physiol. 1999;277(3 Pt 1):L465–71.
147. Tosi MF, Hamedani A, Brosovich J, Alpert SE. ICAM-1-independent, CD18-dependent adhesion between neutrophils and human airway epithelial cells exposed in vitro to ozone. J Immunol. 1994;152(4):1935–42.
148. Wang Q, Teder P, Judd NP, Noble PW, Doerschuk CM. CD44 deficiency leads to enhanced neutrophil migration and lung injury in Escherichia coli pneumonia in mice. Am J Pathol. 2002;161(6):2219–28.
149. Sundd P, Gutierrez E, Koltsova EK, Kuwano Y, Fukuda S, Pospieszalska MK, et al. "Slings" enable neutrophil rolling at high shear. Nature. 2012;488(7411):399–403.
150. Sundd P, Pospieszalska MK, Ley K. Neutrophil rolling at high shear: flattening, catch bond behavior, tethers and slings. Mol Immunol. 2013;55(1):59–69.

Part II
Acute Pulmonary Manifestations Arising From Primary Hematologic Disorders

Chapter 3
Sickle Cell Disease and Acute Chest Syndrome: Mechanisms and Pathogenenesis

Olufolake Adetoro Adisa, Amma Owusu-Ansah, Afua Darkwah Abrahams, Samit Ghosh, and Solomon Fiifi Ofori-Acquah

Introduction

Acute chest syndrome (ACS) is the major lung complication and a leading cause of death in sickle cell disease (SCD). The term ACS was coined in 1979 to describe an unusual, rapidly progressive type of acute lung injury (ALI) that occurs in SCD particularly among adults [1]. Two multicenter prospective studies in the US; the Cooperative Study of Sickle Cell Disease (CSSCD) [2–6], and the National Acute Chest Syndrome Study, and others have defined the incidence, risk factors, clinical presentation, course, etiologies, and outcome of ACS [7–9]. Findings from these large studies underpin the current understanding and clinical management of ACS [10–12]. Chapter 4 contains a detailed discussion of the epidemiology, diagnosis, management, and outcome of ACS. This chapter, after briefly reviewing the salient clinical features, genetic or other risk factors and pathology relevant to our discussion, will focus primarily on pathogenesis of ACS.

O.A. Adisa, MD
Department of Pediatrics, Emory University, Atlanta, GA, USA

A. Owusu-Ansah, MD, MBBS • S. Ghosh, PhD
Division of Hematology/Oncology, Department of Medicine, School of Medicine, University of Pittsburgh, Pittsburgh, PA, USA

A.D. Abrahams, MBChB, FWACP
Department of Pathology, University of Ghana Medical School and Korle Bu Teaching Hospital, University of Ghana, Accra, Ghana

S.F. Ofori-Acquah, PhD (✉)
Department of Pathology, University of Ghana Medical School and Korle Bu Teaching Hospital, University of Ghana, Accra, Ghana

Center for Translational and International Hematology, Pittsburgh Heart, Lung, and Blood Vascular Medicine Institute, University of Pittsburgh, Pittsburgh, PA, USA
e-mail: sfo2@pitt.edu

J.S. Lee, M.P. Donahoe (eds.), *Hematologic Abnormalities and Acute Lung Syndromes*, Respiratory Medicine, DOI 10.1007/978-3-319-41912-1_3

The severity of ACS is highly variable ranging from mild respiratory illness in some patients to acute respiratory distress syndrome (ARDS) requiring intensive care in others. The mean length of hospitalization for all patients with ACS is ~10.5 days, although children typically stay in the hospital ~4 days less than adults [13, 14]. It is the leading reason for admission of SCD patients to the intensive care unit [15]; the most significant predictor of mortality during ACS is the rapid rate of progression to respiratory failure [6].

The presence of a new pulmonary infiltrate in SCD is the major diagnostic criteria for ACS, in association with several symptoms that include fever, chest pain, tachypnea, wheezing, and cough [14]. Children have a higher incidence of fever, cough, and wheezing at diagnosis, while adults are often afebrile, have shortness of breath, chills, and severe pain. Children less than 4 years of age have the highest incidence of ACS [5, 6], and this heightened risk is predictive of future episodes [16, 17], and hospitalizations for VOC within one year of the initial ACS episode [18]. Seasonal variation in incidence, particularly among children is well documented with higher rates during the winter months, attributed to greater episodes of seasonal viral respiratory infections [6, 14]. A comorbid diagnosis of asthma increases the risk of ACS. Children with SCD and asthma or a history of reactive airways disease have increased episodes of VOC and ACS, and present with ACS at a younger age [19–21].

Several other clinical factors exacerbate ACS; they include hypoventilation from pain [22] or over-sedation [14] or fat embolism [23] from marrow infarction or pulmonary thromboembolism. Other factors, include marrow and rib infarction, postoperative atelectasis and airway hyperreactivity, hypoxia, and acute hemolysis [24]. The majority of patients with ACS are hypoxemic, and although the extent of hypoxemia is similar in all ages, children generally have less severe hypoxia. Correction of hypoxia and increasing oxygen carrying capacity to halt progression of ACS are the principal goals of management. Among severely affected patients, these supportive strategies may only temporally calm the underlying disease process. Indeed, repeated ACS episodes are a risk factor for reduced lung function in adults [25]. The diversity of antecedent clinical events that precede ACS suggests that they activate a common downstream pathogenesis pathway.

Clinical Laboratory Predictors of ACS

Blood cell counts and the concentration of many blood constituents that are by-products of vascular inflammation, fat metabolism, oxidative stress, and hemolysis change acutely before the onset of ACS, and during the early phase of the condition. These factors are promising leads to finding specific molecules and cognate pathways that promote the development of the lung injury. Importantly, many of these factors can be measured routinely in the clinical laboratory, and several have been linked to the risk and severity of ACS. Low steady-state hemoglobin (Hb), high fetal Hb (HbF) and low steady-state white blood cell (WBC) count are associated with reduced incidence of ACS [5]. These relationships have, however, become complex in patients receiving hydroxyurea therapy, as some of these hematologic parameters may no longer be predictive of ACS risk [26]. An acute drop in the steady-state hemoglobin concentration is a well-recognized prodrome of ACS, and typically precedes the appearance of a new pulmonary infiltrate on chest X-ray [6, 27]. Patients with multiple ACS episodes have significantly higher concentrations of protein-free plasma heme [26]. A decrease in platelet count to less than 200,000/ mm^3 during ACS is an independent risk factor for neurological event and respiratory failure [14]. Leukocytosis secondary to inflammation or infection is common at ACS diagnosis. Blood cultures are infrequently positive for bacteremia, occurring more in children (38 %), and with a predominance of atypical organisms (*Mycoplasma pneumoniae, Chlamydophila pneumoniae,* and *Legionella pneumophila*) [14]. Transcutaneous pulse oximetry is an appropriate non-invasive measure of oxygen saturation (SpO2) for diagnosis and monitoring of ACS, however arterial blood gas sampling remains the gold standard in determining partial pressure of oxygen and carbon dioxide in patients with impending respiratory failure (PaO_2 <60 mmHg or PCO_2 >50 mmHg). Hypoxia is a significant predictor of ACS severity and outcome [6, 14]; a decrease in SpO2 of 3 % or more from baseline levels or ≤94 % on room air is considered significant with ACS and should prompt early institution of supplemental oxygen therapy.

Postmortem Findings

There is a paucity of postmortem reports of ACS lungs. Several postmortem studies have reported on the pulmonary findings in SCD patients, only one study involved a case of ACS. The autopsy showed the ACS lung was characterized predominantly by edema. In addition, there was evidence of alveolar wall necrosis and fat embolism. A subset of patients develop multiorgan failure syndrome (MOFS)—a syndrome of progressive failure of the coagulation system, liver, kidney, and brain in addition to lung. The pulmonary findings at autopsy in these instances show defective repair of the lung-alveolar epithelium and vascular endothelium of the lung capillaries. The alveoli are filled with mesenchymal cells and their fibrinous products leading to obliteration of alveolar spaces, proliferation of vascular capillary walls with near obliteration of their lumens. The damaged lungs in individuals who die seem incapable of repairing the tissue damage. It has been proposed that tissue necrosis factor α and interleukin-1 are released from damaged lung tissue and initiate a sepsis-like syndrome characterized by fever, need for ionotropic support, and multiorgan failure [28].

Genetic Modifiers

Heme oxygenase-1 (HO-1) is the rate-limiting enzyme of heme degradation. It is encoded by the *HMOX1* gene; the length of a (GT)n dinucleotide repeat in the promoter influences HO-1 gene expression. Shorter length repeats are associated with upregulation of HO-1 gene expression and reduced risk of ACS. A candidate gene association study of the Silent Infarct Transfusion Trial cohort of >900 patients revealed that children with two copies of the short (GT)n allele have lower rates of hospitalization for ACS (incidence rate ratio 0.28, 95 % confidence interval, 0.10–0.81) compared to their counterparts with longer repeats, after adjusting for multiple covariates [29]. This result suggests that short GT repeats in the HO-1 gene promoter confers protection in ACS, presumably due to enhanced HO-1 activity, and is in agreement with increased plasma heme findings by Adisa et al. in children with a history of multiple episodes of ACS [26]. Importantly, the association between ACS risk and *HMOX1* polymorphisms has been replicated in adult and pediatric patients of the Cooperative Study of Sickle Cell Disease (CSSCD) cohort in an independent study [30]. The same study discovered a genome-wide association between rs6141803 located ~8 kb upstream of the *COMMD7* gene and ACS risk [30]. COMMD7 is highly expressed in the lung [31], and it interacts with NF-kB suggesting it may play a role in the inflammation associated with ACS [31, 32]. Interestingly, heme alters the expression of COMMD7 in cultured lung endothelial cells [30]. Heme is therefore functionally linked to the only two large-scale replicated genetic association studies of ACS.

Other smaller studies have identified additional genes that may influence ACS risk. Glutathione-S-transferases [GSTs) are a family of detoxifying enzymes that conjugate glutathione with electrophilic molecules. Glutathione homeostasis is important in maintaining organ integrity from deleterious effect of oxidative stress. Deletion in the GSTM1 gene, located on chromosome 1q13.3 is significantly associated with increased incidence of ACS [33] and severe VOC [34]. VEGFA encodes VEGF and is highly polymorphic with specific mutations influencing the expression of VEGF. Significant differences exists in the VEGFA -583C>T minor allele and genotype frequencies in SCD patients with a history of ACS and in those without ACS, and moreover, these differences are also linked with reduction in serum VEGF levels [35]. Polymorphisms in the β-globin gene cluster including the locus control region, defined by three predominant haplotypes (H1-H3) that account for 96 % of the variation in this region influence the risk of ACS [36]. Individuals carrying one or two copies of H3 haplotype, associated with increased HbF, had a significantly lower rate of hospitalization for ACS after correcting for asthma, alpha thalassemia, and the (GT)n promoter repeat in the HMOX1 gene ($p=0.02$) [37].

Pathogenesis of ACS

Pathogenesis of ACS and acute lung injury (ALI) in SCD generally, has been studied in multiple transgenic SCD mouse strains. The NY1DD and SAD mice express both human and mouse hemoglobins and have consequently a relatively mild disease phenotype. The Berkeley and Townes sickle mice express exclusively human hemoglobin; they were created using knockout and knock-in technologies respectively, and both strains have a severe SCD phenotype. Animal models of ALI and other characteristics in humans with ALI, and acute respiratory distress syndrome have been defined [38]. They include a rapid disease onset and: (a) histological evidence of tissue injury, (b) alterations of the alveolar capillary barrier, (c) an inflammatory response, and (d) evidence of physiological dysfunction. Differences in size and environmental exposure in experimental animals and humans, as well as the comorbidities of SCD patients, preclude full mimicry of all the features of ACS in mice. Nonetheless, transgenic SCD mice offer a powerful tool to unravel the cellular and molecular mechanisms that propagate acute illness on the background of VOC, and intense hemolysis into a lethal ALI.

Hypoxia and Ischemia Reperfusion Injury

Hypoxia causes endothelial activation, increased adhesion of sickle erythrocytes to endothelium, decreased nitric oxide production [39] and upregulated endothelin-1 (ET-1) levels. The activation of NF-kappa B phospho p65 is central in a hypoxia-based VOC-ACS model proposed by Setty and Stuart [40]. It is thought that hypoxia strongly promotes VCAM-1-induced cellular adhesion in the pulmonary microcirculation via two mechanisms; NF-kappa B phospho p65-induced cytokine storm and release of ET-1 to drive VCAM-1 expression. By inhibiting the production of nitric oxide (which downregulates VCAM-1 expression), hypoxia may create an unopposed adhesive endothelial phenotype, which collectively promotes adhesion of sickle-erythrocytes via very-late activation antigen-4 in the pulmonary microvasculature. Together with enhanced vasoconstriction (due to increased ET-1 production), an increase in microvascular sickle erythrocyte sequestration could damage the alveolar capillary barrier to cause the lung injury in ACS.

Soluble vascular cell adhesion molecule-1 (sVCAM-1), nitric oxide (NOx) metabolites, and ET-1 therefore constitute a coalition of ACS surrogate markers with hypoxia as a linchpin. Initial studies showed that sVCAM-1 is increased by a mean of 1.5-fold during ACS [40]. This relationship was confirmed in some studies [41]. However, others found paradoxically low levels of sVCAM-1 in a cohort of pre-transfusion ACS patients [42], and in another study, elevated levels were linked specifically to VOC [43]. These discrepancies may be due to differences in the time blood samples were obtained for interrogation. Plasma NOx concentration decreases [40, 44], while ET-1 is increased by twofold [45] during ACS. The expression pattern of this triad (i.e. VCAM-1, NOx, and ET-1) may reflect an enhanced erythrocyte-endothelial adhesion, vasoconstriction, and increased microvascular sickle erythrocyte sequestration. In the pulmonary vasculature, such perturbations may impact the alveolar capillary barrier and trigger ACS.

Hypoxia/reoxygenation (H/R) is thought to play a central role in the pathogenesis of SCD by causing ischemia reperfusion injury. H/R is used widely as an experimental tool to study SCD pathogenesis in the four common sickle mouse strains (SAD, NY1DD, Berkeley, and Townes). The typical protocol (8 % oxygen for 1–4 h, 1–4 h reoxygenation) causes RBC sickling [46], stasis in dorsal microvessels [47], decrease in mean renal blood velocities [48], endothelial activation [49], increased leukocyte count, leukocyte/endothelial interaction, and emigration across the endothelium [50, 51], conversion of xanthine dehydrogenase to xanthine oxidase [46] activation of nuclear factor NF-kappa B [51, 52] and increased sensitivity to pain [53]. Oxygen concentration (SO_2) is reduced during the hypoxia phase however SO_2 recovers fully when the mice are returned to room air [50, 54]. Consistent with the transient hypoxemia, this protocol does not produce classical ALI in these mice. However, it increases pulmonary congestion by erythrocytes [55] and neutrophils, and it increases BAL protein and pulmonary expression of multiple-hypoxia-responsive genes [56]. A marginally increased hypoxic stress (5–6 % oxygen) is lethal in all sickle mouse strains due to massive congestion in several major organs [48, 57]. This precariously narrow window of hypoxia intolerance may explain why this approach has thus far proved futile to inducing a classical ACS phenotype in sickle mice. Recent studies indicate hemolysis and heme, induce expression of adhesion molecules such as VCAM-1 [58]. Thus, extracellular heme may be the key ingredient missing to effectively induce ACS in hypoxia-based models of sickle lung injury [55].

iNKT Cell Activation

Invariant natural killer T (iNKT) cell depletion or blockade reduces baseline lung dysfunction in the NY1DD mouse [59]. This dysfunction is associated with increased adenosine A(2A) receptor (A(2A)R) mRNA in iNKT cells, and it is reversed by treating these mice with ATL146e, an A(2A)R agonist [60]. A(2A)R agonism attenuates neutrophilic inflammation, ROS generation, and endothelial adherence in several animal models of ischemia-reperfusion injury and A(2A)R agonism signals primarily through cAMP to presumably inhibit NFkB [60]. In a H/R experiment, treatment at the start of reoxygenation reduced congestion and the number of iNKT and polymorphonuclear leukocytes in NY1DD mice. It is unclear whether the untreated control animals in this study developed respiratory distress, though, the absence of lethality indicate none developed respiratory failure [60]. In a phase 1 trial of the A2AR agonist regadenoson in patients with VOC, the proportion of peripheral blood iNKT cells with increased phospho-NF-kB p65 and A2AR expression was significantly higher in VOC compared with steady-state patients [61]. Infusion of regadenoson decreased phospho-NF-kB p65 activation in peripheral blood iNKT cells in patients with VOC. The enhanced systemic baseline inflammation seen in SCD may prime the lung for the more severe injury typical of ACS, in a two-hit model, involving danger associated molecular pattern (DAMP) molecules.

Fat Emboli

Pulmonary fat embolism (PFE) was implicated in ACS pathogenesis based on the discovery of fat-laden bronchoalveolar macrophages in ~50 % of patients [23, 62]. PFE is a common postmortem finding in SCD patients who die of other causes and it is therefore not specific to ACS [63]. Nonetheless, a sharp rise in serum secretory phospholipase A2 (sPLA2) level in ACS patients, and reports that this elevation predicted ACS development bolstered arguments in favor of PFE's causal role [7, 8]. Infarction in the bone marrow during VOC and action of sPLA2 on membrane phospholipids would release lipids into the circulation with subsequent hydrolysis generating free fatty acids that may trigger ACS. Infusion of oleic acid increased myeloperoxidase activity and neutrophil recruitment in the lungs of the Berkeley sickle mouse. However, increased myeloperoxidase activity and airspace neutrophil accumulation did not correlate with each other [64]. Moreover, neutrophil infiltration appears not to be a prominent feature of postmortem human ACS lungs [65]. However, an intronic single nucleotide polymorphism (SNP) rs12720497 in PLA2G4A (the gene encoding cytosolic PLA2) is associated with VOC in a genome-wide association study (GWAS) of the CSSCD cohort. The VOC phenotype in this study, and in others is defined by acute severe unrelenting pain typically associated with hyper-hemolysis even among patients in whom the pain resolves without further complication [66]. Thus, the development of murine models of vasoocclusion and bone marrow infarction that also recapitulate the clinical features of VOC seen in patients may help to unlock the role and mechanism of PFE in ACS development.

Hemolysis

A sharp decrease in total hemoglobin is widely reported prior to and during ACS [5, 6, 14, 24, 27, 65, 67]. The magnitude of the hemoglobin decrease, and its prognostic value are well characterized; patients with the largest drop typically do worse, even in cases where another factor such as PFE is strongly associated with the ACS [23]. Hemolysis is a major source of the oxidant stress in SCD. Plasma concentration of F_2 isoprostanes, an oxidative stress marker is increased by ninefold above baseline during ACS [68]. Marked elevation of LDH [65, 69], and sharp reductions in both L-Arginine and NOx [40, 44], suggests the sharp decrease in hemoglobin in ACS may largely be due to intravascular hemolysis. These studies strongly implicate oxidized byproducts of hemolysis, such as heme, in the pathobiology of ACS. In agreement with this idea, Adisa et al. found increased steady-state plasma-free heme is associated with increased odds of ACS development in children with SCD [$P=0.016$, odds ratio; 2.56, Confidence Interval = 1.19–5.47] [26]. Extracellular heme triggers vascular stasis in sickle mice affirming the central role of this erythroid DAMP molecule in the pathogenesis of SCD [58]. Antibodies to multiple endothelial adhesion molecules, which are induced by heme, blocked this event. In addition, heme rapidly induced P-selectin and vWF expression on the endothelium in vivo. In the CSSCD trial, acute hemolysis that potentially increased extracellular hemoglobin by ~3.6 g/dl was the only predictor of death within 24 h of presentation [6]. VOC and infection are the leading causes of ACS. Together with other ACS etiologies they cause acute hemolysis that ultimately increases the concentration of extracellular heme. Thus heme fulfills the role of a converging pathogenesis axis that links diverse ACS etiologies together.

Extracellular Heme

The heme moiety of Hb is normally secured in a pocket of the constituent globin chains. Oxidation of Hb to metHb destabilizes this interaction and promotes heme loss (Fig. 3.1). Studies of purified solutions of Hb in vitro show that this process is accelerated in the HbS molecule [70]. In addition, intracellular HbS precipitates inside the sickle erythrocyte resulting in the release of up to ~1 μM of heme into the cytosol [71]. This high intracellular heme concentration is consistent with the instability and the consequent enhanced auto-oxidation of Hemoglobin S that promotes

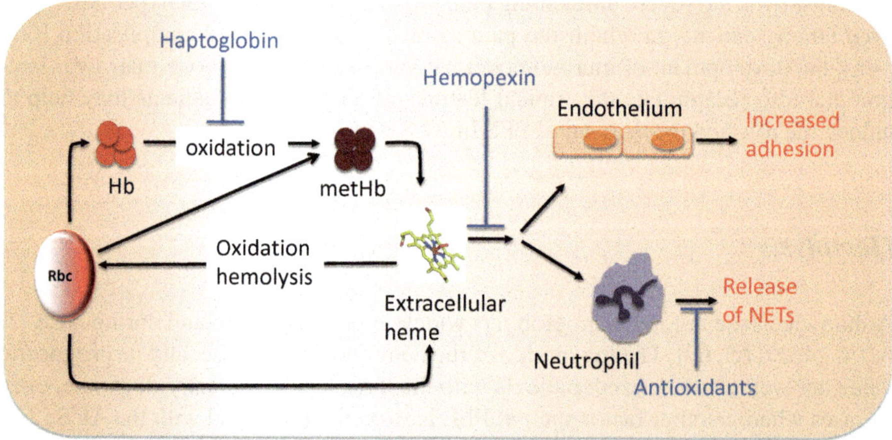

Fig. 3.1 Generation and inflammatory cellular targets of extracellular heme in sickle cell disease. Hemolysis releases cell-free hemoglobin (Hb), which is normally scavenged by haptoglobin and CD163. Free hemoglobin reacts with and scavenges NO via the dioxygenation reaction and also reacts with hydrogen peroxide to generate hydroxyl radicals via the Fenton reaction. Oxidized hemoglobin releases free heme, which can activate the endothelium to increases adhesion molecule expression, and stimulates neutrophils to release NETs

the expulsion of heme from the heme pocket [70, 72–74]. The heme scavenger hemopexin is catabolized at a twofold faster rate in SCD patients, and without a compensatory increase in synthesis [75]. As a result, the steady-state plasma hemopexin level in these patients is ~5-fold lower than normal concomitant with a high level of heme [76, 77]. Thus, in SCD, intravascular hemolysis releases heme directly into the circulation. This notion coupled with the instability of the HbS molecule is consistent with Muller-Eberhard's observation in the late 1960s that SCD patients have extraordinarily high levels of heme in their plasma [76]. This trait is present also in transgenic sickle mice. In the Townes sickle mouse (referred to herein as SS mice), Ghosh et al. and Belcher et al. report mean total plasma heme (TPH) values of 77.9 ± 4.3 μM and 52.6 ± 18.0 μM respectively, while Chen et al. report a mean TPH of ~40 μM in the Berkeley sickle mouse [54, 58, 78].

The role and mechanism of heme in the pathobiology of SCD is complex. Intraperitoneal injections of purified heme exert a salutary effect on vascular stasis in sickle mice by inducing HO-1 [79]. Meanwhile, intravenous injection elevates the extracellular heme pool, depletes plasma hemopexin, and induces a lethal ALI [80]. The latter effect is typical of DAMP molecules—intracellular molecules that elicit robust inflammatory responses when they are released externally by tissue damage [81, 82]. Although heme was already known to be recognized by toll-like receptor 4 (TLR4) [83], elucidation of its ALI inducing effect has helped to define its role as a *bonafide* DAMP molecule. It is arguably the prototypical erythroid DAMP. Intravenous infusion of a modest dose of purified heme caused sudden death in SS mice; autopsies revealed erythrocyte congestion in the lungs suggesting that VOC in the pulmonary microvasculature contributed to this lethality. A model in which the extracellular heme/TLR4 signaling axis activates NF-kappa B phospho p65 to cause VOC through increased adhesion molecule expression and degranulation of Weibel Palade bodies has been proposed [58]. The reverse sequence (i.e. VOC → hemolysis) is well established in humans with SCD, even among those in whom the acute VOC does not progress to a life threatening condition such as ACS [66]. Thus, it appears that VOC and intravascular hemolysis are intertwined in a vicious cycle that drives much of the pathobiology of SCD.

Extracellular Heme Crisis

In a study designed to test the role of extracellular heme in SCD pathogenesis, Ghosh et al. made a serendipitous observation that provides insight into how the concentration of heme is elevated in SCD plasma: heme is amplified. The investigators infused groups of SS, AS, and AA mice with a bolus of purified heme, and as expected this raised the TPH in all the animals to a similar concentration immediately after the challenge. Paradoxically, the TPH in the SS mice continued to increase surpassing the bolus by ~50 % within 30 min. Meanwhile, both control animals (AS and AA) rapidly cleared the exogenous heme from their circulation. This finding showed that there is auto-amplification of extracellular heme in SCD plasma. More importantly, it uncovered for the first time a phenomenon of *extracellular heme crisis*; an acute uncontrolled release of heme into the circulation that was associated with: (a) enhanced oxidation of intracellular HbS, (b) impaired reduction of intracellular metHbS, (c) enhanced heme-induced hemolysis, and (d) rapid depletion of hemopexin. This phenomenon promoted the development of a lethal ALI reminiscent of ACS in the SS mice [54]. Extracellular heme crisis may be inevitable specifically within occluded vascular segments with impaired blood flow in patients with severe VOC who develop acute hemolysis.

Neutrophil Extracellular Traps (NETs)

NETs are released into the plasma by activated neutrophils. They consist of a mesh of extracellular DNA, nucleosomes, and histones decorated with granular enzymes, typically neutrophil elastase. It is thought that NETs trap pathogens with their high concentrations of enzymes. They were first implicated in SCD pathogenesis in a prospective study including 70 patients with VOC [84]. During VOC, levels of both nucleosomes and elastase-α1-antitrypsin complexes increased significantly as compared to steady-state values. Levels of nucleosomes correlated significantly with elastase-α1-antitrypsin complex levels during painful crisis, and the levels were highest in patients with ACS [84]. Extracellular heme stimulates the release of NETs by increasing intracellular neutrophil ROS formation (Fig. 3.1). Plasma from both humans and mice with SCD promotes NET release in vitro, and infusions of hemopexin reduced the number of pulmonary NETs, and the concentration of plasma nucleosomes in the Berkeley sickle mouse. The production of NETs by neutrophils during TNF-α exposure led to an ACS-like condition and sudden death in these animals following cremasteric surgical preparation [78]. DNase I treatment prolonged survival however hemopexin infusions did not, probably, because of the relatively low dose that was used in this study (0.15 mg hemopexin per mouse) [78]. In SCD patients, infections, which increase systemic TNF-α, are important contributing factors to ACS development, thus enhancing the idea that NETs may play an important role in the pathobiology of this lung condition.

Preclinical Murine ACS Model

Complete saturation of hemopexin yielding at least ~1.5 μM of extracellular heme that is seemingly free from other plasma binding partners triggers a lethal ALI in mice [54]. Given the low plasma hemopexin reserve in SCD, this ALI is inducible in ~70 % of sickle mice (Townes and Berkeley) with a relatively low dose of purified heme (i.v. 35 μmol/kg). This preclinical ACS model shares several similarities with the condition in humans. It is characterized by acute onset, acute anemia, pulmonary infiltration, hypoxemia, hypercapnia, acidosis, pulmonary edema, and sudden death (Table 3.1). This model suggests that continuous supply of extracellular heme fuels ACS, and that targeting this supply can avert respiratory failure even

Table 3.1 Characteristics of ACS in patients and in a preclinical mouse model

Parameter	Patients	Mice
Etiology/trigger	Multiple	Extracellular heme
Presentation	Acute onset	Acute onset
Mean hemoglobin loss	0.7–3.6 g/dl	1.4 g/dl
Inflammation	New chest infiltrate	Gross pulmonary infiltrates
Histology	Edema, alveolar wall necrosis, fat emboli	Edema, alveolar wall thickening, hemorrhage
Physiological dysfunction	Hypoxemia, hypercapnia	Hypoxemia, hypercapnia, acidosis
Death due to respiratory failure	Up to 9 % (treated)	0–20 % (treated)[a] 70 % (untreated)[b]
Plasma risk factors	Elevated free heme	Low hemopexin
Genetic modifiers	HMOX1, COMMD7	TLR4
Targeted therapy	None	Hemopexin, TAK-242

[a]Infusion hemopexin provides 100 % survival. TAK-242 provides 85 % survival when given as prophylaxis

[b]Mortality due to infusion of 35 μmol/kg heme

when the initial insult has caused some lung injury. Indeed, this may be one mechanism through which blood transfusion halts ACS, by reducing the concentration of extracellular heme in the intravascular space below the threshold required to cause endothelial barrier disruption.

Directly targeting heme with recombinant hemopexin infusions (1 mg per mouse) produces almost immediate improvement in oxygen saturation, followed steadily by restoration of breath rate in SS mice with hemolytic crisis and respiratory distress [54]. Hemopexin has as unique ability to rapidly squelch the redox activities of heme [85]. This suggests that reactive oxygen species (ROS) signaling contributes to the acute injury in the murine ACS lung, as has previously been suggested for the human ACS lung [68]. In addition, the lethal lung injury in the murine model requires a functional TLR4, which is redox-sensitive. The TLR4 antagonist TAK-242 is effective in preventing lung injury in the murine ACS model [54].

TLR4 mutant mice are protected from respiratory disease when challenged with a high dose of heme that causes a lethal ALI in congenic control mice. This means that the basic mechanism of the ALI, and perhaps other injuries caused by extracellular heme in SCD is mediated by TLR4. Using bone marrow chimeric mice, TLR4 expressed by nonhematopoietic vascular tissues (most likely the endothelium), has been found to mediate heme-induced ALI/ACS [54], and stasis in sickle mice. The receptor had been a major therapeutic target in sepsis resulting in the development of TAK-242 [86, 87] and Eritoran [88]. Both drugs have failed phase III sepsis trials nonetheless they may be ideal candidates for repurposing in SCD [89–91]. In preclinical studies, TAK-242 was effective in preventing respiratory failure in sickle mice only when it was given before or immediately after the induction of hemolytic crisis [54]. Since a majority of ACS patients present initially with well-defined antecedent acute events that are interceded by hemolysis, acute prophylaxis using TLR4 blockade may be an effective strategy to alter the clinical course of this condition.

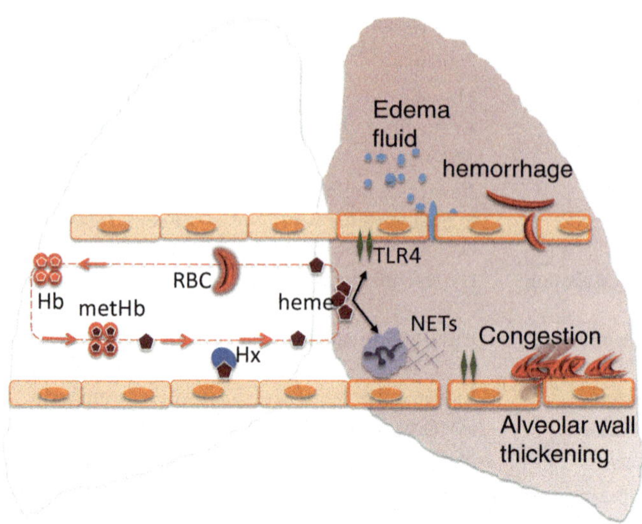

Fig. 3.2 A model of heme-induced acute chest syndrome. The concentration of heme can be auto-amplified in vivo via a phenomenon named extracellular heme crisis (EHC) involving acute hemolysis, release of cell-free hemoglobin, and increased methemoglobin S formation, which ultimately depletes plasma hemopexin reserve. Free extracellular heme interacts with TLR4 on the vessel wall, disrupts the alveolar capillary barrier resulting in acute pulmonary edema, alveolar wall thickening, and microvascular congestion. Collectively these pathologies impair alveolar gas exchange and cause potentially terminal respiratory failure

Conclusion: A Mechanistic Model of ACS Pathogenesis

A mechanism explaining how ACS develops in SCD is proposed (Fig. 3.2). A large proportion of sickle erythrocytes trapped in occlusions with reduced flow, and shielded from the paltry reserve of plasma scavenger molecules is destroyed during acute exacerbations in SCD. In this setting, the acute hemolysis inevitably yields extracellular heme. This heme species can be amplified in vivo generating an excess pool sufficient to trigger and sustain a robust TLR4 mediated inflammation that ultimately causes a lethal ALI. This ACS model is characterized by a diversity of features; clinical, biological, physiological, and pathological, that is common or complementary in humans and mice with SCD (Table 3.1). It is versatile, reproducible, and readily amenable to multiple drug discovery platforms. Studies expanding its conceptual framework may help to further improve our understanding of the pathogenesis of ACS, and to develop effective targeted therapies based on clearly defined mechanism for this devastating lung condition.

Acknowledgements The authors are supported by research funding from the National Heart, Lung and Blood Institute (Award Number: HL106192, HL106192S1, and U01HL117721). The authors thank Sonia Mckoy for comments and proofreading that helped to improve this book chapter.

Authorship
Contribution: OA, AOA, ADA, SG, and SFOA prepared, wrote, and edited the chapter.

Conflict of Interest
The authors OA, AOA, ADA, SG, and SFOA declare that no conflict of interest exists.

References

1. Charache S, Scott JC, Charache P. "Acute chest syndrome" in adults with sickle cell anemia. Microbiology, treatment, and prevention. Arch Intern Med. 1979;139(1):67–9.
2. Platt OS, Brambilla DJ, Rosse WF, Milner PF, Castro O, Steinberg MH, et al. Mortality in sickle cell disease. Life expectancy and risk factors for early death. N Engl J Med. 1994;330(23):1639–44.
3. Gaston M, Rosse WF. The cooperative study of sickle cell disease: review of study design and objectives. Am J Pediatr Hematol Oncol. 1982;4(2):197–201.
4. Gaston M, Smith J, Gallagher D, Flournoy-Gill Z, West S, Bellevue R, et al. Recruitment in the cooperative study of sickle cell disease (CSSCD). Control Clin Trials. 1987;8 Suppl 4:131S–40.
5. Castro O, Brambilla DJ, Thorington B, Reindorf CA, Scott RB, Gillette P, et al. The acute chest syndrome in sickle cell disease: incidence and risk factors. The Cooperative Study of Sickle Cell Disease. Blood. 1994;84(2):643–9.
6. Vichinsky EP, Styles LA, Colangelo LH, Wright EC, Castro O, Nickerson B. Acute chest syndrome in sickle cell disease: clinical presentation and course. Cooperative Study of Sickle Cell Disease. Blood. 1997;89(5):1787–92.
7. Styles LA, Schalkwijk CG, Aarsman AJ, Vichinsky EP, Lubin BH, Kuypers FA. Phospholipase A2 levels in acute chest syndrome of sickle cell disease. Blood. 1996;87(6):2573–8.
8. Styles LA, Aarsman AJ, Vichinsky EP, Kuypers FA. Secretory phospholipase A(2) predicts impending acute chest syndrome in sickle cell disease. Blood. 2000;96(9):3276–8.
9. Bargoma EM, Mitsuyoshi JK, Larkin SK, Styles LA, Kuypers FA, Test ST. Serum C-reactive protein parallels secretory phospholipase A2 in sickle cell disease patients with vasoocclusive crisis or acute chest syndrome. Blood. 2005;105(8):3384–5.
10. Paul RN, Castro OL, Aggarwal A, Oneal PA. Acute chest syndrome: sickle cell disease. Eur J Haematol. 2011;87(3):191–207.
11. Miller ST. How I, treat acute chest syndrome in children with sickle cell disease. Blood. 2011;117(20):5297–305.
12. Desai PC, Ataga KI. The acute chest syndrome of sickle cell disease. Expert Opin Pharmacother. 2013;14(8):991–9.
13. Platt OS. The acute chest syndrome of sickle cell disease. N Engl J Med. 2000;342(25):1904–7.
14. Vichinsky EP, Neumayr LD, Earles AN, Williams R, Lennette ET, Dean D, et al. Causes and outcomes of the acute chest syndrome in sickle cell disease. National Acute Chest Syndrome Study Group. N Engl J Med. 2000;342(25):1855–65.
15. Gladwin MT, Vichinsky E. Pulmonary complications of sickle cell disease. N Engl J Med. 2008;359(21):2254–65.
16. Quinn CT, Shull EP, Ahmad N, Lee NJ, Rogers ZR, Buchanan GR. Prognostic significance of early vaso-occlusive complications in children with sickle cell anemia. Blood. 2007;109(1):40–5.
17. DeBaun MR, Rodeghier M, Cohen R, Kirkham FJ, Rosen CL, Roberts I, et al. Factors predicting future ACS episodes in children with sickle cell anemia. Am J Hematol. 2014;89(11):E212–7.
18. Vance LD, Rodeghier M, Cohen RT, Rosen CL, Kirkham FJ, Strunk RC, et al. Increased risk of severe vaso-occlusive episodes after initial acute chest syndrome in children with sickle cell anemia less than 4 years old: Sleep and asthma cohort. Am J Hematol. 2015;90(5):371–5.

19. Field JJ, DeBaun MR. Asthma and sickle cell disease: two distinct diseases or part of the same process? Hematology Am Soc Hematol Educ Program. 2009:45–53. doi:10.1182/asheducation-2009.1.45.
20. Boyd JH, Macklin EA, Strunk RC, DeBaun MR. Asthma is associated with acute chest syndrome and pain in children with sickle cell anemia. Blood. 2006;108(9):2923–7.
21. Boyd JH, Macklin EA, Strunk RC, DeBaun MR. Asthma is associated with increased mortality in individuals with sickle cell anemia. Haematologica. 2007;92(8):1115–8.
22. Gladwin MT, Rodgers GP. Pathogenesis and treatment of acute chest syndrome of sickle-cell anaemia. Lancet. 2000;355(9214):1476–8.
23. Vichinsky E, Williams R, Das M, Earles AN, Lewis N, Adler A, et al. Pulmonary fat embolism: a distinct cause of severe acute chest syndrome in sickle cell anemia. Blood. 1994;83(11):3107–12.
24. Gladwin MT, Schechter AN, Shelhamer JH, Ognibene FP. The acute chest syndrome in sickle cell disease. Possible role of nitric oxide in its pathophysiology and treatment. Am J Respir Crit Care Med. 1999;159(5 Pt 1):1368–76.
25. Knight-Madden JM, Forrester TS, Lewis NA, Greenough A. The impact of recurrent acute chest syndrome on the lung function of young adults with sickle cell disease. Lung. 2010;188(6):499–504.
26. Adisa OA, Hu Y, Ghosh S, Aryee D, Osunkwo I, Ofori-Acquah SF. Association between plasma free haem and incidence of vaso-occlusive episodes and acute chest syndrome in children with sickle cell disease. Br J Haematol. 2013;162(5):702–5.
27. Davies SC, Luce PJ, Win AA, Riordan JF, Brozovic M. Acute chest syndrome in sickle-cell disease. Lancet. 1984;1(8367):36–8.
28. Snyder LS, Hertz MI, Harmon KR, Bitterman PB. Failure of lung repair following acute lung injury. Regulation of the fibroproliferative response (part 1). Chest. 1990;98(3):733–8.
29. Bean CJ, Boulet SL, Ellingsen D, Pyle ME, Barron-Casella EA, Casella JF, et al. Heme oxygenase-1 gene promoter polymorphism is associated with reduced incidence of acute chest syndrome among children with sickle cell disease. Blood. 2012;120(18):3822–8.
30. Galarneau G, Coady S, Garrett ME, Jeffries N, Puggal M, Paltoo D, et al. Gene-centric association study of acute chest syndrome and painful crisis in sickle cell disease patients. Blood. 2013;122(3):434–42. doi:10.1182/blood-2013-01-478776.
31. Burstein E, Hoberg JE, Wilkinson AS, Rumble JM, Csomos RA, Komarck CM, et al. COMMD proteins, a novel family of structural and functional homologs of MURR1. J Biol Chem. 2005;280(23):22222–32.
32. Zheng L, Liang P, Li J, Huang XB, Liu SC, Zhao HZ, et al. ShRNA-targeted COMMD7 suppresses hepatocellular carcinoma growth. PLoS One. 2012;7(9):e45412.
33. de Oliveira Filho RA, Silva GJ, de Farias Domingos I, Hatzlhofer BL, da Silva Araujo A, de Lima Filho JL, et al. Association between the genetic polymorphisms of glutathione S-transferase (GSTM1 and GSTT1) and the clinical manifestations in sickle cell anemia. Blood Cells Mol Dis. 2013;51(2):76–9.
34. Ellithy HN, Yousri S, Shahin GH. Relation between glutathione S-transferase genes (GSTM1, GSTT1, and GSTP1) polymorphisms and clinical manifestations of sickle cell disease in Egyptian patients. Hematology. 2015;20(10):598–606.
35. Redha NA, Mahdi N, Al-Habboubi HH, Almawi WY. Impact of VEGFA -583C > T polymorphism on serum VEGF levels and the susceptibility to acute chest syndrome in pediatric patients with sickle cell disease. Pediatr Blood Cancer. 2014;61(12):2310–2.
36. Powars DR. Beta s-gene-cluster haplotypes in sickle cell anemia. Clinical and hematologic features. Hematol Oncol Clin North Am. 1991;5(3):475–93.
37. Bean CJ, Boulet SL, Yang G, Payne AB, Ghaji N, Pyle ME, et al. Acute chest syndrome is associated with single nucleotide polymorphism-defined beta globin cluster haplotype in children with sickle cell anaemia. Br J Haematol. 2013;163(2):268–76.
38. Matute-Bello G, Downey G, Moore BB, Groshong SD, Matthay MA, Slutsky AS, et al. An official American Thoracic Society workshop report: features and measurements of experimental acute lung injury in animals. Am J Respir Cell Mol Biol. 2011;44(5):725–38.

39. Sullivan KJ, Kissoon N, Gauger C. Nitric oxide metabolism and the acute chest syndrome of sickle cell anemia. Pediatr Crit Care Med. 2008;9(2):159–68.
40. Stuart MJ, Setty BN. Sickle cell acute chest syndrome: pathogenesis and rationale for treatment. Blood. 1999;94(5):1555–60.
41. Sakhalkar VS, Rao SP, Weedon J, Miller ST. Elevated plasma sVCAM-1 levels in children with sickle cell disease: impact of chronic transfusion therapy. Am J Hematol. 2004;76(1):57–60.
42. Liem RI, O'Gorman MR, Brown DL. Effect of red cell exchange transfusion on plasma levels of inflammatory mediators in sickle cell patients with acute chest syndrome. Am J Hematol. 2004;76(1):19–25.
43. Duits AJ, Pieters RC, Saleh AW, van Rosmalen E, Katerberg H, Berend K, et al. Enhanced levels of soluble VCAM-1 in sickle cell patients and their specific increment during vasoocclusive crisis. Clin Immunol Immunopathol. 1996;81(1):96–8.
44. Morris CR, Kuypers FA, Larkin S, Vichinsky EP, Styles LA. Patterns of arginine and nitric oxide in patients with sickle cell disease with vaso-occlusive crisis and acute chest syndrome. J Pediatr Hematol Oncol. 2000;22(6):515–20.
45. Hammerman SI, Kourembanas S, Conca TJ, Tucci M, Brauer M, Farber HW. Endothelin-1 production during the acute chest syndrome in sickle cell disease. Am J Respir Crit Care Med. 1997;156(1):280–5.
46. Osarogiagbon UR, Choong S, Belcher JD, Vercellotti GM, Paller MS, Hebbel RP. Reperfusion injury pathophysiology in sickle transgenic mice. Blood. 2000;96(1):314–20.
47. Kalambur VS, Mahaseth H, Bischof JC, Kielbik MC, Welch TE, Vilback A, et al. Microvascular blood flow and stasis in transgenic sickle mice: utility of a dorsal skin fold chamber for intravital microscopy. Am J Hematol. 2004;77(2):117–25.
48. Sabaa N, de Franceschi L, Bonnin P, Castier Y, Malpeli G, Debbabi H, et al. Endothelin receptor antagonism prevents hypoxia-induced mortality and morbidity in a mouse model of sickle-cell disease. J Clin Invest. 2008;118(5):1924–33.
49. Solovey A, Kollander R, Shet A, Milbauer LC, Choong S, Panoskaltsis-Mortari A, et al. Endothelial cell expression of tissue factor in sickle mice is augmented by hypoxia/reoxygenation and inhibited by lovastatin. Blood. 2004;104(3):840–6.
50. Kaul DK, Hebbel RP. Hypoxia/reoxygenation causes inflammatory response in transgenic sickle mice but not in normal mice. J Clin Invest. 2000;106(3):411–20.
51. Kaul DK, Liu XD, Choong S, Belcher JD, Vercellotti GM, Hebbel RP. Anti-inflammatory therapy ameliorates leukocyte adhesion and microvascular flow abnormalities in transgenic sickle mice. Am J Physiol Heart Circ Physiol. 2004;287(1):H293–301.
52. Kollander R, Solovey A, Milbauer LC, Abdulla F, Kelm Jr RJ, Hebbel RP. Nuclear factor-kappa B (NFkappaB) component p50 in blood mononuclear cells regulates endothelial tissue factor expression in sickle transgenic mice: implications for the coagulopathy of sickle cell disease. Transl Res. 2010;155(4):170–7.
53. Cain DM, Vang D, Simone DA, Hebbel RP, Gupta K. Mouse models for studying pain in sickle disease: effects of strain, age, and acuteness. Br J Haematol. 2012;156(4):535–44.
54. Ghosh S, Adisa OA, Chappa P, Tan F, Jackson KA, Archer DR, et al. Extracellular hemin crisis triggers acute chest syndrome in sickle mice. J Clin Invest. 2013;123:4809–20.
55. Pritchard Jr KA, Ou J, Ou Z, Shi Y, Franciosi JP, Signorino P, et al. Hypoxia-induced acute lung injury in murine models of sickle cell disease. Am J Physiol Lung Cell Mol Physiol. 2004;286(4):L705–14.
56. de Franceschi L, Baron A, Scarpa A, Adrie C, Janin A, Barbi S, et al. Inhaled nitric oxide protects transgenic SAD mice from sickle cell disease-specific lung injury induced by hypoxia/reoxygenation. Blood. 2003;102(3):1087–96.
57. Iyamu EW, Turner EA, Asakura T. Niprisan (Nix-0699) improves the survival rates of transgenic sickle cell mice under acute severe hypoxic conditions. Br J Haematol. 2003;122(6):1001–8.
58. Belcher JD, Chen C, Nguyen J, Milbauer L, Abdulla F, Alayash AI, et al. Heme triggers TLR4 signaling leading to endothelial cell activation and vaso-occlusion in murine sickle cell disease. Blood. 2014;123(3):377–90.

59. Wallace KL, Marshall MA, Ramos SI, Lannigan JA, Field JJ, Strieter RM, et al. NKT cells mediate pulmonary inflammation and dysfunction in murine sickle cell disease through production of IFN-gamma and CXCR3 chemokines. Blood. 2009;114(3):667–76.
60. Wallace KL, Linden J. Adenosine A2A receptors induced on iNKT and NK cells reduce pulmonary inflammation and injury in mice with sickle cell disease. Blood. 2010;116(23): 5010–20.
61. Field JJ, Lin G, Okam MM, Majerus E, Keefer J, Onyekwere O, et al. Sickle cell vaso-occlusion causes activation of iNKT cells that is decreased by the adenosine A2A receptor agonist regadenoson. Blood. 2013;121(17):3329–34.
62. Godeau B, Schaeffer A, Bachir D, Fleury-Feith J, Galacteros F, Verra F, et al. Bronchoalveolar lavage in adult sickle cell patients with acute chest syndrome: value for diagnostic assessment of fat embolism. Am J Respir Crit Care Med. 1996;153(5):1691–6.
63. Haupt HM, Moore GW, Bauer TW, Hutchins GM. The lung in sickle cell disease. Chest. 1982;81(3):332–7.
64. Hsu L, McDermott T, Brown L, Aguayo SM. Transgenic HbS mouse neutrophils in increased susceptibility to acute lung injury: implications for sickle acute chest syndrome. Chest. 1999;116(1 Suppl):92S.
65. Maitre B, Habibi A, Roudot-Thoraval F, Bachir D, Belghiti DD, Galacteros F, et al. Acute chest syndrome in adults with sickle cell disease. Chest. 2000;117(5):1386–92.
66. Ballas SK, Marcolina MJ. Hyperhemolysis during the evolution of uncomplicated acute painful episodes in patients with sickle cell anemia. Transfusion. 2006;46(1):105–10.
67. Sprinkle RH, Cole T, Smith S, Buchanan GR. Acute chest syndrome in children with sickle cell disease. A retrospective analysis of 100 hospitalized cases. Am J Pediatr Hematol Oncol. 1986;8(2):105–10.
68. Klings ES, Christman BW, McClung J, Stucchi AF, McMahon L, Brauer M, et al. Increased F2 isoprostanes in the acute chest syndrome of sickle cell disease as a marker of oxidative stress. Am J Respir Crit Care Med. 2001;164(7):1248–52.
69. van Agtmael MA, Cheng JD, Nossent HC. Acute chest syndrome in adult Afro-Caribbean patients with sickle cell disease. Analysis of 81 episodes among 53 patients. Arch Intern Med. 1994;154(5):557–61.
70. Hebbel RP, Morgan WT, Eaton JW, Hedlund BE. Accelerated autoxidation and heme loss due to instability of sickle hemoglobin. Proc Natl Acad Sci U S A. 1988;85(1):237–41.
71. Liu SC, Zhai S, Palek J. Detection of hemin release during hemoglobin S denaturation. Blood. 1988;71(6):1755–8.
72. Jeney V, Balla J, Yachie A, Varga Z, Vercellotti GM, Eaton JW, et al. Pro-oxidant and cytotoxic effects of circulating heme. Blood. 2002;100(3):879–87.
73. Umbreit J. Methemoglobin—it's not just blue: a concise review. Am J Hematol. 2007;82(2):134–44.
74. Hebbel RP. Reconstructing sickle cell disease: a data-based analysis of the "hyperhemolysis paradigm" for pulmonary hypertension from the perspective of evidence-based medicine. Am J Hematol. 2011;86(2):123–54.
75. Foidart M, Liem HH, Adornato BT, Engel WK, Muller-Eberhard U. Hemopexin metabolism in patients with altered serum levels. J Lab Clin Med. 1983;102(5):838–46.
76. Muller-Eberhard U, Javid J, Liem HH, Hanstein A, Hanna M. Plasma concentrations of hemopexin, haptoglobin and heme in patients with various hemolytic diseases. Blood. 1968;32(5):811–5.
77. Wochner RD, Spilberg I, Iio A, Liem HH, Muller-Eberhard U. Hemopexin metabolism in sickle-cell disease, porphyrias and control subjects—effects of heme injection. N Engl J Med. 1974;290(15):822–6.
78. Chen G, Zhang D, Fuchs TA, Wagner DD, Frenette PS. Heme-induced neutrophil extracellular traps contribute to the pathogenesis of sickle cell disease. Blood. 2014;123(24):3818–27.
79. Belcher JD, Mahaseth H, Welch TE, Otterbein LE, Hebbel RP, Vercellotti GM. Heme oxygenase-1 is a modulator of inflammation and vaso-occlusion in transgenic sickle mice. J Clin Invest. 2006;116(3):808–16.

80. Ghosh S, Ofori-Acquah SF. Acute chest syndrome in transgenic mouse models of sickle cell disease triggered by free heme. Blood. 2010;116 Suppl 1:944.
81. Bianchi ME. DAMPs, PAMPs and alarmins: all we need to know about danger. J Leukoc Biol. 2007;81(1):1–5.
82. Lotze MT, Deisseroth A, Rubartelli A. Damage associated molecular pattern molecules. Clin Immunol. 2007;124(1):1–4.
83. Figueiredo RT, Fernandez PL, Mourao-Sa DS, Porto BN, Dutra FF, Alves LS, et al. Characterization of heme as activator of Toll-like receptor 4. J Biol Chem. 2007;282(28):20221–9.
84. Schimmel M, Nur E, Biemond BJ, van Mierlo GJ, Solati S, Brandjes DP, et al. Nucleosomes and neutrophil activation in sickle cell disease painful crisis. Haematologica. 2013;98(11): 1797–803.
85. Grinberg LN, O'Brien PJ, Hrkal Z. The effects of heme-binding proteins on the peroxidative and catalatic activities of hemin. Free Radic Biol Med. 1999;27(1-2):214–9.
86. Ii M, Matsunaga N, Hazeki K, Nakamura K, Takashima K, Seya T, et al. A novel cyclohexene derivative, ethyl (6R)-6-[N-(2-Chloro-4-fluorophenyl)sulfamoyl]cyclohex-1-ene-1-carboxylate (TAK-242), selectively inhibits toll-like receptor 4-mediated cytokine production through suppression of intracellular signaling. Mol Pharmacol. 2006;69(4):1288–95.
87. Sha T, Sunamoto M, Kitazaki T, Sato J, Ii M, Iizawa Y. Therapeutic effects of TAK-242, a novel selective Toll-like receptor 4 signal transduction inhibitor, in mouse endotoxin shock model. Eur J Pharmacol. 2007;571(2–3):231–9.
88. Tidswell M, Tillis W, Larosa SP, Lynn M, Wittek AE, Kao R, et al. Phase 2 trial of eritoran tetrasodium (E5564), a toll-like receptor 4 antagonist, in patients with severe sepsis. Crit Care Med. 2010; 38(1):72–83.
89. Rice TW, Wheeler AP, Bernard GR, Vincent JL, Angus DC, Aikawa N, et al. A randomized, double-blind, placebo-controlled trial of TAK-242 for the treatment of severe sepsis. Crit Care Med. 2010;38(8):1685–94.
90. Opal SM, Laterre PF, Francois B, LaRosa SP, Angus DC, Mira JP, et al. Effect of eritoran, an antagonist of MD2-TLR4, on mortality in patients with severe sepsis: the ACCESS randomized trial. JAMA. 2013;309(11):1154–62.
91. Tse MT. Trial watch: sepsis study failure highlights need for trial design rethink. Nat Rev Drug Discov. 2013;12(5):334.

Chapter 4
Sickle Cell Disease and Acute Chest Syndrome: Epidemiology, Diagnosis, Management, Outcomes

Justin R. Sysol and Roberto Machado

Introduction

Sickle cell disease (SCD) is an autosomal recessive disorder affecting millions of individuals worldwide, making it one of the most common monogenetic diseases. Sickle cell anemia, the most common and severe form of SCD, occurs in patients with a single amino acid substitution of glutamic acid for valine in the β-globin gene, resulting in an abnormal hemoglobin form called hemoglobin S (HbS) within the erythrocytes. Mutant HbS has reduced solubility when deoxygenated compared to normal hemoglobin A (HbA), leading to polymerization and aggregation of sickle erythrocytes in the microvasculature. Structural abnormalities and cumulative damage to the cellular membrane of sickled erythrocytes results in hemolysis and the development of chronic hemolytic anemia, as well as vaso-occlusion and multiorgan pathology. Compound heterozygosity of HbS with other β-globin gene mutations results in additional types of SCD, such as hemoglobin SC or hemoglobin S-β-thalassemia [1]. Despite significant improvements in the life expectancy of patients with sickle cell disease, estimates of the median age at death range from 42 to 53 years for men and 48 to 58.5 years for women [2, 3].

The pathology of SCD is multifactorial and results from the structural and functional changes of sickled erythrocytes. Deoxygenated HbS polymerizes and aggregates inside erythrocytes, forming rigid, sickled cells. The abundance of polymerized HbS is strongly influenced by both the level of deoxygenation and the concentration of intracellular HbS [4], and determines the severity of SCD [5]. Pathologic sickled erythrocytes have increased adherence to the vascular endothelium, leading to

J.R. Sysol, BS • R. Machado, MD (✉)
Division of Pulmonary, Critical Care, Sleep and Allergy, Department of Medicine, University of Illinois College of Medicine at Chicago, Chicago, IL, USA

Department of Pharmacology, University of Illinois at Chicago, Chicago, IL, USA
e-mail: machador@uic.edu

J.S. Lee, M.P. Donahoe (eds.), *Hematologic Abnormalities and Acute Lung Syndromes*, Respiratory Medicine, DOI 10.1007/978-3-319-41912-1_4

microvasculature occlusion and subsequent multiorgan damage. Vaso-occlusion often manifests as episodic pain crises in SCD patients, a disease hallmark, as well as a high frequency of acute chest syndrome (ACS) [2, 6]. Due to chronically low Hb levels in SCD, patients rely on an overproduction of erythrocytes. Acute splenic sequestration and infectious and inflammatory processes, such as ACS, can interfere with erythropoiesis and trigger reticulocytopenia, or "aplastic crisis" in patients.

Sickled erythrocytes navigating the microcirculation are continually exposed to mechanical and oxidant injury, damaging the cell membrane and leading to a shortened erythrocyte lifespan, increased hemolysis and the development of chronic hemolytic anemia in patients. Importantly, intravascular hemolysis depletes the bioavailability of nitric oxide (NO) levels through the abundant release of both cell-free Hb, an NO scavenger, and arginase, which catabolizes arginine, a substrate necessary for NO synthesis [7]. Reduction in NO disrupts vascular homeostasis, leading to endothelial dysfunction, proliferation of cells within the vascular wall, thrombosis, and inflammatory stress [8–11]. Ischemia-reperfusion injury at sites of vessel occlusion can also promote inflammation and oxidative stress [12–15].

The low pressure and oxygen-tension within the pulmonary arterial bed can promote enhanced HbS polymerization and erythrocyte sickling [16]. Both acute and chronic pulmonary complications occur commonly in SCD and are a major cause of morbidity and mortality among these patients [2, 16–18]. Acute complications of SCD include asthma and ACS, while chronic complications can include pulmonary hypertension, restrictive lung disease (fibrosis), and corpulmonale [8, 19, 20]. In the Cooperative Study of Sickle Cell Disease (CSSCD) [21], a prospective, multi-institutional study of 3764 patients, over 20 % of adults with SCD likely had fatal pulmonary complications [2]. In another long-term, follow-up study of 299 SCD patients who participated in the Multicenter Study of Hydroxyurea in Sickle Cell Anemia (MSH), pulmonary complications were found to account for 24 % of deaths [22]. Though these results demonstrate the increasing recognition of pulmonary disease in SCD, there remains an imperative need for improved mechanistic understanding of these disease processes and novel therapeutic strategies.

Acute Chest Syndrome

The acute chest syndrome (ACS) is a lung injury syndrome of multiple etiologies first described in 1979 to describe a cohort of SCD patients presenting with fever, chest pain, increased white blood cell count, and pulmonary infiltrates [23]. The pathogenic mechanisms and epidemiology of ACS in SCD has been further studied since that time, and is currently defined as the development of a new pulmonary infiltrate, involving at least one complete lung segment, that is accompanied by fever, chest pain, tachypnea, wheezing, or cough [6, 24–26]. The pulmonary infiltrate appearing on chest radiography must be consistent with alveolar consolidation and not atelectasis [27]. ACS can affect both children and adults with any type of sickle hemoglobinopathy, but is more prevalent in individuals with homozygous sickle cell disease (HbSS) [28].

Three major mechanisms are known to be involved in the vaso-occlusive pathogenesis of ACS in SCD: infection, bone marrow and/or fat embolization, and direct pulmonary microvascular infarction due to red blood cell (RBC) sequestration [24, 29] (Fig. 4.1). The National Acute Chest Syndrome Study Group analyzed 671 episodes of ACS in 538 patients with SCD to determine the cause, outcome, and response to therapy [6]. Respiratory samples obtained from sputum and bronchoalveolar lavage

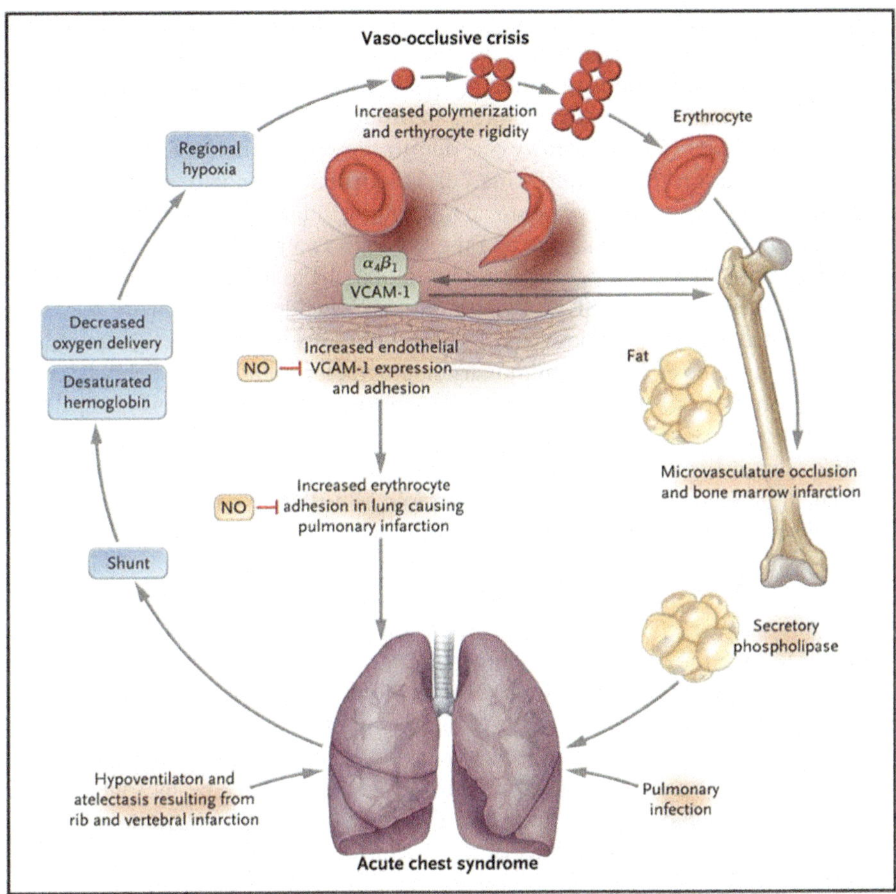

Fig. 4.1 Pathologic mechanisms of acute chest syndrome. *(From: Gladwin MT and Vichinsky E. Pulmonary complications of sickle cell disease. New England Journal of Medicine.2008; 359(21):2254–65. [PMID:19020327])*. The acute chest syndrome in sickle cell disease is a lung injury syndrome known to be initiated by three major mechanisms, including infection, bone marrow and/or fat embolization, and direct pulmonary microvascular infarction due to red blood cell sequestration. The mechanisms lead to vaso-occlusion by sickle cells with resulting infarction and lung injury. Ventilation–perfusion mismatch and hypoxemia due to lung injury leads to increased deoxygenation and polymerization of hemoglobin S, and erythrocyte vaso-occlusion. This pathologic mechanism promotes bone marrow infarction and pulmonary vaso-occlusion. *NO* nitric oxide; *VCAM-1* vascular cell adhesion molecule 1

were analyzed for viral and bacterial infections. A specific pathogen could not be identified in the majority of cases, however numerous different pathogens were identified, including *Chlamydia pneumoniae* (29 % of patients), *Mycoplasma pneumoniae* (20 %), and respiratory syncytial virus (10 %). Cases of severe ACS related to seasonal influenza have also been described [30, 31].

Bone marrow ischemia and necrosis are characteristic of vaso-occlusion in SCD and can lead to the release of fat and bone marrow into the circulation. ACS due to pulmonary fat and bone marrow embolizationhas a distinct and severe clinical course, associated with a high prevalence of bone and chest pain, neurologic symptoms, and decreased time to recovery [29, 32], and may be involved in up to 77 % of ACS episodes in adults [33]. Fat embolization can be diagnosed by the presence of lipid-laden macrophages in bronchoalveolar lavage fluid (BALF) from ACS patients [32–34]. However, due to the requirement of bronchoscopy, this method is not routinely performed and the true incidence of embolization is unknown. Since chest and rib pain are common manifestations of SCD, non-sickle pulmonary conditions such as fat embolism can be difficult to diagnose.

Direct pulmonary vaso-occlusion and infarction due to adhesion of sickled RBCs also contributes to ACS in SCD, though the exact incidence or primary causative nature of these events is unknown. A study in 144 cases of ACS to evaluate pulmonary artery thrombosis by CT–pulmonary angiography found a 17 % prevalence of pulmonary thrombosis without associated peripheral venous thrombosis [35]. These events occurred in patients with higher platelet counts and lower hemolytic rates during ACS, suggestive of in situ thrombosis. It is important to note that other causes of ACS, including infection and fat or bone emboli, as well as hypoxemia, may contribute to the development of pulmonary thrombosis in ACS. Prophylactic therapy for venous thromboembolism with low molecular weight or unfractionated heparin is therefore commonly used in adults with ACS, unless otherwise contraindicated.

In addition, severe acute hemolysis has been identified as a predictor of sudden death due to ACS [36]. The role of hemolysis-derived plasma-free Hb and its byproducts, including hemin (the oxidized prosthetic moiety of Hb), have been proposed as a novel inflammatory mechanism in ACS [37], and this may directly contribute to lung injury in the context of vaso-occlusive crisis. In support of the role of hemolysis in ACS, genetic variants in inducible hemeoxygenase 1 (HO-1), the rate-limiting enzyme in heme catabolism, are associated with ACS incidence in children [38].

Other pulmonary complications of SCD can be modulated by ACS, including pulmonary hypertension [39]. Pulmonary pressures can rise during episodes of ACS, leading to the development of acute right heart failure and increased mortality following the ACS event [17]. Therefore, prevention of ACS may reduce mortality in SCD patients with PH [40].

Epidemiology and Clinical Presentation

ACS is the second most common cause of hospitalization in SCD, second only to vaso-occlusive pain crisis, and is a leading cause of admission to an intensive care unit and premature death [2, 27]. Ten to twenty percent of patients admitted with acute vaso-occlusive pain crisis develop ACS in the first 3 days of hospitalization, and the mean duration of hospitalization for patients with ACS is 10.5 days [6]. While most cases are self-limited, some progress rapidly to acute respiratory failure with high rates of morbidity and mortality [41]. Overall mortality is 3 % in all ACS patients and 9 % in adults [6]. ACS therefore requires rapid management to prevent clinical decompensation and death. Recent increased awareness, the chronic use of hydroxyurea, and the aggressive use of early transfusion therapy, collectively, have led to a decrease in ACS-related mortality [42]. For example, a multicenter trial of inhaled NO for vaso-occlusive crisis found that only 10 % of patients in the placebo and treatment arm developed ACS and none required mechanical ventilation or died [42].

A natural history study by the CSSCD in both adults and children found that 29 % of all SCD patients will have at least one episode of ACS, and approximately half of those patients will have more than one ACS episode [28]. In patients with ACS, up to 78 % of episodes are associated with vaso-occlusive pain crisis, and the majority of patients also have chest pain, cough, and fever [33, 36]. The incidence of ACS in SCD is dependent on the subtype present. ACS episodes can affect patients with any type of SCD, but is most prevalent in individuals with HbSS (12.8 per 100 patient-years) compared to those with HbS-β^0-thalassemia (9.4 per 100 patient-years), HbSC (5.2 per 100 patient-years), or HbS-β^+-thalassemia (3.9 per 100 patient-years) [28]. The presence of α-thalassemia does not alter the ACS incidence rate in HbSS patients [28].

There are significant differences in the incidence and clinical presentation of ACS between adults and children with SCD, likely reflecting the differing etiologies in these age groups (Table 4.1). The incidence of ACS is higher in children (2–4 years of age) than adults (>20 years of age) with HbSS, with 25.3 events vs. 8.8 events per 100 patient-years, respectively [28, 36]. The course of disease tends to be milder in children, with higher rates of infectious causes. Adult cases of ACS are more severe, associated with pain, and have higher rates of mortality, with a higher incidence of pulmonary fat and bone marrow emboli [6, 29]. Adults with greater ACS incidence have a higher rate of all-cause mortality than those with low ACS incidence, and this increased rate of mortality may contribute to the decline in ACS incidence with age [28]. Despite these important differences between age groups, the clinical management is similar in both children and adults.

Numerous risk factors are associated with increased frequency of ACS. In children, asthma has been identified as an important modifiable risk factor. A CSSCD study in 291 African American children with HbSS followed beyond age 5 years found that asthma was significantly associated with more frequent ACS episodes (0.39 vs. 0.20 events per patient-year) and painful episodes (1.39 vs. 0.47 events per patient-year) [43]. Other clinical events that increase the risk of ACS include major surgical procedures, hypoxemia, a vascular necrosis of the hips, acute rib infarcts, pregnancy, use of narcotics, acute anemic events (aplastic crises), and previous pulmonary events [28, 36]. Active cigarette smoking or environmental smoke exposure are associated with more than twice the rate of ACS episodes, though no dose effect has been determined [44]. Significantly higher rates of ACS have also been reported following influenza infection [30, 31] and in winter months [36], findings most evident in children but present in all age groups.

Table 4.1 Characteristics of patients with acute chest syndrome[a]

Characteristic	All patients (*N*=537 1	Age at first episode of acute chest syndrome			*P* value[b]
		0–9 Years (*N*=264)	10–19 Years (*N*=145)	≥20 Years (*N*=128)	
Sex (%)					
Male	58	63	57	48	0.02
Female	42	38	43	53	
Hemoglobinopathy (%)					
SS	82	83	81	83	0.94
Other	18	17	19	17	
Mean age at first episode of acute chest syndrome (year)	13.8	5.4	14.6	30.2	<0.001
Medical history (%)					
Vaso-occlusive event	80	72	85	89	<0.001
Transfusion	74	63	84	86	<0.001
Acute chest syndrome or pneumonia	67	63	66	76	0.03
Prophylactic antibiotic therapy	57	81	51	13	<0.001
Major surgery	40	26	48	61	<0.001
Neurologic disease	16	10	17	29	<0.001
Sleep apnea	14	14	17	11	0.41
Red-cell antibodies	12	7	14	21	<0.001
Aseptic necrosis or fracture	12	5	11	26	<0.001
Asthma	11	14	9	5	0.01
Smoking	10	0	4	36	<0.001
Renal disease or urinary tract infection	7	3	7	14	<0.001
Chronic transfusion therapy	5	5	5	7	0.64
Cardiac disease	4	1	3	12	<0.001
Chronic lung disease	4	3	4	5	0.46
Pulmonary edema	4	1	3	9	<0.001
Clubbing	2	1	0	5	0.002
Deep-vein thrombosis	1	<1	0	3	0.01
Tuberculosis	<1	0	0	1	0.20
Reason for current admission (%)					
Acute chest syndrome	52	61	46	42	<0.001
Other[c]	48	39	54	58	
Symptoms at diagnosis of acute chest syndrome (%)					
Fever	80	86	78	70	<0.001
Cough	62	69	58	54	0 006
Chest pain	44	27	67	55	<0.001
Tachypnea	45	47	47	39	0.27

(continued)

Table 4.1 (continued)

Characteristic	All patients (*N*=537 1	Age at first episode of acute chest syndrome			*P* value[b]
		0–9 Years (*N*=264)	10–19 Years (*N*=145)	≥20 Years (*N*=128)	
Shortness of breath	41	31	44	58	<0.001
Pain in arms and legs	37	22	44	59	<0.001
Abdominal pain	35	38	36	29	0.24
Rib or sternal pain	21	14	26	30	<0.001
Reactive airway disease	13	17	12	6	0.01
Neurologic dysfunction	4	3	3	7	0.11
Cyanosis	2	1	3	3	0.24
Heart failure	1	2	1	1	0.49

From: Vichinsky EP et al. Causes and outcomes of the acute chest syndrome in sickle cell disease. National Acute Chest Syndrome Study Group. New England Journal of Medicine. 2000; 342(25):1855–65. Table 1. [PMID: 10861320]

[a]Because of rounding, percentages may not total 100. Data on one patient were excluded because the patient's birth date was not known

[b]*P* values were calculated by chi-square analyses

[c]Other reason s included a vaso-occlusive event, anemia, fever, infection, gastrointestinal or abdominal pain, asthma, urologic and orthopedic conditions, heart failure, and surgery

Several laboratory parameters are associated with the development of ACS. Rates of ACS are positively correlated with non-vaso-occlusive crisis, steady-state white blood cell counts and Hb concentration and inversely correlated with fetal Hb (HbF) levels [28]. Though higher steady-state Hb levels are associated with ACS, during acute hospitalization for vaso-occlusive crisis, the development of ACS is often preceded by an abrupt drop in Hb levels (mean decrease of 0.78 g/dL from steady-state levels) and increases in markers of hemolysis, such as lactate dehydrogenase (LDH) [6, 27]. A drop in platelet count also has been shown to precede ACS, with levels <200,000 cells/mm^3, and is an independent predictor of neurologic complications during hospitalization and need for mechanical ventilation [6, 45]. Understanding the epidemiology and complex etiologies of ACS in SCD, which differ among age groups, is critically important to diagnosing and treating this devastating disease manifestation.

Diagnosis

ACS is currently defined as an acute illness in SCD patients presenting with radiographic evidence of a new pulmonary infiltrate, involving at least one complete lung segment, that is accompanied by fever, chest pain, tachypnea, wheezing, or cough [6, 24–26] (Fig. 4.2a). Abdominal, limb, rib, or sternal pain is also common, along with intercostal retractions, nasal flaring, the use of accessory muscles for

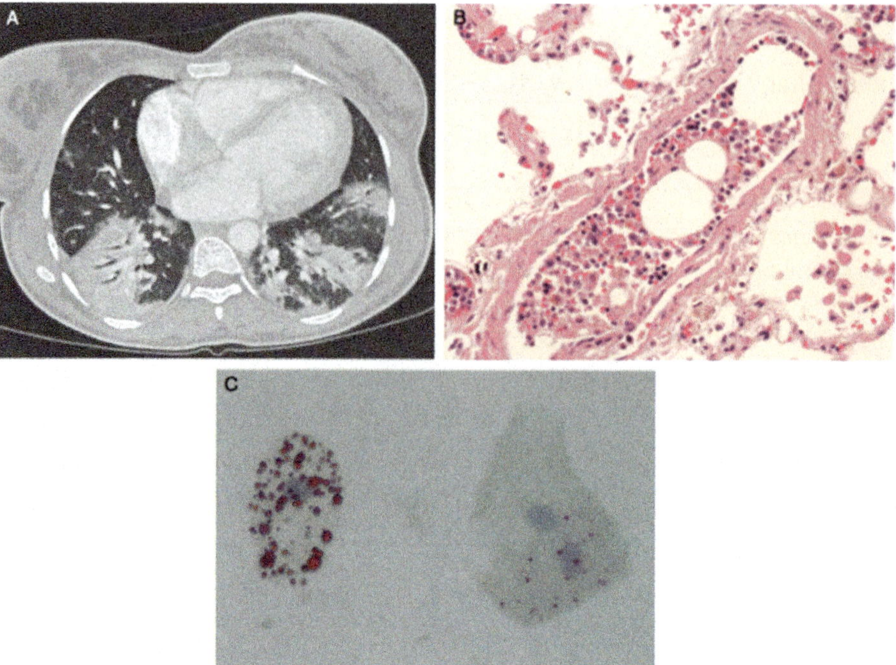

Fig. 4.2 (**a–c**): Radiographic and pathologic findings in acute chest syndrome. *(From: Vij R and Machado RF. Pulmonary Complications of Hemoglobinopathies. Chest. 2010;138(4):973–983. [PMID:20923801]).* (**a**) Chest CT scan of a 27-year-old woman with multifocal bilateral consolidations due to acute chest syndrome. (**b**) Post mortem specimen of a patient who died during an episode of vaso-occlusive crisis and acute chest syndrome depicting bone marrow emboli within a small pulmonary artery (hematoxylin and eosin stain, original magnification 40×). (**c**) Lipid inclusions within alveolar macrophages obtained by sputum induction in a patient with acute chest syndrome (oil-red O stain, original magnification 40×)

respiration, and decreased SpO2 (>2 % from steady-state). The clinical presentation, epidemiology, risks, and outcomes of ACS are variable, and the syndrome can often be diagnosed as pneumonia due to the number of shared features. Many of the clinical features of ACS are also age-dependent, reflecting differences in etiology among age groups, with adults having more causative fat embolization and children with a higher proportion of infectious causes and reactive airway disease.

The diagnosis of ACS in SCD patients requires a high index of suspicion, and there are a number of recommended diagnostic approaches. Since the development of ACS often occurs 24–72 h after the onset of severe vaso-occlusive pain symptoms, it is critical that vigilance be kept during hospitalization of SCD patients, as they may be in the prodromal stages of ACS [25]. A thorough history and physical exam is required for all patients with SCD who present clinically with suspected signs of ACS, along with assessment of vital signs including oxygen saturation. Respiratory rate, pulse rate, and body temperature values have been shown to be higher in children than adults with ACS [36]. Patients with evidence of oxygen desaturation should have arterial blood gas measurements obtained to confirm the hypoxia [46], since pulse oximetry can be inaccurate in the presence of significant anemia. It is important to note that hypoventilation due to pain crisis or over-sedation can contribute to hypoxemia and exacerbation of ACS.

Chest radiography is required for all suspected ACS cases presenting with chest pain and/or fevers, though the findings may differ between adults and children. The CSSCD found that young children had more frequent infiltrates in the upper and middle lung lobes, while adults had more frequent lower and multiple lobe involvement and pleural effusion. However, another large, multicenter study found similar radiographic findings between adults and children with ACS [6, 36]. Radiologic signs are often absent early in development of ACS and may underestimate the severity of hypoxia [47], therefore treatment should not be delayed in the absence of significant findings and repeated chest X-rays should be obtained in suspected ACS cases.

Obtaining complete blood counts with white blood cell (WBC) differential, reticulocyte counts, and cultures of blood and sputum are also recommended for workup of suspected ACS cases. As mentioned above, an abrupt decrease in Hb concentration and platelet number often precede the development of ACS and are markers of disease severity [6, 45]. Reticulocyte counts can be used to assess for adequate bone marrow function and exclude red cell aplasia due to erythrovirus B19 infection [48]. ACS is associated with a systemic inflammatory state, with a mean peak temperature of 38.9 °C during hospitalization and a mean WBC count of 23,000 cell/mm^3 [6]. Biochemical testing for C-reactive protein (CRP) can be useful in monitoring the inflammatory state of ACS patients, especially given the risk of multiorgan failure syndrome (discussed below), though the sensitivity and specificity of this test may be decreased if an infectious agent is present. Elevation in secretory phospholipase A2, a potent inflammatory mediator, occurs early in the course of ACS, before radiographic changes are detected, and has been shown to predict ACS onset [49].

Serological testing for infectious agents should also be considered in patients with ACS, both acutely and throughout illness, including detection of atypical respiratory organisms associated with ACS, such as *Chlamyophila pneumoniae*, *Mycoplasma pneumoniae*, and *Legionella* [48]. Pneumococcal and *Legionella* antigens may be detected in the urine. Testing for viral agents within sputum and nasopharyngeal samples via PCR and immunofluorescence staining, including influenza, respiratory syncytial virus, and erythrovirus B19, may also be indicated in ACS based on clinical and hematological findings [6, 48]. Identification of infective organisms can guide therapeutic treatment and/or the use of isolation facilities.

Bone marrow ischemia and necrosis lead to systemic fat and marrow embolization and contribute to a multiorgan failure syndrome with high clinical overlap and association with ACS (Fig. 4.2b). Patients with this syndrome can present with acute dysfunction of the lung, kidney, or liver, along with fever, alterations in mental status, seizures, decreased hemoglobin levels, thrombocytopenia, and coagulopathy. The similar presentation of multiorgan failure syndrome and ACS demonstrates a shared underlying etiology, with ACS predominantly affecting the lung [50]. Since the clinical manifestations of pulmonary fat embolization can be indistinguishable from other ACS causes, the diagnosis requires the identification of lipid-laden alveolar macrophages using Oil Red O staining (Fig. 4.2c). Bronchoscopy with BALF collection can be used for diagnosis, including identification of bacterial and viral agents, however this technique has been associated with an increased risk of requiring mechanical ventilation [6]. A significant correlation between results from the bronchoscopy method and induced sputum sampling of alveolar macrophages has been reported, and ACS patients with the presence of lipid-ladenalveolar macrophages in induced sputum have more extra-thoracic pain, neurological symptoms, thrombocytopenia, and elevated transaminase levels [51].

Other diagnostic procedures for ACS could include chest CT, ventilation-perfusion scanning, and angiographic imaging techniques to evaluate for pulmonary emboli, which have been shown to occur in the lungs due to both in situ vaso-occlusion of sickled erythrocytes and also secondary to pulmonary artery thrombosis in ACS [6]. Pulmonary artery filling defects are expected in these studies due to sickle cell vaso-occlusion [47, 52]. Though the extent of vascular occlusion identified by chest CT has been shown to correlate with clinical severity and degree of hypoxia in contrast to chest X-ray [47], it is not routinely recommended due to the high radiation exposure and the recurrence rate of ACS [48]. A recent study comparing the diagnostic performance and reproducibility of CT and bedside chest radiography during ACS found that CT more frequently identified lung consolidation patterns predominating in the lung bases and correlated with severity and disease course, however bedside chest radiography using CT as a reference had high sensitivity but low specificity [53].

Blood type should be determined for all patients at risk of ACS, given the potential requirement of emergency transfusion [48]. Erythrocyte alloimmunization is a serious complication in SCD patients and may result in delayed hemolytic transfusion reactions and difficulty finding compatible units [54]. Erythrocyte alloantibodies also may become undetectable over time in SCD patients, posing an even greater risk for adverse reactions during transfusion [54].

When SCD patients present with symptoms of ACS, several other life-threatening conditions should be considered in the differential diagnosis, as mentioned previously. These include pneumonia, pulmonary embolus, and acute coronary syndrome. Pneumonia cannot be distinguished clinically from ACS, therefore empirical antibiotic therapy is administered upon presentation. Pulmonary emboli originating from deep vein thrombosis are difficult to distinguish from in situ pulmonary thrombi or fat or bone marrow emboli occurring frequently in ACS, which do not respond to anti-coagulation therapy [24, 29]. Signs and symptoms of vaso-occlusive pain crisis and evidence of new pulmonary radiographic densities can assist in ruling out pulmonary embolus. Testing for D-dimers is unhelpful in SCD patients due to basally elevated levels [55]. ACS symptoms along with the detection of deep vein thrombosis in the lower extremities by ultrasound imaging, recent surgery, or extended periods of immobility suggest the presence of pulmonary emboli.

Acute coronary syndrome due to the rupture and dislodging of an atherosclerotic plaque within a coronary artery should also be considered with ACS symptom presentation, though coronary artery disease is uncommon in SCD [56]. Depending on clinical suspicion and patient history, electrocardiography and serum troponin levels can also be measured to evaluate for myocardial damage, since acute multiorgan failure may be present when vaso-occlusive pain crisis and myocardial damage are both present.

As described above, the diagnostic evaluation of ACS in SCD requires a high degree of clinical suspicion. Though most cases are self-limited, rapid progression to acute respiratory failure can occur with high rates of morbidity and mortality [41]. ACS therefore requires aggressive management in order to minimize poor clinical outcomes. All patients suspected of having ACS should receive chest radiography, complete blood counts with WBC differential, blood oxygen saturation testing (ABG), standard biochemistry testing, and blood group and screen [48]. Clinical indications may warrant the use of diagnostic blood cultures, sputum bacterial cultures, nasopharyngeal and sputum testing for viruses, and serology and urine testing. Other procedures and testing described should be carefully considered based on the clinical presentation and identification of potential differential diagnoses.

Management

Acute care for patients with ACS focuses on the prevention and reversal of acute respiratory failure, and will potentially mitigate irreversible lung damage. This includes immediate pain control, fluid management, supplemental oxygen, blood transfusion, antibiotic therapy, and prophylaxis for deep vein thromboembolism. These measures will typically result in the rapid resolution of symptoms in the majority of patients. However, it is imperative to recognize the course of ACS development differs among age groups, as ACS in adult cases can occur acutely or may evolve several days after admission for severe pain crisis, versus children who more often present acutely. Therefore, clinical suspicion for ACS in SCD patients should be high following any vaso-occlusive pain episode.

Vaso-occlusive pain crisis in SCD affecting the thorax can lead to severe discomfort and alveolar hypoventilation. Proper pain control with parenteral opioids is imperative during ACS episodes, and is often delivered by patient-controlled analgesia in adults. Continuous cardiorespiratory monitoring is required to avoid over-sedation and narcosis, which can lead to hypoventilation and subsequent hypoxemia, worsening ACS outcomes [6].

The severity of ACS often limits oral hydration in patients. Therefore, fluid management must be utilized to prevent hypovolemia and should be individualized based on the cardiopulmonary status of the patient. Though fluid replacement therapy is important in the management of ACS, care must be taken to prevent overhydration, which can result in pulmonary vascular congestion and edema, exacerbating the course of ACS [48]. It is also important to recognize that a substantial proportion of patients with ACS develop right ventricular dysfunction and in these patients aggressive IV fluid therapy could lead to worsening cor pulmonale.

Supplemental oxygen therapy is delivered to adults with ACS with oxygen saturation (SaO_2) <90 % or arterial oxygen partial pressure (PaO_2) <60 mmHg [6]. SaO_2 levels estimated by pulse oximetry should be confirmed with ABG analysis, and baseline values may be helpful in determining desaturation (decrease >3 % from baseline) when available. Co-oximetry provides the most accurate measure of SaO_2 in patients with SCD, as vasoconstriction, hypotension, and hypothermia can affect pulse oximetry values. It is important to note that patients with SCD have a right-shifted oxyhemoglobin dissociation curve due to the presence of HbS. The need for supplemental oxygen should be continuously monitored in ACS.

Incentive spirometry, used to improve lung function and prevent atelectasis and pulmonary infiltrates, has been shown to decrease the rate of ACS in children admitted to the hospital for vaso-occlusive pain crisis [57]. While no studies to date have determined the benefit of this therapy in preventing the worsening of ACS in SCD patients, it is likely to be an important adjunct therapy. The use of this intervention may be limited by pain and should be tailored to the individual patient with the help of a respiratory physiotherapist [48].

Empirical antibiotic therapy is administered to patients suspected of having ACS, though infectious causes are less common in adults than children with SCD and respiratory samples from sputum and BALF do not identify a causative pathogen in the majority of ACS cases [6]. The most commonly identified organisms are atypical bacteria, including *Chlamydia pneumoniae* and *Mycoplasma pneumoniae*, along with *Streptococcus pneumoniae* and *Haemophilus influenzae* [6] (Table 4.2). Therefore, a typical antibiotic regimen may consist of a cephalosporin and a macrolide intravenously until fever subsides for at least 24 h, followed by oral administration for 7–10 days [6]. The antibiotics used should be tailored to culture results, when available, and local antibiotic resistance profiles should be considered [48]. There are currently no randomized control trials for antibiotic treatment regimens in the management of ACS.

Transfusion therapy is a mainstay treatment for patients with ACS despite the absence of any prospective cohort studies to demonstrate a change in patient outcomes. One large study found an increase in $PaO_2$of 8 mmHg and increase in SaO_2 of 3 % following transfusion in ACS patients, with an even greater improvement in SaO_2 in patients who had demonstrated hypoxia prior to transfusion [6]. The oxygenation benefits of transfusion are due to a left-shift in the oxyhemoglobin dissociation curves, which is usually right-shifted at baseline in SCD due to the presence of HbS. Sickle-negative, leukocyte-depleted packed RBCs with extensive matching to Rhesus D, C, and E, as well as Kell antigens should be used for transfusion [58]. Since SCD patients often receive transfusions for many acute and chronic complications throughout the course of their disease, there is a risk for iron overload and alloimmunization. Therefore even with the use of antigen-matched and cross match-compatible blood, transfusions may pose a risk to patients with ACS.

The need for transfusion and the modality of simple versus exchange transfusion should be individualized based on ACS severity and the risk for developing acute

Table 4.2 Infectious pathogens isolated in 671 episodes of the acute chest syndrome[a]

Pathogen	No. of episodes
Chlamydia pneumoniae	71
Mycoplasma pneumoniae	51
Respiratory syncytial virus	26
Coagulase-positive *Staphylococcus aureus*	12
Streptococcus pneumoniae	11
Mycoplasma hominis	10
Parvovirus	10
Rhinovirus	8
Parainfluenza virus	6
Haemophilus influenzae	5
Cytomegalovirus	4
Influenza A virus	4
Legionella pneumophila	4
Escherichia coli	3
Epstein–Barr virus	3
Herpes simplex virus	3
Pseudomonas species	3
Adenovirus	2
Branhamella species	2
Echovirus	2
Beta-hemolytic streptococcus	2
Mycobacterium tuberculosis	2
Enterobacter species	1
Klebsiella pneumoniae	1
Mycobacterium avium complex	1
Salmonella species	1
Serratia marcescens	1
Total	249

From: Vichinsky EP et al. *Causes and outcomes of the acute chest syndrome in sickle cell disease. National Acute Chest Syndrome Study Group. New England Journal of Medicine. 2000; 342(25):1855–65. [PMID: 10861320]*

[a]All infectious agents isolated during episodes of the acute chest syndrome are included

respiratory failure [58]. Transfusion is required less often in children with ACS, who tend to have shorter, self-limited episodes due mainly to respiratory infections [6]. Simple RBC transfusion decreases the concentration of HbS by dilution, and should be considered in more stable patients with single-lobe involvement, mild hypoxemia responsive to low-flow oxygen, and worsening anemia [58]. Exchange transfusion performed by automated erythrocytapheresis can rapidly reduce the percentage of

HbS without the risks of iron overload or hyperviscosity, but the risk of alloimmunization remains. This modality is often reserved for ACS patients with multilobar involvement, refractory hypoxemia, and imminent or rapidly progressing lung injury, or in less severe patients with high Hb concentrations (≥9 g/dL) to avoid hyperviscosity [58]. It has been demonstrated that conservative transfusion regimens are as effective as aggressive regimens in preventing perioperative complications in SCD, with the conservative regimen resulting in significantly fewer transfusion-associated complications [59]. Additionally, similar improvements in oxygen saturation were observed in a large cohort of ACS patients receiving either simple or exchange transfusions [6].

Bronchodilator therapy is often used in the treatment of ACS, however, there is a need for a randomized control trial to assess the risks and benefits of this therapy for ACS in SCD patients. Since wheezing occurs more often in children during ACS episodes compared to adults [6], and an association between ACS and asthma is known in children [43], the use of bronchodilators in ACS in this patient population may have increased benefit. Patients with evidence of reactive airway disease, acute bronchospasm, or the development of progressive respiratory distress during ACS should be considered for this therapy [48].

Advanced respiratory support in a critical care setting is needed for some ACS patients, indicated by worsening hypoxemia, severe dyspnea, and respiratory acidosis due to hypoventilation and hypercapnia [48]. The use of noninvasive ventilation (NIV) support to improve patient outcomes in ACS has been explored. A prospective, randomized study of 71 ACS episodes in 67 patients at one center demonstrated that NIV more rapidly decreased respiratory rate and improved gas exchange in ACS compared to oxygen alone [41]. However, NIV did not significantly reduce the number of hypoxemic patients at day 3 and was associated with decreased patient satisfaction and compliance. No differences were observed in pain relief, transfusions, or length of stay.

The National Acute Chest Syndrome Study Group found that 13 % of all ACS patients and 22 % of adults with ACS required the use of invasive mechanical ventilation (MV) during hospitalization, with a mean duration of MV of 4.6 days [6]. As previously discussed, there are several important risk factors influencing the need for invasive MV in ACS. These include platelet counts less than 200,000 cells/ mm^3 (likely indicative of the fat embolization syndrome), the number of lobes involved on chest radiography, and a self-reported or medical record history of cardiac disease [6]. The complications of heart disease are now thought to reflect the presence of occult pulmonary hypertension and cor pulmonale, as a recent study in 84 patients hospitalized with ACS found that 13 % manifested right heart failure [17]. Strikingly, this patient subgroup had the highest need for invasive MV and death, suggesting that pulmonary hypertension and right heart dysfunction is a major comorbidity during ACS.

Despite the aggressive nature of ACS, outcomes of patients requiring invasive MV are generally positive, with 81 % of patients recovering [6], compared to significantly lower recovery rates reported in patients with acute respiratory distress syndrome (ARDS). Strategies for the use of MV in ACS should follow similar strategies to treat acute respiratory distress syndrome (ARDS), including minimizing tidal volumes to prevent alveolar over-distension [60].

Given the significant morbidity and mortality associated with the development of ACS in SCD, significant measures can be taken to prevent the onset of ACS. These include the use of hydroxyurea therapy, chronic transfusion therapy, and hematopoietic cell transplantation.

The benefits of hydroxyurea therapy in SCD are far-reaching and well established, and were first demonstrated by the Multicenter Study of Hydroxyurea in Sickle Cell Anemia, a double-blind, placebo controlled trial in 299 adults with SCD [61]. Hydroxyurea has been shown to decrease the incidence of vaso-occlusive pain crises in SCD and reduce the risk ACS development by approximately 50 % when administered in the outpatient setting, and may also prevent splenic dysfunction, cerebral-artery damage, and secondary stroke [61, 62]. Importantly, hydroxyurea also significantly reduces the need for transfusion therapy and has been demonstrated to reduce overall mortality by 40 % in SCD. The beneficial mechanisms of hydroxyurea include increasing the number of RBCs containing high levels of HbF, (via stimulation of soluble guanylatecyclase and killing of cycling cells through inhibition of ribonucleotidereductase), as well as decreasing RBC membrane damage, sickling and vaso-occlusion [62] (Fig. 4.3). These factors can result in a significant reduction in ischemia, necrosis, hemolysis, and vascular damage. Given the known teratogenic effects of hydroxyurea, patients should not be treated during pregnancy or breast-feeding, and contraception should be used in patients receiving therapy. Before initiation of hydroxyurea therapy, baseline measures of complete blood counts, hepatic function, and renal function should be established to determine appropriate dosing. The myelosuppressive effects of hydroxyurea therapy should also be monitored with routine peripheral blood counts, and dose adjustment should be made as needed [62].

As the natural history of ACS in SCD has evolved with modern diagnostic and therapeutic approaches, it has been established that a subset of patients are at very high risk for poor long-term outcomes and death. In addition to the described acute care strategies for ACS, several preventative measures may be employed in these patients. Hydroxyurea therapy is recommended for adult SCD patients with a history of ACS or frequent vaso-occlusive pain episodes, unless otherwise contraindicated, as described above [62]. In patients with multiple moderate to severe ACS episodes despite maximal hydroxyurea therapy, the use of chronic transfusion therapy to maintain a low percentage of RBCs containing HbS has been shown to decrease the rate of ACS and vaso-occlusive pain crises in SCD [63]. Careful risk-benefit assessments must be made in patients considered for chronic transfusion given the association of this therapy with a wide variety of adverse reactions. Myeloablative hematopoietic cell transplantation, currently the only cure for SCD, may be recommended for patients with severe symptoms that are unresponsive to hydroxyurea therapy or have a history of ACS and have a HLA-matched sibling available as a donor [64]. Despite the potentially curative outcome of transplantation

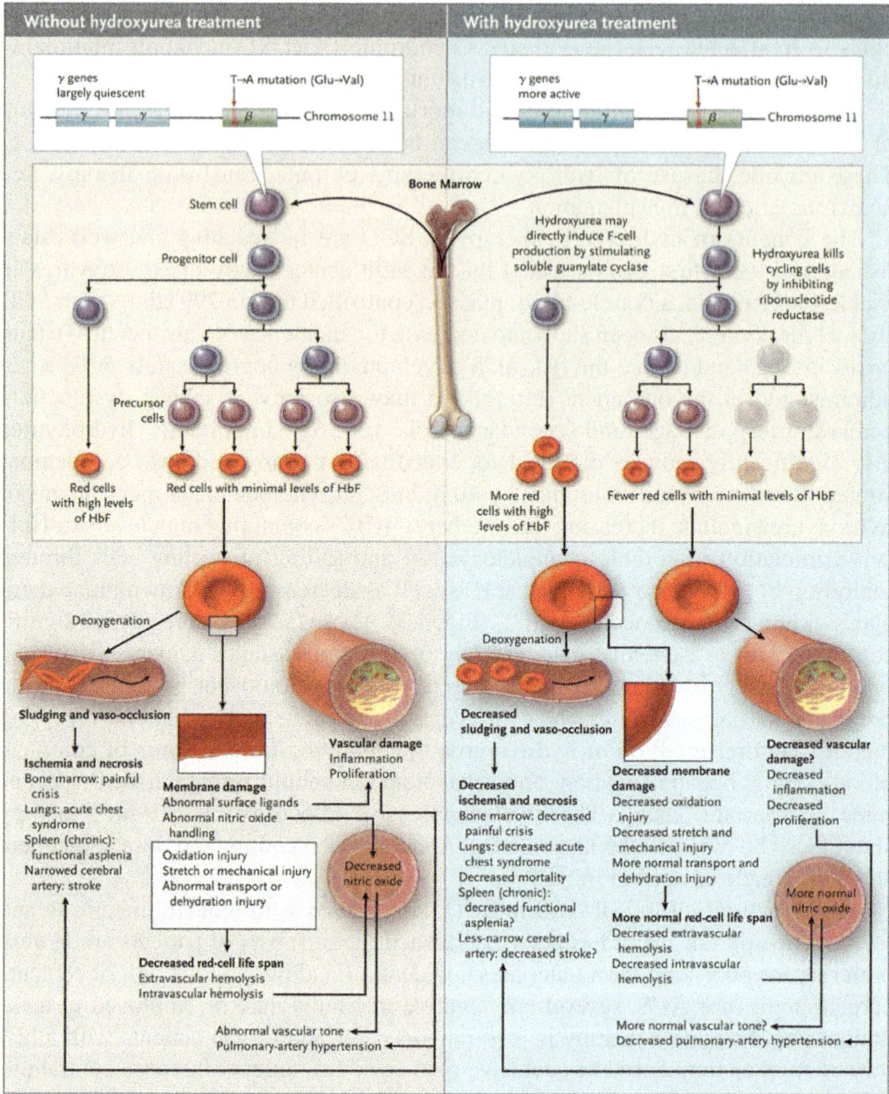

Fig. 4.3 The pathophysiological effects of hydroxyurea therapy in sickle cell disease. *(From: Platt OS. Hydroxyurea for the treatment of sickle cell anemia. New England Journal of Medicine. 2008;358(13):1362–9. [PMID: 18367739])*. Mutations within the β-globin gene in sickle cell disease result in the production of sickle hemoglobin (HbS) within red blood cells (RBCs). Most RBCs produced in the bone marrow are derived from mature precursor cells and contain mostly HbS. Deoxygenation conditions induce HbS polymerization and morphological sickling of RBCs within the circulation, leading to pathologic vaso-occlusion and acute chest syndrome. HbS damages the RBC membrane through several mechanisms resulting in hemolysis, depletion of nitric oxide, and increased adherence to and damage of vascular cells. Hydroxyurea therapy induces γ-globin gene expression and can kill cycling cells, forcing more RBCs called F-cells to be produced, which are derived directly from primitive progenitor cells and contain high fetal hemoglobin (HbF) content. This can reduce pathologic RBC membrane damage, vaso-occlusion,

in SCD, there is an associated risk of mortality of 7–10 % and relatively few studies done to address patient selection and criteria for transplant. The use of alternative donor sources and non-myeloablative transplant regimens are currently under investigation, but their utility in ACS remains uncertain.

Outcomes

Despite advances in therapy and our understanding of the pathophysiological mechanisms underlying ACS, it remains a leading cause of morbidity and mortality in patients with SCD.A higher incidence rate of ACS in adults with SCD is associated with an increased risk of death [2]. Multiorgan complications during ACS episodes are also prevalent, including vaso-occlusive crises, abdominal pain, and neurological, cardiac, gastrointestinal, and renal events [6]. The clinical features of ACS at the time of presentation are age-dependent due to differences in etiologies among age groups, with a striking difference in the overall rate of death per ACS episode between adults (4.3 %) and children (1.1 %) [36]. The onset of ACS is often preceded by vaso-occlusive crisis, chest pain, and dyspnea in adults, while fever and cough are more common in children. Though the majority of ACS cases occur in HbSS patients, a comparable rate of death per ACS episode has been observed in both HbSS and HbSC patients (1.9 and 1.6 %, respectively) [36].

In a large study conducted by the National Acute Chest Syndrome Study Group, the mean hospital stay for all ACS patients was found to be 10.5 days (12.8 days in adults), and that prolonged hospitalization was independently associated with an age of 20 years or more, a history of vaso-occlusive events, a platelet count of <200,000 cells/mm^3 at diagnosis, pain in the arms and legs at presentation, extensive radiographic abnormalities, evidence of effusion on chest radiography, fever, transfusion therapy, and evidence of respiratory failure [6]. Of the 3 % of patients that died from ACS in this study, the most common causes of death were pulmonary emboli and infectious bronchopneumonia. Older patients were more likely to have complications and die during hospitalization for ACS, and respiratory failure, defined by the need for mechanical ventilation, occurred in 13 % of patients. The development of neurological events, including altered mental status, seizures, and neuromuscular abnormalities, occurred in 11 % of ACS patients, and 46 % of these patients had respiratory failure. Of the subset of patients with neurological complications and respiratory failure, 92 % received transfusion therapy and 23 % died [6]. Together, these findings highlight the significant sequelae associated with ACS, which contribute to poor patient outcomes.

Fig 4.3 (continued) ischemia, and necrosis. Hydroxyurea also produces nitric oxide, which may help to regulate vascular tone, and directly stimulates HbF production. Overall, hydroxyurea therapy leads to fewer symptoms in patients, less severe hemolytic anemia, fewer cases of acute chest syndrome, and lower mortality

Conclusion

ACS is a major cause of morbidity and mortality in adults and children with SCD and is associated with a multitude of multiorgan complications. The burden of this condition is likely to become more prevalent as the life expectancy of these patients continues to improve. A high index of suspicion is required to correctly diagnose ACS in SCD patients and improve outcomes. Though both acute and long-term strategies for the clinical management of ACS continue to advance, there is an imperative need for novel therapeutics, preventative strategies, and predictive measures for this devastating condition.

References

1. Ashley-Koch A, Yang Q, Olney RS. Sickle hemoglobin (HbS) allele and sickle cell disease: a HuGE review. Am J Epidemiol. 2000;151(9):839–45.
2. Platt OS, Brambilla DJ, Rosse WF, Milner PF, Castro O, Steinberg MH, et al. Mortality in sickle cell disease. Life expectancy and risk factors for early death. N Engl J Med. 1994;330(23):1639–44.
3. Wierenga KJ, Hambleton IR, Lewis NA. Survival estimates for patients with homozygous sickle-cell disease in Jamaica: a clinic-based population study. Lancet. 2001;357(9257):680–3.
4. Bunn HF. Pathogenesis and treatment of sickle cell disease. N Engl J Med. 1997;337(11):762–9.
5. Brittenham GM, Schechter AN, Noguchi CT. Hemoglobin S polymerization: primary determinant of the hemolytic and clinical severity of the sickling syndromes. Blood. 1985;65(1):183–9.
6. Vichinsky EP, Neumayr LD, Earles AN, Williams R, Lennette ET, Dean D, et al. Causes and outcomes of the acute chest syndrome in sickle cell disease. National Acute Chest Syndrome Study Group. N Engl J Med. 2000;342(25):1855–65.
7. Rother RP, Bell L, Hillmen P, Gladwin MT. The clinical sequelae of intravascular hemolysis and extracellular plasma hemoglobin: a novel mechanism of human disease. JAMA. 2005;293(13):1653–62.
8. Gladwin MT, Sachdev V, Jison ML, Shizukuda Y, Plehn JF, Minter K, et al. Pulmonary hypertension as a risk factor for death in patients with sickle cell disease. N Engl J Med. 2004;350(9):886–95.
9. Frei AC, Guo Y, Jones DW, Pritchard Jr KA, Fagan KA, Hogg N, et al. Vascular dysfunction in a murine model of severe hemolysis. Blood. 2008;112(2):398–405.
10. Hsu L, McDermott T, Brown L, Aguayo SM. Transgenic HbS mouse neutrophils in increased susceptibility to acute lung injury: implications for sickle acute chest syndrome. Chest. 1999;116(1 Suppl):92S.
11. Gladwin MT. Role of the red blood cell in nitric oxide homeostasis and hypoxic vasodilation. Adv Exp Med Biol. 2006;588:189–205.
12. Platt OS. Sickle cell anemia as an inflammatory disease. J Clin Invest. 2000;106(3):337–8.
13. Kaul DK, Hebbel RP. Hypoxia/reoxygenation causes inflammatory response in transgenic sickle mice but not in normal mice. J Clin Invest. 2000;106(3):411–20.
14. Klings ES, Farber HW. Role of free radicals in the pathogenesis of acute chest syndrome in sickle cell disease. Respir Res. 2001;2(5):280–5.
15. Hebbel RP. Ischemia-reperfusion injury in sickle cell anemia: relationship to acute chest syndrome, endothelial dysfunction, arterial vasculopathy, and inflammatory pain. Hematol Oncol Clin North Am. 2014;28(2):181–98.

16. Powars D, Weidman JA, Odom-Maryon T, Niland JC, Johnson C. Sickle cell chronic lung disease: prior morbidity and the risk of pulmonary failure. Medicine. 1988;67(1):66–76.
17. Mekontso Dessap A, Leon R, Habibi A, Nzouakou R, Roudot-Thoraval F, Adnot S, et al. Pulmonary hypertension and cor pulmonale during severe acute chest syndrome in sickle cell disease. Am J Respir Crit Care Med. 2008;177(6):646–53.
18. Thomas AN, Pattison C, Serjeant GR. Causes of death in sickle-cell disease in Jamaica. Br Med J. 1982;285(6342):633–5.
19. Minter KR, Gladwin MT. Pulmonary complications of sickle cell anemia. A need for increased recognition, treatment, and research. Am J Respir Crit Care Med. 2001;164(11):2016–9.
20. Siddiqui AK, Ahmed S. Pulmonary manifestations of sickle cell disease. Postgrad Med J. 2003;79(933):384–90.
21. Gaston M, Rosse WF. The cooperative study of sickle cell disease: review of study design and objectives. Am J Pediatr Hematol Oncol. 1982;4(2):197–201.
22. Steinberg MH, McCarthy WF, Castro O, Ballas SK, Armstrong FD, Smith W, et al. The risks and benefits of long-term use of hydroxyurea in sickle cell anemia: A 17.5 year follow-up. Am J Hematol. 2010;85(6):403–8.
23. Charache S, Scott JC, Charache P. "Acute chest syndrome" in adults with sickle cell anemia. Microbiology, treatment, and prevention. Arch Intern Med. 1979;139(1):67–9.
24. Ballas SK, Lieff S, Benjamin LJ, Dampier CD, Heeney MM, Hoppe C, et al. Definitions of the phenotypic manifestations of sickle cell disease. Am J Hematol. 2010;85(1):6–13.
25. Gladwin MT, Vichinsky E. Pulmonary complications of sickle cell disease. N Engl J Med. 2008;359(21):2254–65.
26. Platt OS. The acute chest syndrome of sickle cell disease. N Engl J Med. 2000;342(25):1904–7.
27. Miller AC, Gladwin MT. Pulmonary complications of sickle cell disease. Am J Respir Crit Care Med. 2012;185(11):1154–65.
28. Castro O, Brambilla DJ, Thorington B, Reindorf CA, Scott RB, Gillette P, et al. The acute chest syndrome in sickle cell disease: incidence and risk factors. The Cooperative Study of Sickle Cell Disease. Blood. 1994;84(2):643–9.
29. Dang NC, Johnson C, Eslami-Farsani M, Haywood LJ. Bone marrow embolism in sickle cell disease: a review. Am J Hematol. 2005;79(1):61–7.
30. George A, Benton J, Pratt J, Kim MO, Kalinyak KA, Kalfa TA, et al. The impact of the 2009 H1N1 influenza pandemic on pediatric patients with sickle cell disease. Pediatr Blood Cancer. 2011;57(4):648–53.
31. Strouse JJ, Reller ME, Bundy DG, Amoako M, Cancio M, Han RN, et al. Severe pandemic H1N1 and seasonal influenza in children and young adults with sickle cell disease. Blood. 2010;116(18):3431–4.
32. Vichinsky E, Williams R, Das M, Earles AN, Lewis N, Adler A, et al. Pulmonary fat embolism: a distinct cause of severe acute chest syndrome in sickle cell anemia. Blood. 1994;83(11):3107–12.
33. Maitre B, Habibi A, Roudot-Thoraval F, Bachir D, Belghiti DD, Galacteros F, et al. Acute chest syndrome in adults with sickle cell disease. Chest. 2000;117(5):1386–92.
34. Godeau B, Schaeffer A, Bachir D, Fleury-Feith J, Galacteros F, Verra F, et al. Bronchoalveolar lavage in adult sickle cell patients with acute chest syndrome: value for diagnostic assessment of fat embolism. Am J Respir Crit Care Med. 1996;153(5):1691–6.
35. Mekontso Dessap A, Deux JF, Abidi N, Lavenu-Bombled C, Melica G, Renaud B, et al. Pulmonary artery thrombosis during acute chest syndrome in sickle cell disease. Am J Respir Crit Care Med. 2011;184(9):1022–9.
36. Vichinsky EP, Styles LA, Colangelo LH, Wright EC, Castro O, Nickerson B. Acute chest syndrome in sickle cell disease: clinical presentation and course. Cooperative Study of Sickle Cell Disease. Blood. 1997;89(5):1787–92.
37. Ghosh S, Adisa OA, Chappa P, Tan F, Jackson KA, Archer DR, et al. Extracellular hemin crisis triggers acute chest syndrome in sickle mice. J Clin Invest. 2013;123(11):4809–20.

38. Bean CJ, Boulet SL, Ellingsen D, Pyle ME, Barron-Casella EA, Casella JF, et al. Heme oxygenase-1 gene promoter polymorphism is associated with reduced incidence of acute chest syndrome among children with sickle cell disease. Blood. 2012;120(18):3822–8.
39. Potoka KP, Gladwin MT. Vasculopathy and pulmonary hypertension in sickle cell disease. Am J Physiol Lung Cell Mol Physiol. 2015;308(4):L314–24.
40. Klings ES, Machado RF, Barst RJ, Morris CR, Mubarak KK, Gordeuk VR, et al. An official American Thoracic Society clinical practice guideline: diagnosis, risk stratification, and management of pulmonary hypertension of sickle cell disease. Am J Respir Crit Care Med. 2014;189(6):727–40.
41. Fartoukh M, Lefort Y, Habibi A, Bachir D, Galacteros F, Godeau B, et al. Early intermittent noninvasive ventilation for acute chest syndrome in adults with sickle cell disease: a pilot study. Intensive Care Med. 2010;36(8):1355–62.
42. Gladwin MT, Kato GJ, Weiner D, Onyekwere OC, Dampier C, Hsu L, et al. Nitric oxide for inhalation in the acute treatment of sickle cell pain crisis: a randomized controlled trial. JAMA. 2011;305(9):893–902.
43. Boyd JH, Macklin EA, Strunk RC, DeBaun MR. Asthma is associated with acute chest syndrome and pain in children with sickle cell anemia. Blood. 2006;108(9):2923–7.
44. Cohen RT, DeBaun MR, Blinder MA, Strunk RC, Field JJ. Smoking is associated with an increased risk of acute chest syndrome and pain among adults with sickle cell disease. Blood. 2010;115(18):3852–4.
45. Velasquez MP, Mariscalco MM, Goldstein SL, Airewele GE. Erythrocytapheresis in children with sickle cell disease and acute chest syndrome. Pediatr Blood Cancer. 2009;53(6):1060–3.
46. Desai PC, Ataga KI. The acute chest syndrome of sickle cell disease. Expert Opin Pharmacother. 2013;14(8):991–9.
47. Bhalla M, Abboud MR, McLoud TC, Shepard JA, Munden MM, Jackson SM, et al. Acute chest syndrome in sickle cell disease: CT evidence of microvascular occlusion. Radiology. 1993;187(1):45–9.
48. Howard J, Hart N, Roberts-Harewood M, Cummins M, Awogbade M, Davis B. Guideline on the management of acute chest syndrome in sickle cell disease. Br J Haematol. 2015;169(4):492–505.
49. Styles LA, Aarsman AJ, Vichinsky EP, Kuypers FA. Secretory phospholipase A(2) predicts impending acute chest syndrome in sickle cell disease. Blood. 2000;96(9):3276–8.
50. Hassell KL, Eckman JR, Lane PA. Acute multiorgan failure syndrome: a potentially catastrophic complication of severe sickle cell pain episodes. Am J Med. 1994;96(2):155–62.
51. Lechapt E, Habibi A, Bachir D, Galacteros F, Schaeffer A, Desvaux D, et al. Induced sputum versus bronchoalveolar lavage during acute chest syndrome in sickle cell disease. Am J Respir Crit Care Med. 2003;168(11):1373–7.
52. Feldman L, Gross R, Garon J, Nallari A, Kaur N, Motwani B, et al. Sickle cell patient with an acute chest syndrome and a negative chest X-ray: potential role of the ventilation and perfusion (V/Q) lung scan. Am J Hematol. 2003;74(3):214–5.
53. Mekontso Dessap A, Deux JF, Habibi A, Abidi N, Godeau B, Adnot S, et al. Lung imaging during acute chest syndrome in sickle cell disease: computed tomography patterns and diagnostic accuracy of bedside chest radiograph. Thorax. 2014;69(2):144–51.
54. Vichinsky EP. Current issues with blood transfusions in sickle cell disease. Semin Hematol. 2001;38(1 Suppl 1):14–22.
55. Francis Jr RB. Elevated fibrin D-dimer fragment in sickle cell anemia: evidence for activation of coagulation during the steady state as well as in painful crisis. Haemostasis. 1989;19(2):105–11.
56. Manci EA, Culberson DE, Yang YM, Gardner TM, Powell R, Haynes Jr J, et al. Causes of death in sickle cell disease: an autopsy study. Br J Haematol. 2003;123(2):359–65.
57. Bellet PS, Kalinyak KA, Shukla R, Gelfand MJ, Rucknagel DL. Incentive spirometry to prevent acute pulmonary complications in sickle cell diseases. N Engl J Med. 1995;333(11):699–703.
58. Melton CW, Haynes Jr J. Sickle acute lung injury: role of prevention and early aggressive intervention strategies on outcome. Clin Chest Med. 2006;27(3):487–502. vii.
59. Vichinsky EP, Haberkern CM, Neumayr L, Earles AN, Black D, Koshy M, et al. A comparison of conservative and aggressive transfusion regimens in the perioperative management of sickle

cell disease. The Preoperative Transfusion in Sickle Cell Disease Study Group. N Engl J Med. 1995;333(4):206–13.
60. The Acute Respiratory Distress Syndrome Network. Ventilation with lower tidal volumes as compared with traditional tidal volumes for acute lung injury and the acute respiratory distress syndrome. New Engl J Med. 2000;342(18):1301–8.
61. Charache S, Terrin ML, Moore RD, Dover GJ, Barton FB, Eckert SV, et al. Effect of hydroxyurea on the frequency of painful crises in sickle cell anemia. Investigators of the Multicenter Study of Hydroxyurea in Sickle Cell Anemia. N Engl J Med. 1995;332(20):1317–22.
62. Platt OS. Hydroxyurea for the treatment of sickle cell anemia. N Engl J Med. 2008;358(13):1362–9.
63. Alvarez O, Yovetich NA, Scott JP, Owen W, Miller ST, Schultz W, et al. Pain and other nonneurological adverse events in children with sickle cell anemia and previous stroke who received hydroxyurea and phlebotomy or chronic transfusions and chelation: results from the SWiTCH clinical trial. Am J Hematol. 2013;88(11):932–8.
64. Shenoy S. Hematopoietic stem cell transplantation for sickle cell disease: current practice and emerging trends. Hematology. 2011;2011:273–9.

Chapter 5
Thrombophilias and Acute Pulmonary Thromboembolic Disease

Shani Gunning-Carter, Gregory J. Kato, and Belinda Rivera-Lebron

Inherited Thrombophilias

Virchow in the 1800s postulated that changes in the flow of blood, the vessel wall, and blood composition resulted in thrombus formation (Fig. 5.1). It is the changes in the composition of blood that is often referred to as thrombophilia, inherited or acquired. Thrombophilia may be recognized in approximately 50 % of patients with venous thromboembolism (VTE) [1]. Factor V Leiden (FVL), prothrombin G20210A mutation, deficiencies of protein C, protein S, or antithrombin are the most common inherited thrombophilias (Fig. 5.2).

Factor V Leiden (FVL), the most common inherited thrombophilia, is prevalent in 4–7 % of the Caucasian American population, 2 % Hispanic-Americans and 1 % African-Americans [2]. It is rare in native African and Asian populations [3]. FVL is characterized by a poor anticoagulant response to activated protein C (APC). APC is a natural anticoagulant that degrades activated factors V and VIII (FVa and FVIIIa). The FVL mutation is due to a single point mutation in the factor V gene affecting the first APC cleavage site of FVa, where arginine is replaced by gluta-

S. Gunning-Carter, MD
Division of Hematology-Oncology, Department of Medicine, Monongahela Valley Hospital, Monongahela, PA, USA

G.J. Kato, MD (✉)
Division of Hematology-Oncology, Department of Medicine, Monongahela Valley Hospital, Monongahela, PA, USA

Division of Hematology/Oncology, Pittsburgh Heart, Lung, and Blood Vascular Medicine Institute, Department of Medicine, University of Pittsburgh School of Medicine, Pittsburgh, PA, USA
e-mail: katogj@upmc.edu

B. Rivera-Lebron, MD, MS
Division of Pulmonary, Allergy, and Critical Care Medicine, Department of Medicine, University of Pittsburgh School of Medicine, Pittsburgh, PA, USA

J.S. Lee, M.P. Donahoe (eds.), *Hematologic Abnormalities and Acute Lung Syndromes*, Respiratory Medicine, DOI 10.1007/978-3-319-41912-1_5

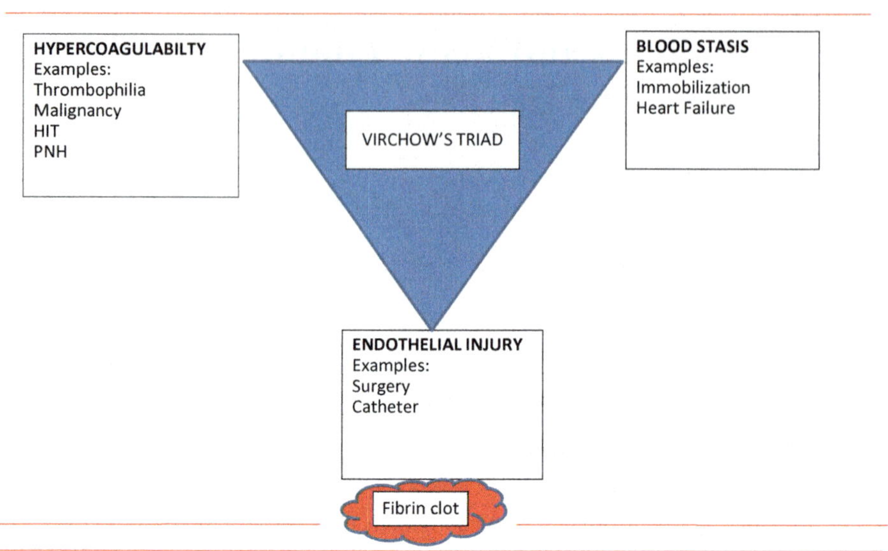

Fig. 5.1 Virchow's triad. Virchow's triad describes the three main factors that predispose thrombosis

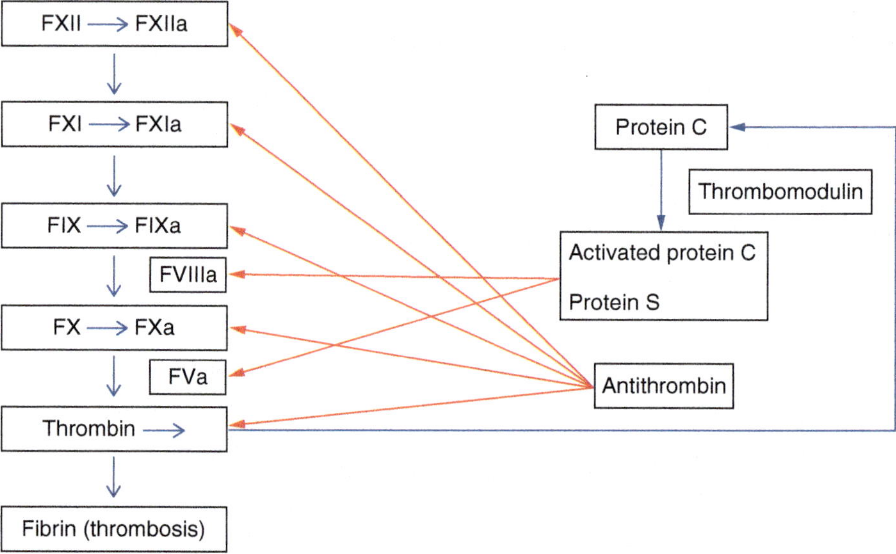

Fig. 5.2 Coagulation cascade. The intrinsic pathway of the coagulation cascade includes the most common inherited thrombophilias

mine at position 506. This mutated cleavage site is less susceptible to proteolytic inactivation by APC, known as APC resistance (APCR). Less common causes of APCR include other rare factor V mutations, antiphospholipid antibodies, increased estrogen states, and cancers. APCR is detected by functional activated partial thromboplastin time-based coagulation assays using factor V-deficient plasma. The FVL gene is confirmed by genetic polymerase chain reaction (PCR) testing.

Prothrombin G20210A mutation (PG) is the second most common inherited thrombophilia, occurring in 2% of the Caucasian population and is rare in non-Caucasians [4]. It results from a substitution of guanine for adenine at nucleotide 20210 in the prothrombin gene leading to increased prothrombin plasma levels. The mutant prothrombin gene is diagnosed by genetic testing.

Protein C (PC) and protein S (PS) are vitamin K-dependent glycoproteins. APC and its cofactor PS inhibit FVa and FVIIIa and suppress thrombin generation. PS additionally inhibits the prothrombinase and tenase complexes. PC deficiency affects 0.2–0.4% of the general population [4] and PS deficiency 0.16–0.21% [5]. Acquired protein C and S deficiencies occur in disseminated intravascular coagulation (DIC), liver disease, and with the use of vitamin K antagonist therapy (usually warfarin). Increased estrogen states, such as pregnancy or oral contraceptive use, may also decrease Protein S levels. Functional assays are used to detect Protein C and S deficiencies and immunoassays detect PC, free and total PS antigen levels.

Antithrombin (AT) is a natural anticoagulant that inhibits thrombin and activated factors IX, X XI, and XII. AT inhibition is markedly enhanced 1000-fold by heparin. AT deficiency has a prevalence of 0.02% in the general population [4, 6]. Functional assays and immunoassays are available to detect AT deficiency. Acquired AT deficiency is seen in DIC, liver disease, nephrotic syndrome, surgery, asparaginase therapy, and heparin use.

Thrombophilia testing is recommended in patients suspected of having an inherited thrombophilia: unexplained thrombosis at young age (<50 years), recurrent thrombosis, family history of thrombosis, and thrombosis at unusual locations. Timing of testing is important as various factors can result in misleading results, for example anticoagulant therapy or acute thrombosis may lower PS and AT levels. Ideally, testing should be performed once off anticoagulation therapy for at least 2–3 weeks at the completion of the initial 3 month anticoagulation period. The aim of testing is to detect individuals at increased risk for recurrent disease and to determine if extended anticoagulation is required. Any abnormal results should be confirmed on repeat testing using an independent blood sample.

Individuals with any inherited thrombophilia and acute pulmonary embolism are treated with standard therapeutic anticoagulation for a minimum of 3 months. Precautions for anticoagulation include overlapping parenteral anticoagulant for at least 5 days with initial vitamin K antagonist therapy to prevent warfarin-induced skin necrosis in PC and PS deficiency and AT replacement may be required to achieve adequate anticoagulation with heparin therapy in AT deficiency. Individuals found to have more than one inherited thrombophilia, homozygous FVL or PG, or PC, PS, or AT deficiency are more prone to recurrent disease (than heterozygous FVL or PG) and should be considered for long-term anticoagulation.

Acquired Thrombophilic States and Thromboembolism

Paroxysmal Nocturnal Hemoglobinuria

Paroxysmal nocturnal hemoglobinuria (PNH) is a rare acquired clonal stem cell disorder characterized by intravascular hemolysis, thrombosis, and bone marrow failure. PNH affects 1–5 cases per million population [7] and is usually seen in young adults (median age 42 years) of both genders, but may affect all ages. The median survival is 10–15 years, with a French group reporting median survival of 22 years [8]. Spontaneous remission occurs in about 10–15 % of patients at any time [9].

PNH results from an acquired somatic mutation in the X-linked phosphatidylinositol glycan-class A (*PIGA*), resulting in deficiency of surface proteins attached by the glycosylphosphatidylinositol (GPI) anchor. More than 180 *PIGA* gene mutations have been identified in patients with PNH. Both CD55 and CD59 are among the missing GPI-anchored proteins. CD55 regulates the formation and stability of the C3 and C5 convertases and CD59 prevents the formation of the membrane attack complex (MAC). Complement activation occurs through a series of reactions that leads to formation of the MAC, which results in lysis of the target cell. Absent complement regulatory proteins on PNH erythrocytes accounts for terminal complement mediated hemolysis.

PNH results in variety of clinical features, ranging from asymptomatic disease to life-threatening thrombosis (Table 5.1).

The severity of hemolysis is related to the size of the PNH cell clonal population. Complications related to the presence of free hemoglobin in the plasma include renal toxicity and nitric oxide depletion. Nitric oxide regulates smooth muscle tone and its depletion leads to smooth muscle contraction, including vasoconstriction, contraction of gastrointestinal tract smooth muscle and pulmonary hypertension.

Table 5.1 Clinical manifestations of PNH

Intravascular hemolysis	Thrombosis	Bone marrow failure
Anemia Fatigue Shortness of breath Hemoglobinuria Renal failure Abdominal pain Back pain Chest pain Erectile dysfunction Esophagospasm Dysphagia Cholelithiasis Jaundice	Deep venous thrombosis Pulmonary emboli Intra-abdominal: hepatic, splenic, mesenteric, and renal vein thrombosis Cerebral vein thrombosis Retinal vein thrombosis Dermal vein thrombosis Arterial thrombosis (less common)	Anemia Neutropenia-infections Thrombocytopenia—bleeding Aplastic anemia Myelodysplastic syndrome Progression to AML (rare)

Patients with a hemolytic crisis present with fatigue, dyspnea, chest pain, abdominal pain, esophageal spasms, dysphagia, back pain, erectile dysfunction, and renal failure. Most patients with PNH have some degree of bone marrow failure, even if there are no cytopenias present. Other bone marrow disorders may present with PNH, such as aplastic anemia (AA) or myelodysplastic syndrome (MDS), and are usually associated with a hypocellular marrow, pancytopenia, less intravascular hemolysis, and a smaller PNH clone.

Hemolysis is possibly an important contributing factor to the development of thrombosis as an increased incidence of thrombosis is seen in patients with larger PNH clones and thrombosis frequently follows a hemolytic episode [10]. The mechanism of thrombosis in PNH is not well understood but is possibly related to platelet activation initiated by hemolysis and complement, and increased procoagulant and fibrinolytic activity. Approximately 40 % of patients develop thrombosis, mostly venous, especially in the hepatic, portal, splenic, or cerebral veins [11]. The leading cause of death in PNH patients is thrombosis and the initial thrombotic event increases the relative risk of death in PNH five to tenfold [12].

Laboratory findings consistent with hemolytic anemia include increased reticulocyte count and LDH, decreased haptoglobin, hemoglobinuria, and hemosiderinuria, in addition to a negative direct Coombs test. Iron deficiency may result from urine-related iron losses. A bone marrow biopsy is not essential but may be helpful in evaluating patients with pancytopenia or suspected bone marrow disorders. The marrow may appear hypocellular, normocellular, or hypercellular, and erythroid hyperplasia is common. Appropriate imaging studies, such as abdominal ultrasound or magnetic resonance imaging, are obtained to evaluate any worrisome symptoms or signs.

Historically, the Ham test was used to diagnose PNH, where increased red cell lysis after exposure to acidified serum denoted a positive result. Low sensitivity and specificity were major limitations of this study, as well as the inability to determine the size of the PNH clone. Flow cytometry of peripheral blood is the preferred diagnostic test. Flow cytometry detects reduced levels of GPI-anchored proteins (CD55 and CD59), and measures the presence and size of the PNH clonal population. PNH type III cells express complete deficiency of GPI-linked proteins, PNH type II cells show partial deficiency, and PNH type I cells have normal protein levels.

Patients with PNH are classified into clinical subcategories: (1) classic PNH (intravascular hemolysis without another bone marrow abnormality, and usually a large clone >50 %), (2) PNH in the setting of other bone marrow failure disorders, such as AA/PNH or MDS/PNH, or (3) subclinical PNH (very small PNH clone without hemolysis).

Treatment depends on the severity of disease. Allogeneic hematopoietic cell transplantation and eculizumab are the only established therapies for treatment of classic PNH. Eculizumab is approved for treatment of PNH and is indicated in patients with significant hemolysis and symptomatic disease. Eculizumab is a humanized monoclonal antibody that blocks complement C5 and prevents formation of the membrane attack complex (Fig. 5.3). Eculizumab reduced hemolysis and thrombotic risk, and improved anemia, fatigue, and quality of life in PNH patients

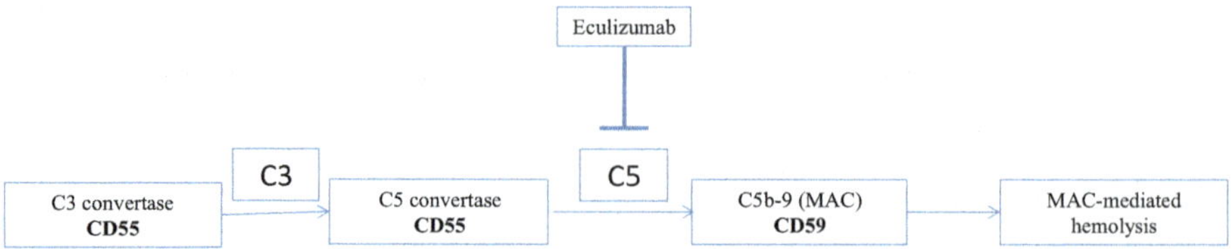

Fig. 5.3 PNH complement activation. CD55- and CD59-deficient red cells in PNH are lysed by activated complement. Complement C5 is inhibited by the drug eculizumab

[10]. Treatment with eculizumab is continued indefinitely as it does not impact the underlying stem cell disorder or any associated BM failure syndromes. Eculizumab increases the risk of *Neisseria meningitidis* with chronic use but is otherwise well tolerated.

Allogeneic hematopoietic cell transplantation (HCT) is the only cure for PNH. However, HCT is associated with significant morbidity and mortality compared to the relatively safe eculizumab. The decision for HCT should be made by physicians experienced in transplantation and PNH, and may be reserved for patients for whom eculizumab fails, or with associated severe aplastic anemia or high risk MDS.

Patients with associated BM failure disorders do not require PNH-specific therapy and treatment should be aimed at the underlying BM failure disorder. Asymptomatic patients (subclinical PNH) do not need any treatment for PNH. Other supportive therapies include red blood cell transfusions for severe anemia, and supplementation with iron for iron deficiency and folate for hemolysis. Prophylactic anticoagulation is not needed for patients without prior thrombosis. However, PNH patients treated with eculizumab and history of prior thrombosis should continue anticoagulation due to the increased risk of a recurrent event [13].

Heparin-Induced Thrombocytopenia

Heparin-induced thrombocytopenia (HIT) is a potentially life-threatening condition that occurs following exposure to heparin and affects approximately 1–5 % of patients on heparin. Venous and/or arterial thrombosis is the major clinical finding in HIT. Mortality rates up to 20 % were seen in patients with HIT, but have improved with early recognition and intervention.

Two forms of HIT are recognized. Type I HIT (nonimmune heparin-associated thrombocytopenia) is characterized by a mild, transient fall in platelet count (rarely <100,000/μL) that typically develops within the first 2 days of heparin exposure and resolves with continued heparin use. Type I HIT is not associated with thrombosis and is of no clinical significance. Type II HIT is immune-mediated and associated with thrombosis. Type II HIT will be discussed from hereon.

HIT is caused by IgG autoantibodies directed against complexes of platelet factor 4 (PF4) and heparin. Platelet Fc receptors bind the antibody-heparin-PF4 complex, resulting in activation of platelets and subsequent procoagulant response with thrombin generation. HIT antibodies also bind to endothelial cells, leading to endothelial cell activation with increased tissue factor and thrombin generation [14]. Thrombocytopenia occurs when the IgG-coated platelets are removed by the macrophages of the reticuloendothelial system and during platelet consumption for thrombi formation.

The majority of HIT patients (85–90 %) present with thrombocytopenia, less than 150,000/μL, 5–14 days after exposure to heparin, regardless of the dose or route of administration. HIT occurs predominantly with exposure to unfractionated heparin, and is more common in women and surgical patients [15, 16]. The platelet count falls greater than 50 % from baseline with a mean nadir of 60,000/μL. However, 5 % of patients may not develop thrombocytopenia but demonstrate a 30–50 % drop in platelet count. Platelet counts rarely fall below 20,000/μL and bleeding is hardly seen. Rapid onset HIT (within the first 24 h of exposure) occurs in patients previously exposed to heparin within the previous 100 days secondary to the presence of HIT antibodies already in the patient's plasma. Delayed onset HIT has been described and is seen up to 3 weeks after heparin exposure, caused by high titers of platelet-activating heparin-induced IgG resulting in heparin-independent platelet activation, in addition to heparin-dependent activation [17].

Thrombosis is seen in up to 50 % of patients with HIT. Thrombocytopenia often precedes thrombosis. Venous thromboembolism occurs more frequently than arterial thrombi. Pulmonary embolism was the most common life-threatening thrombotic event, occurring in 25 % of all patients [18]. Complications of HIT include ischemic limb gangrene resulting in amputation, skin necrosis, myocardial infarction, stroke, organ infarction, or post-intravenous heparin anaphylaxis. The increased thrombotic risk persists for days to weeks after discontinuation of heparin [19].

The initial suspicion of HIT is clinical. A clinical scoring system, such as the 4T's score, is used to guide the determination of HIT and need for further investigation. The 4T's score has been validated and assesses the degree of Thrombocytopenia, Timing relative to heparin exposure, presence of Thrombosis, and other causes for thrombocytopenia. One study reported a negative predictive value of a low 4T's score of 0.998 and positive predictive value of an intermediate and high score of 0.14 and 0.64, respectively [20, 21]. Essentially, a low 4T's score rules out HIT and intermediate or high scores require further testing for HIT.

HIT antibodies can be demonstrated by immunoassays (enzyme-linked immunosorbent assays [ELISA]) that detect anti-PF4/heparin antibodies or functional assays (serotonin-release assay [SRA]) that detect heparin-dependent platelet activation by patient serum. It is important to note that all cases of HIT are caused by platelet-activating antibodies, but not all PF4/heparin complex antibodies result in HIT (some antibodies are clinically insignificant). There is data showing clinical correlation between immunoassays and SRAs. A weakly positive ELISA (OD 0.40 to <1.00) was associated with a less than 5 % low probability of a strongly positive SRA and increased to approximately 90 % with an OD greater than 2.00 [22]. The SRA is more specific and is considered the "gold standard" for diagnosing HIT, but it is less widely available, more complex and may take up to several days. The SRA is especially useful in cases of indeterminate immunoassays (OD 0.4 to 2.0).

Patients with HIT (presumptive due to intermediate or high 4T score, or confirmed by SRA) should have all heparin products stopped, including heparin flushes. A non-heparin anticoagulant should then be substituted due to the increased thrombotic risk, unless there is bleeding or a high risk of bleeding. Treatment should not be delayed while awaiting confirmative laboratory testing. Early intervention may prevent thrombotic events and subsequent morbidity and mortality [23]. Alternative anticoagulants used to treat HIT include direct thrombin inhibitors (argatroban, bivalirudin), fondaparinux (anti-factor Xa inhibitor), and danaparoid. The choice of anticoagulant agent depends on the patient's renal and hepatic function. Vitamin K antagonists (VKA) such as warfarin should not be given in acute HIT and should only be started when the platelet count has recovered to at least 150,000/μL due to the increased risk of venous limb gangrene and skin necrosis [24]. The non-heparin anticoagulant should be continued for a minimum overlap of at least 5 days with VKAs and the target international normalized ratio (INR) has been reached. If the patient had been on VKA therapy at the time HIT was diagnosed, Vitamin K should be given. Target-specific oral anticoagulants, such as rivaroxaban and dabigatran, should be effective treatment for HIT based on principle, however, clinical data is limited and their off-label use is considered on a case by case basis [25]. Anticoagulation with a non-heparin anticoagulant should be continued for at least 2–3 months in patients with HIT, and for at least 3–6 months in patients with associated thrombosis. If the diagnosis of HIT is excluded, heparin may be resumed. Patients with confirmed HIT should avoid heparin, including low molecular weight heparin (LMWH) due to strong cross-reactivity of the HIT antibody, for life.

Antiphospholipid Syndrome

Antiphospholipid syndrome (APS) is an acquired thrombophilic state characterized by venous and arterial thrombosis, as well as recurrent miscarriages and pregnancy complications, in the presence of antiphospholipid antibodies [26]. Antiphospholipid antibodies (APL) are autoantibodies directed against phospholipids and phospholipid-binding proteins. APL may occur in the absence of disease (primary APS), or are often seen in association with other diseases, especially systemic lupus erythematosus. They occur in other rheumatologic conditions, or may be associated with infections—bacterial or viral, medications such as hydralazine and phenytoin, and malignancy. APL may be seen in healthy individuals, up to 5 %, but these are usually transient and of no clinical significance. Thrombosis appears to occur through various mechanisms including activation of platelets and endothelial cells, increased tissue factor and thrombin generation, and interference with antithrombotic pathways [27].

APS is diagnosed based on the revised Sapporo classification, which requires at least one clinical and one laboratory criteria [28]. Clinical criteria include either the confirmed presence of venous, arterial, or small vessel thrombosis in any tissue or organ, or pregnancy complications such as three or more unexplained early pregnancy losses, one or more unexplained fetal death of at least 10 weeks gestation, or one or more preterm delivery prior to 34 weeks of gestation due to eclampsia, preeclampsia, or placental insufficiency. The persistence of the following APL on two or more occasions at least 12 weeks apart must be demonstrated on laboratory testing: lupus anticoagulant (LA), anticardiolipin antibodies (ACL) immunoglobulin G (IgG) and immunoglobulin M (IgM) in moderate or high titers, or anti-β_2-glycoprotein-I antibodies (anti-β_2GPI) in moderate or high titers. Lupus anticoagulants are detected by various functional coagulation assays that result in prolonged clotting times. ACL and β_2GPI antibodies are detected by ELISA. Triple positivity is associated with a higher risk of thrombosis. Testing for additional antibodies, such as antiphosphatidylserine antibodies, is not recommended as their association with thrombosis is not well established.

Venous thromboembolism is the most common clinical manifestation of APS. Other clinical findings that do not meet criteria include thrombocytopenia, livedo reticularis, valvular disease, neurological manifestations such as memory impairment and white matter lesions on MRI, and rare episodes of bleeding due to prothrombin antibodies. Catastrophic APS may be seen in a small proportion of patients who develop widespread thrombosis with multiorgan failure.

Patients with APS and venous thromboembolism are treated using standard anticoagulation with unfractionated heparin or LMWH, followed by warfarin targeting an INR of 2–3 [29]. LA may interfere with PTT and PT/INR anticoagulation assays and in such cases other studies are employed, such as anti-factor-Xa, chromogenic factor X, or factor II activity, to determine the level of anticoagulation. The recommendation is to continue anticoagulation indefinitely in patients with confirmed APS due to the high risk of recurrence [30]. Target specific oral anticoagulants are not recommended for treating VTE in APS until more evidence becomes available for their use in such patients. The treatment of arterial thrombosis is controversial and options include antiplatelet therapy, anticoagulant therapy, or both. Treatment for catastrophic APS includes anticoagulation and glucocorticoids, and possibly IVIG, plasma exchange, and other immunosuppressants such as cyclophosphamide [31]. Pregnant women with APS should be treated with LMWH and/or low-dose aspirin based on their history and clinical presentation.

Myeloproliferative Neoplasms

Myeloproliferative neoplasms (MPNs) are hematopoietic stem cell clonal disorders characterized by the overproduction of one or more of hematopoietic cells. MPNs have the potential to evolve into myelofibrosis or acute myeloid leukemia. The four most common MPNs are polycythemia vera (PV), essential thrombocythemia (ET), primary myelofibrosis (PMF), and chronic myeloid leukemia (CML). Other MPNs include chronic neutrophilic leukemia, chronic eosinophilic leukemia, and mastocytosis. CML is associated with a balanced translocation between 9 and 22 [t(9;22)9q34;11)] called the Philadelphia chromosome. PV, ET, and MF are Philadelphia chromosome negative and in many cases are characterized by JAK2 mutations. These mutations cause constitutive activation of the JAK2 tyrosine kinase (gain of function) resulting in increased cell proliferation and survival. Almost all patients with PV have a JAK2 V617F or exon 12 mutation, whereas ET and PMF display 50–60 % JAK2 V617F mutations [32]. Additional mutations, such as CALR and MPL, are detected in patients with JAK-2 negative MPNs.

MPNs are rare and seen in approximately 0.5–3 per 100,000 persons depending on the subtype [33]. MPNs, especially PV and ET, are associated with an increased risk of thrombosis, both venous and arterial. Thrombosis in unusual locations, such as the splanchnic circulation and cerebral veins, should raise the suspicion for an underlying MPN. MPNs accounted for 40 % of Budd Chiari syndrome and 31 % of portal vein thrombosis [34]. The pathogenesis of thrombosis is complex and involves various processes, such as increased inflammatory cytokines, leukocyte-derived proteases, and endothelial adhesion molecules, leading to a procoagulant environment. Patients may present with fatigue, fever, night sweats, pruritus, early satiety due to splenomegaly, erythromelalgia, headaches, vision changes, and bleeding due to acquired von Willebrand disease.

Treatment depends on the underlying disease and aims to prevent or minimize complications, especially thrombotic risk in ET and PV [35]. Low dose aspirin, with or without hydroxyurea (an antimetabolite), is recommended in patients at high thrombotic risk, those with prior thrombosis and age greater than 60 years [36]. Phlebotomy and/ or hydroxyurea are used to control hematocrit in PV. Platelet lowering agents, such as hydroxyurea or anagrelide, are used in ET patients at increased thrombotic risk. Low risk or asymptomatic patients with MPN may be observed. Supportive measures such as red blood cell or platelet transfusions are used for significant cytopenias. Hematopoietic cell transplantation is the only curative treatment for PMF but is associated with significant transplant-related mortality and so is reserved for specific patients. Ruxolitinib is a JAK1/JAK2 inhibitor approved for treatment of certain MPNs, for whom hydroxyurea has failed or those with high risk MF.

Acute Pulmonary Thromboembolic Disease

Introduction

Venous thromboembolism (VTE) includes deep vein thrombosis (DVT) and pulmonary embolism (PE). The exact incidence of VTE is unknown but it is estimated at 300,000–600,000 cases each year in the United States [37]. VTE is responsible for the hospitalization of 150,000–250,000 patients annually and 100,000–200,000 deaths each year in the United States [38]. PE is the third most frequent cardiovascular disease [39, 40] and the most common preventable cause of hospital death.

Acute PE is the most serious presentation of VTE . It is a potentially life-threatening disease and up to 25 % of cases present as sudden death. Acute PE spans a wide spectrum of clinical outcomes mainly based on the right ventricle's (RV) capacity to tolerate strain. Increased RV afterload causes RV dilation that then incites cardiac ischemia, coronary hypoperfusion, and hypotension that can progress to cardiogenic shock.

Pathogenesis

The three mechanisms of Virchow's triad, blood stasis, endothelial injury, and blood hypercoagulability, are the basis of thrombus development (Fig. 5.1). First, blood stasis plays a major role in the pathogenesis of VTE, as thrombosis usually starts in the deep veins of the lower extremities, where blood flow is decreased. Thrombi, however, may also originate from higher in the pelvic and renal veins, inferior vena cava, upper extremity veins, and right heart. PE occurs when thrombi break off, travel to the lung, and occlude the main pulmonary artery, lobar branches, or more distal smaller vessels in the periphery. However, not all PE originates from DVT, but may arise in the pulmonary vasculature, which have been termed de novo PE [41, 42]. Second, endothelial injury and vessel-wall damage, more predominant in arterial thrombosis, results in collagen and tissue factor exposure, followed by events leading to thrombus formation. Exposed collagen recruits circulating platelets, which are subsequently activated and become a major component of the developing thrombus. Tissue factor initiates the coagulation cascade and generates thrombin and fibrin (Fig. 5.2) [43]. Last, conditions that shift the balance between natural anticoagulant and procoagulant processes may result in hypercoagulable states and thrombus formation.

Risk Factors and Stratification

A list of predisposing risk factors for VTE is in Table 5.2. Pulmonary embolism is associated with genetic and acquired risk factors. However, VTE can also occur in the absence of these factors.

Massive or *high-risk* PE is defined as an acute PE with sustained hypotension (systolic blood pressure <90 mmHg for at least 15 min or requiring inotropic support), pulselessness, or persistent profound bradycardia [44, 45]. Approximately 5 % of patients with PE are categorized as massive. In the International Cooperative Pulmonary Embolism Registry (ICOPER), the 90-day mortality rate for patients with *high-risk* PE at presentation was 52 % [45–47].

Forty percent of patients with PE present as submassive or *intermediate-risk* PE. These patients have an acute PE without systemic hypotension (systolic blood pressure >90 mmHg) but have either RV dysfunction and/or myocardial necrosis.

Table 5.2 Risk factors for venous thromboembolism (VTE)

Inherited	Acquired
Factor V Leiden	Immobilization
Prothrombin G20210A	Acute medical illness
Protein C deficiency	Trauma
Protein S deficiency	Major surgery, especially orthopedic
Antithrombin deficiency	Malignancy
Dysfibrinogenemia	Pregnancy
Hypoplasminogenemia	Estrogen-containing contraceptives or hormone replacement therapy
Factor XII deficiency	Medications, such as Tamoxifen, Thalidomide
Sickle cell disease	Central venous catheters
	Congestive heart failure
	Chronic lung diseases, such as chronic obstructive pulmonary disease (COPD)
	Nephrotic syndrome
	Liver disease
	Obesity
	Inflammatory bowel disease
	Sepsis
	Myeloproliferative neoplasm
	Antiphospholipid syndrome
	Paroxysmal nocturnal hemoglobinuria
	Heparin-induced thrombocytopenia
	Advanced age

RV dysfunction is defined by presence of at least one of the following: RV dilation (apical 4-chamber RV diameter divided by LV diameter >0.9) or RV systolic dysfunction on echocardiography; RV dilation (4-chamber RV diameter divided by LV diameter >0.9) on CT; elevation of BNP (>90 pg/mL); elevation of N-terminal pro-BNP (>500 pg/mL); or electrocardiographic changes (new complete or incomplete right bundle-branch block, anteroseptal ST elevation or depression, or anteroseptal T-wave inversion). Myocardial necrosis is defined by either of the following: elevation of troponin I (>0.4 ng/mL); or elevation of troponin T (>0.1 ng/mL) [45]. In patients who have evidence of both RV dysfunction and myocardial necrosis, 30-day mortality can reach 24.5 % [48]. Close monitoring of this group is recommended for early detection of hemodynamic decompensation and change in management.

Hemodynamically stable patients with preserved RV size and function are classified as *low-risk* PE and have excellent prognosis once anticoagulation therapy is established [45].

The PE score index (PESI) is a validated clinical prediction rule that classifies patients with PE into categories of increasing risk of mortality and other adverse medical outcomes [48, 49]. The full version includes 11 patient characteristics that are independently associated with mortality and stratifies patients with pulmonary embolism into five severity classes, with a 30-day mortality rates ranging between 0 and 1.6 % in class I to 10.0–24.5 % in class V. The simplified PESI version includes six of the clinical characteristics and stratifies patients into low 30-day mortality of 1.0 % compared with 10.9 % in the high-risk group.

Diagnosis

Signs and symptoms of PE are nonspecific and can include dyspnea, pleuritic chest pain, cough, hemoptysis, lightheadedness, syncope, tachypnea, and tachycardia. Cardiac examination can reveal a left parasternal heave, a third heart sound or an early systolic murmur at the left lower sternal border that intensifies during inspiration and diminishes with expiration.

A thrombophilia evaluation is recommended for recurrent VTE. This includes lupus anticoagulant, anticardiolipin antibody, beta-2-glycoprotein, antiprothrombin, Factor V Leiden, prothrombin gene mutation, antithrombin III, protein C and protein S levels. Timing of this work up depends on current anticoagulation, as some results are altered by heparin and/or Coumadin and are ideally ordered at time of thrombosis prior to initiating these medications.

Following clinical and laboratory assessment in patients whom PE is suspected will allow classification of patients into categories of pre-test probability of diagnosis (PE likely or PE unlikely). The Wells rule and Geneva score are the most widely used and validated [50–52] (see Table 5.3) [52, 53]. For example, if PE is "likely" using modified Wells criteria, a CT scan is warranted next to diagnose PE. If after calculating Wells score, PE is "unlikely," obtaining a D-dimer level may be used to determine if diagnostic imaging is necessary. D-dimer is elevated in presence of acute thrombosis. A low D-dimer (<500 μg/L) has a high negative predictive value and suggests VTE is unlikely. However, presence of elevated D-dimer does not confirm presence of PE. If PE is likely, computed tomographic (CT) pulmonary angiogram or CTPA is the imaging modality of first choice. Even though pulmonary angiography is the gold standard for the diagnosis of PE, CTPA has become the preferred method for the diagnosis of PE, due to its widespread availability. The PIOPED II trial showed that CT scans have a sensitivity of 83 % and specificity of 96 % [54].

Echocardiogram can be used to determine presence of RV strain and provide real-time information on risk-stratification. RV dilation, dysfunction or hypokinesis and elevated tricuspid regurgitation velocity (TRV) or pulmonary artery systolic pressure (PASP) could be consistent with a PE. These changes can be seen with a 25 % or greater occlusion of the pulmonary artery [55]. Thrombi can also be seen in heart chambers on echocardiogram, this is called "thrombus-in-transit." It has a prevalence of 4 % and is associated with increased RV hypokinesis [56]. Overall, transthoracic echocardiogram has a sensitivity of 50–70 % [55].

Ventilation/perfusion scintigraphy (V/Q scan) may be used in patients with a normal chest x-ray, in pregnant women, or in patients with contraindications to con-

Table 5.3 Clinical prediction rules for diagnosing PE

Wells rule		Geneva rule	
Characteristics	Points	Characteristics	Points
Clinical signs and symptoms of symptoms of DVT	3.0	Age	
		60–79 Years	1
		≥80 Years	2
PE is the most likely diagnosis	3.0	Findings on chest radiograph	
		Plate-like atelectasis	1
		Elevated hemidiaphragm	1
Tachycardia (HR > 100 bpm)	1.5	Tachycardia (HR > 100 bpm)	1
Immobilization or surgery in the previous 4 weeks	1.5	Recent surgery	3
Previous DVT or PE	1.5	Previous DVT or PE	2
Hemoptysis	1.0	$PaCO_2$	
		<36 mmHg	2
		36–38.9 mmHg	1
Active malignancy	1.0	PaO_2	
		<48.7 mmHg	4
		48.7–59.9 mmHg	3
		60–71.2 mmHg	2
		71.3–82.4 mmHg	1
Traditional wells criteria		*Clinical probability*	
High probability	>6	High probability	>8
Moderate probability	2-6	Moderate probability	5-8
Low probability	<2	Low probability	<5
Modified wells criteria		*Revised geneva rule*	
PE likely	>4	Age >65 years	1
PE unlikely	≤4	Previous DVT or PE	3
		Surgery or fracture in the past month	2
		Active malignancy or cured <1 year	2
		Unilateral lower limb pain	3
		Hemoptysis	2
		HR	
		75–94 bpm	3
		≥95	5
		Pain on deep palpation of lower limb and unilateral edema	4
		Clinical probability	
		High probability	>10
		Moderate probability	4–10
		Low probability	<4

PE pulmonary embolism, *DVT* deep venous thrombosis, *HR* heart rate, *Bpm* beats per minute trast, such as contrast-induced anaphylaxis or significant renal insufficiency [44]. V/Q scans are the gold-standard diagnosis of chronic thromboembolic disease.

Lower extremity Doppler can be used to diagnose the presence of DVT. Lower extremity Doppler has a sensitivity of >90 % and specificity of 95 % for symptomatic DVT [57]. Presence of DVT seen on lower extremity Doppler can be suggestive of a PE, however the absence of clot cannot rule it out.

Management

Systemic thrombolysis is the recommended treatment for *high-risk* PE [44, 45]. It improves hemodynamic parameters, reverses RV dysfunction, and improves survival in patients with acute PE. However is associated with increased risk of major bleeding, including intracranial hemorrhage [58, 59]. Contraindications to thrombolysis would be active bleeding or high-risk of bleeding, such as brain or major organ surgery. In-hospital all-cause mortality in hemodynamically unstable patients who received thrombolytic therapy was 15 % versus 47 % without thrombolytic therapy ($p < 0.0001$) [60].

The use of systemic thrombolysis for patients without hemodynamic compromise remains controversial. The recently published Pulmonary Embolism Thrombolysis (PEITHO) trial studied the role of fibrinolytic therapy in patients with *intermediate-risk* PE [61]. Its primary outcome, a composite of all-cause death or hemodynamic decompensation within 7 days after randomization, was significantly reduced with thrombolysis (2.6 % vs. 5.6 %; odds ratio 0.44; 95 % CI 0.23–0.87; $p = 0.02$). However, an increased risk of major hemorrhage (6.3 % vs. 1.5 %; $p < 0.001$) and stroke (2 % vs. 0.2 %; $p = 0.003$) was observed. An alternative strategy using reduced-dose tissue plasminogen activator (tPA) (50 mg) in patients with "moderate PE" may be as effective as full dose (100 mg), but reported no significant bleeding or differences in mortality [62]. Current guidelines recommend against the routine use of systemic thrombolysis in these patients [44, 63].

The use of catheter-directed thrombolysis is emerging as an effective alternative in patients with *intermediate* or *high-risk* PE, using small doses of thrombolytic agent [15]. In a randomized, controlled clinical trial of 59 *intermediate-risk* patients, heparin plus ultrasound-guided catheter-directed thrombolysis was compared to heparin alone [16]. Ultrasound-guided catheter-directed tPA significantly reversed RV dilatation at 24 h by echocardiogram, without an increased risk of bleeding.

For *intermediate* or *high-risk* PE, surgical embolectomy may be an alternative, especially if thrombolysis is contraindicated or has failed. A perioperative mortality of <6 % has been reported for embolectomy before hemodynamic collapse [17].

Acute RV failure is the leading cause of death in patients with *high-risk* PE. Supportive treatment with volume expansion, vasopressors, oxygenation, and intubation, when necessary, may help sustain the cardiac output and prevent hemodynamic collapse. There have been no randomized trials to determine the optimal vasopressor support in this patient population; however norepinephrine alone seems to improve RV function. The addition of dobutamine can be considered when a patient has a low cardiac index to increase myocardial contractility. Extracorporeal membrane oxygenation (ECMO) may rescue those in critical situations, ensuring circulation, and oxygenation until definitive management is provided.

Anticoagulation initially with low molecular weight or unfractionated heparin transitioned to vitamin K antagonists (warfarin in the U.S., phenprocoumon and acenocoumarol in some European countries) or new direct oral anticoagulants (DOA) is recommended for all acute PE patients. It prevents early death and recurrent symptomatic or fatal VTE [44]. The standard anticoagulation should be at least 3 months. After withdrawal of anticoagulant treatment, the risk of recurrence if anticoagulants are stopped after 6 or 12 months can be expected to be similar to that after 3 months [44]. Indefinite treatment reduces the risk for recurrent VTE by about 90 %, but this benefit is partially offset by a 1 % annual risk of major bleeding [44].

IVC filter placement may be indicated in patients with absolute contraindication to anticoagulation and in patients with recurrent PE despite adequate anticoagulation [44, 45].

Prognosis

Recurrent VTE, bleeding risks associated with anticoagulation and pulmonary hypertension (PH) contribute to the chronic morbidity associated with PE [64]. VTE recurrence has been reported to reach 10 % at 2 years, 20 % at 5 years and 30 % at 10 years [65]. Elevated D-dimer levels after discontinuation of anticoagulation may indicate increased risk of recurrence [66].

PE resolves in most cases after treatment with anticoagulation for PE and patients are able to return to their previous quality of life. However, it has been estimated than in approximately 0.1–0.5 % of patients who survive PE go on to develop chronic thromboembolic pulmonary hypertension (CTEPH) [67], and in fact this may be higher. In a single center prospective study of patients who had PE and developed symptomatic CTEPH, the cumulative incidence was reported at 3.8 % at 2 years [65]. If we extrapolate these data, the numbers could be almost 20,000 cases per year. Furthermore in another study it was found that in patients diagnosed with CTEPH, as many as 25 % had no known previous history of PE or DVT [68].

CTEPH symptoms are similar to those with PE or PH due to other causes. Symptoms can include dyspnea on exertion, fatigue, palpitations, lightheadedness, or syncope. Often the disease is indolent and if gone unsuspected, diagnosis can be delayed.

The most sensitive diagnostic test for the diagnosis of CTEPH is the ventilation/perfusion scintigraphy (V/Q scan) obtained after at least 3 months of effective anticoagulation for a VTE. This is considered the gold standard and is more sensitive (96–95 %) than CT angiogram (51 %) as a screening test for CTEPH [69]. An echocardiogram is routinely performed as a screening test for PH, followed by a confirmatory right heart catheterization (RHC). The diagnosis of CTEPH is based on a mean pulmonary arterial pressure ≥25 mmHg with a pulmonary arterial wedge pressure ≤15 mmHg on a RHC and at least one perfusion defect detected by VQ scan [44].

Pulmonary endarterectomy (PTE) is the treatment of choice for CTEPH. The operability of patients is determined mostly by clot accessibility, patient comorbidities, and expertise of the surgical team. At experienced centers, this procedure is associated with low mortality (<5 %).

Medical therapy with a new medication, riociguat (Adempas®) has been recently approved for treatment of nonoperable, persistent, or recurrent PH after PTE [70]. Riociguat is a soluble guanylate cyclase stimulator that works by augmenting nitric oxide signaling through the soluble guanylate cyclase–cyclic guanosine monophosphate pathway. Riociguat increases the level of cyclic guanosine monophosphate, resulting in vasorelaxation and antiproliferative and antifibrotic effects. It has been shown to significantly improve exercise capacity and pulmonary vascular resistance in patients with chronic thromboembolic pulmonary hypertension [70]. However, in cases where the patient is deemed operable, it is recommended not to delay surgery, for a trial of medical therapy. All patients with CTEPH are recommended to be treated with lifelong anticoagulation.

References

1. Middeldorp S, van Hylckama Vlieg A. Does thrombophilia testing help in the clinical management of patients? Br J Haematol. 2008;143(3):321–35.
2. Ridker PM, Miletich JP, Hennekens CH, Buring JE. Ethnic distribution of factor V Leiden in 4047 men and women. Implications for venous thromboembolism screening. JAMA. 1997;277(16):1305–7.
3. Rees DC, Cox M, Clegg JB. World distribution of factor V Leiden. Lancet. 1995;346 (8983):1133–4.
4. Seligsohn U, Lubetsky A. Genetic susceptibility to venous thrombosis. N Engl J Med. 2001;344(16):1222–31.
5. ten Kate MK, van der Meer J. Protein S deficiency: a clinical perspective. Haemophilia. 2008;14(6):1222–8.
6. Tait RC, Walker ID, Perry DJ, Islam SI, Daly ME, McCall F, et al. Prevalence of antithrombin deficiency in the healthy population. Br J Haematol. 1994;87(1):106–12.
7. Risitano AM, Rotoli B. Paroxysmal nocturnal hemoglobinuria: pathophysiology, natural history and treatment options in the era of biological agents. Biologics. 2008;2(2):205–22.
8. de Latour RP, Mary JY, Salanoubat C, Terriou L, Etienne G, Mohty M, et al. Paroxysmal nocturnal hemoglobinuria: natural history of disease subcategories. Blood. 2008;112(8): 3099–106.
9. Bessler M, Hiken J. The pathophysiology of disease in patients with paroxysmal nocturnal hemoglobinuria. ASH Educ Prog Book. 2008;2008(1):104–10.
10. Hillmen P, Muus P, Duhrsen U, Risitano AM, Schubert J, Luzzatto L, et al. Effect of the complement inhibitor eculizumab on thromboembolism in patients with paroxysmal nocturnal hemoglobinuria. Blood. 2007;110(12):4123–8.
11. Hillmen P, Lewis SM, Bessler M, Luzzatto L, Dacie JV. Natural history of paroxysmal nocturnal hemoglobinuria. N Engl J Med. 1995;333(19):1253–8.

12. Moyo VM, Mukhina GL, Garrett ES, Brodsky RA. Natural history of paroxysmal nocturnal haemoglobinuria using modern diagnostic assays. Br J Haematol. 2004;126(1):133–8.
13. Kelly RJ, Hill A, Arnold LM, Brooksbank GL, Richards SJ, Cullen M, et al. Long-term treatment with eculizumab in paroxysmal nocturnal hemoglobinuria: sustained efficacy and improved survival. Blood. 2011;117(25):6786–92.
14. Greinacher A. Heparin-induced thrombocytopenia. J Thromb Haemost. 2009;7 Suppl 1:9–12.
15. Warkentin TE, Sheppard JA, Sigouin CS, Kohlmann T, Eichler P, Greinacher A. Gender imbalance and risk factor interactions in heparin-induced thrombocytopenia. Blood. 2006;108(9):2937–41.
16. Warkentin TE. Heparin-induced thrombocytopenia: a clinicopathologic syndrome. Thromb Haemost. 1999;82(2):439–47.
17. Warkentin TE, Kelton JG. Delayed-onset heparin-induced thrombocytopenia and thrombosis. Ann Intern Med. 2001;135(7):502–6.
18. Warkentin TE, Kelton JG. A 14-year study of heparin-induced thrombocytopenia. Am J Med. 1996;101(5):502–7.
19. Arepally GM, Ortel TL. Heparin-induced thrombocytopenia. N Engl J Med. 2006;355 (8):809–17.
20. Cuker A, Gimotty PA, Crowther MA, Warkentin TE. Predictive value of the 4Ts scoring system for heparin-induced thrombocytopenia: a systematic review and meta-analysis. Blood. 2012;120(20):4160–7.
21. Lo GK, Juhl D, Warkentin TE, Sigouin CS, Eichler P, Greinacher A. Evaluation of pretest clinical score (4T's) for the diagnosis of heparin-induced thrombocytopenia in two clinical settings. J Thromb Haemost. 2006;4(4):759–65.
22. Warkentin TE, Sheppard JI, Moore JC, Sigouin CS, Kelton JG. Quantitative interpretation of optical density measurements using PF4-dependent enzyme-immunoassays. J Thromb Haemost. 2008;6(8):1304–12.
23. Wallis DE, Workman DL, Lewis BE, Steen L, Pifarre R, Moran JF. Failure of early heparin cessation as treatment for heparin-induced thrombocytopenia. Am J Med. 1999;106 (6):629–35.
24. Srinivasan AF, Rice L, Bartholomew JR, Rangaswamy C, La Perna L, Thompson JE, et al. Warfarin-induced skin necrosis and venous limb gangrene in the setting of heparin-induced thrombocytopenia. Arch Intern Med. 2004;164(1):66–70.
25. Linkins LA, Dans AL, Moores LK, Bona R, Davidson BL, Schulman S, et al. Treatment and prevention of heparin-induced thrombocytopenia: Antithrombotic Therapy and Prevention of Thrombosis, 9th ed., American College of Chest Physicians Evidence-Based Clinical Practice Guidelines. Chest. 2012;141(2 Suppl):e495S–530S.
26. Ruiz-Irastorza G, Crowther M, Branch W, Khamashta MA. Antiphospholipid syndrome. Lancet. 2010;376(9751):1498–509.
27. Hoffman M, Monroe DM, Roubey RA. Links between the immune and coagulation systems: how do "antiphospholipid antibodies" cause thrombosis? Immunol Res. 2000;22(2-3):191–7.
28. Miyakis S, Lockshin MD, Atsumi T, Branch DW, Brey RL, Cervera R, et al. International consensus statement on an update of the classification criteria for definite antiphospholipid syndrome (APS). J Thromb Haemost. 2006;4(2):295–306.
29. Crowther MA, Ginsberg JS, Julian J, Denburg J, Hirsh J, Douketis J, et al. A comparison of two intensities of warfarin for the prevention of recurrent thrombosis in patients with the antiphospholipid antibody syndrome. N Engl J Med. 2003;349(12):1133–8.
30. Ruiz-Irastorza G, Cuadrado MJ, Ruiz-Arruza I, Brey R, Crowther M, Derksen R, et al. Evidence-based recommendations for the prevention and long-term management of thrombosis in antiphospholipid antibody-positive patients: report of a task force at the 13th International Congress on antiphospholipid antibodies. Lupus. 2011;20(2):206–18.
31. Cervera R, Rodriguez-Pinto I, Colafrancesco S, Conti F, Valesini G, Rosario C, et al. 14th international congress on antiphospholipid antibodies task force report on catastrophic antiphospholipid syndrome. Autoimmun Rev. 2014;13(7):699–707.

32. Baxter EJ, Scott LM, Campbell PJ, East C, Fourouclas N, Swanton S, et al. Acquired mutation of the tyrosine kinase JAK2 in human myeloproliferative disorders. Lancet. 2005;365 (9464):1054–61.
33. Price GL, Davis KL, Karve S, Pohl G, Walgren RA. Survival patterns in United States (US) medicare enrollees with non-CML myeloproliferative neoplasms (MPN). PLoS One. 2014;9(3), e90299.
34. Smalberg JH, Arends LR, Valla DC, Kiladjian JJ, Janssen HL, Leebeek FW. Myeloproliferative neoplasms in Budd-Chiari syndrome and portal vein thrombosis: a meta-analysis. Blood. 2012;120(25):4921–8.
35. Tefferi A, Vainchenker W. Myeloproliferative neoplasms: molecular pathophysiology, essential clinical understanding, and treatment strategies. J Clin Oncol. 2011;29(5):573–82.
36. Barbui T, Finazzi G, Falanga A. Myeloproliferative neoplasms and thrombosis. 2013. 2013-09-26 00:00:00. 2176–84 p.
37. Heit JA. The epidemiology of venous thromboembolism in the community. Arterioscler Thromb Vasc Biol. 2008;28(3):370–2.
38. Lloyd-Jones D, Adams RJ, Brown TM, Carnethon M, Dai S, De Simone G, et al. Heart disease and stroke statistics—2010 update: a report from the American Heart Association. Circulation. 2010;121(7):e46–215.
39. Tapson VF. Acute pulmonary embolism. N Engl J Med. 2008;358(10):1037–52.
40. Mozaffarian D, Benjamin EJ, Go AS, Arnett DK, Blaha MJ, Cushman M, et al. Heart disease and stroke statistics—2015 update: a report from the American Heart Association. Circulation. 2015;131(4):e29–322.
41. Velmahos GC, Spaniolas K, Tabbara M, Abujudeh HH, de Moya M, Gervasini A, et al. Pulmonary embolism and deep venous thrombosis in trauma: are they related? Arch Surg. 2009;144(10):928–32.
42. Van Gent JM, Zander AL, Olson EJ, Shackford SR, Dunne CE, Sise CB, et al. Pulmonary embolism without deep venous thrombosis: de novo or missed deep venous thrombosis? J Trauma Acute Care Surg. 2014;76(5):1270–4.
43. Furie B, Furie BC. Mechanisms of thrombus formation. N Engl J Med. 2008;359(9):938–49.
44. Konstantinides SV, Torbicki A, Agnelli G, Danchin N, Fitzmaurice D, Galie N, et al. 2014 ESC Guidelines on the diagnosis and management of acute pulmonary embolism: The Task Force for the Diagnosis and Management of Acute Pulmonary Embolism of the European Society of Cardiology (ESC) Endorsed by the European Respiratory Society (ERS). Eur Heart J. 2014.
45. Jaff MR, McMurtry MS, Archer SL, Cushman M, Goldenberg N, Goldhaber SZ, et al. Management of massive and submassive pulmonary embolism, iliofemoral deep vein thrombosis, and chronic thromboembolic pulmonary hypertension: a scientific statement from the American Heart Association. Circulation. 2011;123(16):1788–830.
46. Kucher N, Rossi E, De Rosa M, Goldhaber SZ. Massive pulmonary embolism. Circulation. 2006;113(4):577–82.
47. Kasper W, Konstantinides S, Geibel A, Olschewski M, Heinrich F, Grosser KD, et al. Management strategies and determinants of outcome in acute major pulmonary embolism: results of a multicenter registry. J Am Coll Cardiol. 1997;30(5):1165–71.
48. Aujesky D, Obrosky DS, Stone RA, Auble TE, Perrier A, Cornuz J, et al. Derivation and validation of a prognostic model for pulmonary embolism. Am J Respir Crit Care Med. 2005;172(8):1041–6.
49. Jimenez D, Aujesky D, Moores L, Gomez V, Lobo JL, Uresandi F, et al. Simplification of the pulmonary embolism severity index for prognostication in patients with acute symptomatic pulmonary embolism. Arch Intern Med. 2010;170(15):1383–9.
50. Wells PS, Anderson DR, Rodger M, Ginsberg JS, Kearon C, Gent M, et al. Derivation of a simple clinical model to categorize patients probability of pulmonary embolism: increasing the models utility with the SimpliRED D-dimer. Thromb Haemost. 2000;83(3):416–20.
51. Aujesky D, Fine MJ. Does guideline adherence for empiric antibiotic therapy reduce mortality in community-acquired pneumonia? Am J Respir Crit Care Med. 2005;172(6):655–6.

52. Le Gal G, Righini M, Roy PM, Sanchez O, Aujesky D, Bounameaux H, et al. Prediction of pulmonary embolism in the emergency department: the revised Geneva score. Ann Intern Med. 2006;144(3):165–71.
53. van Belle A, Buller HR, Huisman MV, Huisman PM, Kaasjager K, Kamphuisen PW, et al. Effectiveness of managing suspected pulmonary embolism using an algorithm combining clinical probability, D-dimer testing, and computed tomography. JAMA. 2006;295(2):172–9.
54. Stein PD, Fowler SE, Goodman LR, Gottschalk A, Hales CA, Hull RD, et al. Multidetector computed tomography for acute pulmonary embolism. N Engl J Med. 2006;354 (22):2317–27.
55. Goldhaber SZ. Echocardiography in the management of pulmonary embolism. Ann Intern Med. 2002;136(9):691–700.
56. Torbicki A, Galie N, Covezzoli A, Rossi E, De Rosa M, Goldhaber SZ. Right heart thrombi in pulmonary embolism: results from the International Cooperative Pulmonary Embolism Registry. J Am Coll Cardiol. 2003;41(12):2245–51.
57. Kearon C, Ginsberg JS, Hirsh J. The role of venous ultrasonography in the diagnosis of suspected deep venous thrombosis and pulmonary embolism. Ann Intern Med. 1998;129 (12):1044–9.
58. Tebbe U, Graf A, Kamke W, Zahn R, Forycki F, Kratzsch G, et al. Hemodynamic effects of double bolus reteplase versus alteplase infusion in massive pulmonary embolism. Am Heart J. 1999;138(1 Pt 1):39–44.
59. Konstantinides S, Tiede N, Geibel A, Olschewski M, Just H, Kasper W. Comparison of alteplase versus heparin for resolution of major pulmonary embolism. Am J Cardiol. 1998;82(8):966–70.
60. Stein PD, Matta F. Thrombolytic therapy in unstable patients with acute pulmonary embolism: saves lives but underused. Am J Med. 2012;125(5):465–70.
61. Meyer G, Vicaut E, Danays T, Agnelli G, Becattini C, Beyer-Westendorf J, et al. Fibrinolysis for patients with intermediate-risk pulmonary embolism. N Engl J Med. 2014;370(15): 1402–11.
62. Sharifi M, Bay C, Skrocki L, Rahimi F, Mehdipour M. Moderate pulmonary embolism treated with thrombolysis (from the "MOPETT" trial). Am J Cardiol. 2013;111(2):273–7.
63. Torbicki A, Perrier A, Konstantinides S, Agnelli G, Galie N, Pruszczyk P, et al. Guidelines on the diagnosis and management of acute pulmonary embolism: the Task Force for the Diagnosis and Management of Acute Pulmonary Embolism of the European Society of Cardiology (ESC). Eur Heart J. 2008;29(18):2276–315.
64. Beckman MG, Hooper WC, Critchley SE, Ortel TL. Venous thromboembolism: a public health concern. Am J Prev Med. 2010;38(4 Suppl):S495–501.
65. Pengo V, Lensing AW, Prins MH, Marchiori A, Davidson BL, Tiozzo F, et al. Incidence of chronic thromboembolic pulmonary hypertension after pulmonary embolism. N Engl J Med. 2004;350(22):2257–64.
66. Cosmi B, Legnani C, Tosetto A, Pengo V, Ghirarduzzi A, Testa S, et al. Usefulness of repeated D-dimer testing after stopping anticoagulation for a first episode of unprovoked venous thromboembolism: the PROLONG II prospective study. Blood. 2010;115(3):481–8.
67. Auger WR, Fedullo PF. Chronic thromboembolic pulmonary hypertension. Semin Respir Crit Care Med. 2009;30(4):471–83.
68. Pepke-Zaba J, Delcroix M, Lang I, Mayer E, Jansa P, Ambroz D, et al. Chronic thromboembolic pulmonary hypertension (CTEPH): results from an international prospective registry. Circulation. 2011;124(18):1973–81.
69. Tunariu N, Gibbs SJ, Win Z, Gin-Sing W, Graham A, Gishen P, et al. Ventilation-perfusion scintigraphy is more sensitive than multidetector CTPA in detecting chronic thromboembolic pulmonary disease as a treatable cause of pulmonary hypertension. J Nucl Med. 2007;48 (5):680–4.
70. Ghofrani HA, D'Armini AM, Grimminger F, Hoeper MM, Jansa P, Kim NH, et al. Riociguat for the treatment of chronic thromboembolic pulmonary hypertension. N Engl J Med. 2013;369(4):319–29.

Chapter 6
Bleeding Disorders: Diagnosis and Treatment of Hemorrhagic Complications in the Intensive Care Unit

Craig D. Seaman and Margaret V. Ragni

Inherited Bleeding Disorders

The two most common bleeding disorders likely to be encountered in the ICU setting are von Willebrand disease (VWD) and hemophilia. The essentials necessary for the prompt recognition, diagnosis, and treatment of these disorders are discussed below.

von Willebrand Disease

Background

VWD is a heterogeneous disease caused by deficient or defective von Willebrand factor (VWF). VWD disease subtypes are associated with specific VWF structural-related defects, most of which have a genetic basis. VWD is the most commonly inherited bleeding disorder affecting as many as 1 % of the population [1]. Bleeding is usually mucocutaneous in origin, commonly manifesting as menorrhagia, epistaxis, ecchymosis, or postoperative bleeding. Ascertaining a definitive diagnosis of VWD is difficult as VWD exhibits variable penetrance and clinical severity varies from individual to individual, unrelated to VWF level. Furthermore, VWF levels vary considerably from person to person, even within the same person over time, and are affected by extra genic factors, including stress, trauma, infection, estrogen, and ABO blood types. VWF levels do not always correlate with clinical symptoms; therefore, many affected persons go undiagnosed.

C.D. Seaman, MD, MS (✉) • M.V. Ragni, MD, MPH
Division of Hematology/Oncology, Department of Medicine, University of Pittsburgh School of Medicine, Pittsburgh, PA, USA
e-mail: seamanc@upmc.edu

J.S. Lee, M.P. Donahoe (eds.), *Hematologic Abnormalities and Acute Lung Syndromes*, Respiratory Medicine, DOI 10.1007/978-3-319-41912-1_6

VWF is a large multimeric glycoprotein synthesized in endothelial cells and megakaryocytes. It is stored in Weibel-Palade bodies in endothelial cells and alpha-granules in platelets. Circulating VWF, whose half-life is approximately 12 h, binds to factor VIII (FVIII) providing stability for FVIII and preventing proteolytic degradation of FVIII. VWF binds to subendothelial collagen at the sites of vascular injury. There, it facilitates platelet adhesion by binding to the platelet glycoprotein Ib-IX-V receptor complex. VWF binding leads to platelet activation and aggregation, which is termed primary hemostasis. This process is most effective at high shear rates, where a conformational change in VWF multimers enhances platelet binding [2].

Classification

There are several VWD variants, which result in quantitative (types 1 and 3) or qualitative (types 2A, 2B, 2M, and 2N) VWF defects (Table 6.1) [2]. Type 1 VWD is characterized by reduced levels of VWF. This is the most common VWD variant representing roughly 70–80 % of VWD diagnoses [3]. Type 2 VWD variants represent approximately 20–30 % of VWD diagnoses. Type 2A is the most common type 2 VWD variant, while types 2B, 2M, and 2N VWD occur infrequently. Type 2 VWD variants are characterized by reduced VWF activity with normal or near normal VWF levels. Type 2A VWD results in the loss of large molecular weight multimers through defects in intracellular transport and processing or increased susceptibility to proteolysis in the circulation [4]. Type 2B VWD is characterized by increased VWF-platelet binding resulting in thrombocytopenia and loss of large molecular weight multimers. Type 2M VWD results in decreased VWF-platelet binding. VWF-FVIII binding is defective in type 2N VWD resulting in mildly reduced FVIII levels. Type 3, a rare VWD variant occurring as infrequently as 0.5 per 1,000,000 persons, is the most severe form of VWD [5]. It is characterized by very low or undetectable VWF levels and, consequently, significantly reduced FVIII levels (anywhere from 1 to 10 %). There are other rare variants, such as platelet-type VWD and Vicenza VWD that can occur.

Genetics

The VWF gene is located near the short arm of chromosome 12. It spans 178 kb and contains 52 exons [6]. VWF mutations that cause VWD include large deletions, frameshift mutations, nonsense mutations, and missense mutations. Mature VWF consists of 3 A and B domains, 2 C domains, and 4 D domains. The specific domain location of the VWF gene mutation often correlates with a particular VWD variant [7]. To date, 70 % of those with type 1 VWD, and nearly all of those with type 2 and 3 VWD, have detectable genetic abnormalities that cause the disease. Type 1 VWD usually involves single amino acid substitutions in the D3 domain. Type 2A VWD involves mutations in the D3 or A2 domains. Types 2B, 2M, and 2N VWD include

Table 6.1 Classification and diagnosis of von Willebrand disease

	VWF:Ag	VWF:RCo	VWF:RCo/VWF:Ag	FVIIII	Multimer pattern	LD-RIPA	Platelet count	Other specialized testing
Type 1	Mild decrease	Mild decrease	>0.5–0.7	Normal or mild decrease	Normal	Absent	Normal	
Type 1C	Mild decrease	Mild decrease	>0.5–0.7	Normal or mild decrease	Normal	Absent	Normal	Increased VWFpp/VWF:Ag
Type 2A	Absent	Moderate decrease	<0.5–0.7	Normal or mild decrease	Loss of HMW multimers	Absent	Normal	Abnormal VWF:collagen binding assay
Type 2B	Mild decrease	Moderate decrease	<0.5–0.7	Normal or mild decrease	Loss of HMW multimers	Increased	Decreased	Abnormal VWF:platelet binding assay
Type 2M	Mild decrease	Moderate decrease	<0.5–0.7	Normal or mild decrease	Normal	Normal	Normal	
Type 2N	Normal or mild decrease	Normal or mild decrease	<0.5–0.7	Moderate decrease	Normal	Normal	Normal	Abnormal VWF:FVIII binding assay
Type 3	Absent	Absent	>0.5–0.7	Absent	Absent		Normal	
Platelet type	Mild decrease	Moderate decrease	<0.5–0.7	Normal or mild decrease	Loss of HMW multimers		Decreased	Normal VWF:platelet binding assay

HMW high molecular weight, *FVIII* factor VIII, *LD-RIPA* low dose ristocetin induced platelet aggregation, *VWF:Ag* von Willebrand factor antigen, *VWFpp* von Willebrand factor propeptide, *VWF:RCo* von Willebrand factor ristocetin cofactor mutations in the A1, A3, and D3 domains, respectively. Types 3 VWD usually involves nonsense and frameshift mutations and occurs throughout the VWF gene [3]. All VWD variants are inherited in an autosomal dominant fashion except for type 2N VWD and type 3 VWD, which are inherited autosomal recessively.

Clinical Manifestations

VWD is a disorder of primary hemostasis; therefore, bleeding manifestations are primarily mucocutaneous in origin. The most common bleeding symptoms include epistaxis, easy bruising, menorrhagia, gingival bleeding, gastrointestinal bleeding, and postoperative bleeding. VWD is often overlooked as a cause of menorrhagia; however, it is a common presenting symptom in women with VWD and should be considered in the appropriate clinical context. Angiodysplasia is uncommon, but usually associated with type 2 or 3 VWD, and should be considered in any VWD patient with chronic gastrointestinal bleeding [8]. The occurrence of hemarthroses and hematomas is uncommon except in the more severe forms of the disease, such as type 3 VWD. Bleeding commonly occurs following hemostatic challenge, such as surgery, dental extractions, menarche, and childbirth. With the latter, it is critical to recognize that while bleeding occurs early, it may persist as long as 6 weeks postpartum. Clinical bleeding symptoms are often variable within families, and even within the same person at different times.

Diagnostic Studies

Laboratory testing for the diagnosis and classification of VWD is imperfect (Table 6.1) [2]. VWF and FVIII are acute phase reactants; therefore, levels are increased with inflammation, trauma, and stress. Several other factors affect VWF levels, including estrogen, pregnancy, and blood type. In the appropriate clinical scenario, normal testing does not necessarily exclude the presence of VWD and may need to be repeated on multiple occasions.

Assays to measure VWF antigen (VWF:Ag), VWF ristocetin cofactor (VWF:RCo), and FVIII levels are the initial tests performed when VWD is suspected. These tests are commonly available at most hospitals. VWF:Ag is an immunoassay used to the measure the concentration of VWF in plasma. Most laboratories used enzyme-linked immunosorbent assay (ELISA) or automated latex immunoassay (LIA). VWF:RCo is an assay performed to measure the functional activity of VWF based on ristocetin-induced platelet agglutination (RIPA). Ristocetin is an antibiotic that triggers VWF-platelet binding. Despite significant intra- and inter-laboratory variation, VWF:RCo is still the most sensitive and specific test available for measuring VWF function [9]. FVIII levels are measured in a functional assay based on the activated partial thromboplastin time (aPTT) to determine coagulant activity. For all of the above tests, reference ranges vary by laboratory but the normal range is generally considered to be 0.50 IU/dL to 2.00 IU/dL.

Depending on the results of the above tests, further testing may be indicated. While VWF:Ag and VWF:RCo levels less than 0.30 IU/dL are indicative of VWD based on the higher presence of genetic mutations in patients with these levels, generally VWF:Ag and VWF:RCo levels less than 0.50 IU/dL are considered clinically diagnostic of VWD. Decreased VWF:Ag levels and normal or comparably decreased VWF:RCo levels are consistent with type 1 VWD. Undetectable or nearly undetectable VWF:Ag and VWF:RCo levels along with significantly reduced FVIII levels are consistent with type 3 VWD. Type 2 VWD is suspected when VWF:RCo levels are decreased out of proportion to VWF:Ag levels. A ratio less than 0.5 to 0.7 can help distinguish type 2 VWD from type 1 VWD [10]. If type 2 VWD is suspected, multimer analysis is helpful in determining the specific subtype of type 2 VWD. Multimer analysis is done using agarose gel electrophoresis to separate out VWF proteins (multimers) by molecular weight followed by visualization with immunostaining. Loss of high molecular weight multimers is consistent with type 2A or 2B VWD. Type 2M and 2N have normal multimer analyses. Type 1 VWD has a reduced staining intensity, which affects all markers. In type 3 VWD, all markers are absent or barely visible. Differentiating between type 2A and 2B VWD can be done using the platelet count, which is often decreased in type 2B VWD, and RIPA. Ristocetin does cause VWD-platelet binding at low concentrations, less than 0.6 mg/mL; however, VWF hyperresponsiveness to ristocetin at these low concentrations in type 2B VWD results in increased VWF-platelet binding and platelet agglutination at rest. Other less commonly used tests, include the VWF: platelet binding assay, which will help distinguish type 2B VWD from platelet-type VWD; the VWF:collagen binding assay to assist in differentiating type 2A VWD from type 2M VWD; and the VWF:factor VIII binding assay to aid in diagnosing type 2N VWD.

Treatment

Therapy for VWD is generally aimed at increasing VWF levels in type 1 VWD and replacing abnormal VWF in types 2 and 3 VWD. In type 1 VWD, VWF can be increased by stimulating the release of endogenous VWF from endothelial stores with DDAVP (1-desamino-8-D-arginine vasopressin) or by providing VWF replacement with the use of VWF-containing plasma concentrates. DDAVP is a synthetic analogue of vasopressin. It can be administered intranasally or intravenously. Nasal administration of DDAVP in the form of Stimate is indicated for minor bleeding, such as epistaxis, or minor wounds. One spray of 150 μg in one nostril is administered to patients weighing less than 50 kg, and one spray of 150 μg in each nostril (totaling 300 μg) is given for those weighing 50 kg or more. Intravenous DDAVP is administration in 50 mL of normal saline over 30 min at a dose of 0.3 μg/kg. This is reserved for more significant minor bleeding or minor surgical procedures, such as uncomplicated dental extractions. The maximum response to DDAVP is seen 30–90 min following administration. DDAVP is generally given every 24 h for a maximum of three doses before clinical responsiveness disappears due to exhaustion of endogenous VWF stores. Potential adverse effects of DDAVP include flushing, headache, nausea, allergic reaction, thrombosis, and water retention. In individuals receiving more than 1.5 L of fluids daily, such as in the postoperative setting, and more commonly in children, water retention can result in hyponatremia and seizures; therefore, it is very important to limit fluid intake to 1.5 L for 24 h after receiving DDAVP [11]. DDAVP is usually indicated for mild type 1 VWD. It is less commonly effective in type 2 VWD and is ineffective in type 3 VWD. Approximately 20 % of type 1 VWD and most type 2 and 3 VWD patients do not respond to DDAVP; therefore, it is recommended that all patients with type 1 VWD undergo a "DDAVP challenge" to assess response to DDAVP, in terms of VWF:Ag, VWF:RCo, and FVIII levels [12]. This should be done at least 3 weeks before anticipation of using DDAVP for a surgery. If the DDVAP challenge is undertaken in less than 3 weeks, VWF stores will not be able to replenished (tachyphylaxis), and response will be limited when it is needed.

Plasma-derived, virus-inactivated VWF-containing concentrates are indicated for VWD in patients unresponsive to DDAVP as well as significant bleeding or major surgical procedures, which will require treatment for longer than 3 days (due to tachyphylaxis). The most commonly used VWF-containing concentrates are Humate-P and Alphanate (Antihemophilic factor/von Willebrand complex [human]). The dosing and duration of therapy is largely empiric and based on expert opinion. Usual practice for surgery involves administering VWF concentrate 80 units/kg by IV slow push, followed by 50 units/kg every 8–12 h for 3–5 days thereafter. Potential adverse effects are uncommon but may include allergic reaction and thrombosis. Recently, the first plasma-free recombinant version of VWF has been studied in clinical trials with promising results and is currently awaiting FDA approval [13].

Other potential therapy includes antifibrinolytic agents, ε-aminocaproic acid and tranexamic acid, which are usually given as adjunctive therapy to DDAVP or VWF concentrates for effective control of mucosal bleeding, especially for menorrhagia or dental surgery. Their use may be limited by the potential to cause nausea.

Hemophilia

Background

Hemophilia is an X-linked hereditary bleeding disorder characterized by deficient or defective coagulation factors VIII (FVIII), in hemophilia A, and IX (FIX), in hemophilia B. Hemophilia A is more common than hemophilia and accounts for 80–85 % of the hemophilia population. Hemophilia A occurs in 1 in every 5000–7000 live male births, and hemophilia B occurs in 1 in every 25,000 to 30,000 live male births [14]. There are approximately 400,000 individuals worldwide affected by hemophilia [15]. Both diseases occur in all races and ethnicities and have no geographic predilection.

FVIII acts as a cofactor for FIX in the coagulation cascade. Following activation by thrombin, activated FVIII (FVIIIa) associates with activated FIX (FIXa) forming the "tensase" complex with factor X (FX). FVIIIa functions to increase the rate of FX activation by FIXa [16]. FX ultimately activates prothrombin, generating thrombin and promoting clot formation. Both FVIII and FIX deficiency leads to reduced thrombin generation and weak and unstable clots.

Genetics

Hemophilia is a classic example of an X-linked recessive disorder. FVIII and FIX genes are located on the long arm of the X chromosome. All female offspring of affected males will inherit the defective X chromosome, and all male offspring will be unaffected. Females inheriting one affected X chromosome are obligate carriers and generally do not develop bleeding manifestations except in the presence of lionization, which results in a greater percentage of the normal FVIII allele being inactivated. 50 % of male offspring of female carriers will have hemophilia, and 50 % of female offspring will be carriers themselves. Approximately, one-third of hemophilia cases result from a spontaneous mutation and no known family history of hemophilia or abnormal bleeding can be identified [17].

The FVIII gene spans 186KB and contains 26 exons [18]. The FIX gene is much smaller, comprised of 33KB with 8 exons [19]. More than 1000 disease-causing mutations have been identified in each gene [20, 21]. The type of mutation often correlates with the severity of disease. Large deletions are associated with severe hemophilia. Alternatively, point mutations are more likely to result in moderate or mild hemophilia. One of the most commonly identified FVIII gene mutations is the intron 22 inversion. Mutations involving CpG dinucleotides account for a significant number of disease-causing mutations involving the FIX gene [22].

Clinical Manifestations

Hemophilia is categorized into three levels of severity: mild (baseline factor level 5–40 %), moderate (baseline factor level 1–5 %), and severe (baseline factor level <1 %). Individuals with mild or moderate hemophilia usually experience bleeding following provocation only, such as trauma or surgery. Severe hemophilia is associated with spontaneous bleeding.

Hemarthroses

The most common bleeding manifestation experienced in hemophilia is joint bleeding, referred to as hemarthrosis, which accounts for 75 % of bleeds [23]. Bleeding most commonly involves large, weight-bearing joints, such as the knees. Other commonly affected joints are the ankles and elbows. Intraarticular bleeding originates from blood vessels in the synovial lining of the joint. Bleeding results in an inflammatory response, and patients initially experience a tingling sensation, referred to as an aura, followed by the development of pain. Physical examination most often reveals a warm and swollen joint with reduced range of motion. Left untreated, pain will progressively worsen. Complications include the potential for recurrent spontaneous bleeding in the affected joint over a short period of time, referred to as a target joint. Other complications of hemarthroses include the potential for chronic hemophilic arthropathy (CHA). Residual intraarticular blood results in chronic inflammation, synovitis, and synovial hypertrophy. This predisposes to further bleeding, loss of articular cartilage, and progressive joint destruction. Along with damage of adjacent bony structures, CHA manifests with chronic joint pain, loss of motion, muscle atrophy, and contractures.

Soft-Tissue Hematomas

Another common manifestation of hemophilia is bleeding into subcutaneous tissues and muscle. The most commonly affected areas are the calves, thighs, and forearms although spontaneous bleeding may occur at any location. If not promptly treated, hemorrhage may have devastating consequences, such as neurovascular compromise and compartment syndrome in extremity bleeds, and life-threatening airway compromise in pharyngeal hematomas, among others. Iliopsoas bleeding is possible and manifests as pain in the groin, back, and/or abdomen. Recurrent hemorrhages may lead to muscle atrophy and contractures.

Other Bleeding Manifestations

While hemarthroses and soft tissue hematomas are the most commonly encountered manifestations of bleeding in hemophilia, spontaneous bleeding may occur at any location. Life-threatening bleeding includes central nervous system hemorrhage, gastrointestinal bleeding, retroperitoneal hematoma, and hemorrhage involving the neck and/or pharynx. Other non-life threatening bleeding includes oral mucosal bleeding, epistaxis, and hematuria.

Diagnosis

The aPTT is prolonged in hemophilia except in mild cases where factor levels are greater than 20–25 %. A mixing study is performed in the initial evaluation of an isolated prolonged aPTT. Correction of the prolonged aPTT is indicative of an underlying factor deficiency, whereas failure of the prolonged aPTT to correct is worrisome for the presence of a factor inhibitor. Once a factor deficiency is suspected, specific factor assays can identify the deficient factor. A one-stage clotting assay will reveal decreased FVIII and FIX levels in hemophilia A and B, respectively.

Treatment

Recombinant factor FVIII (rFVIII) and IX (rFIX) are the preferred treatments for hemophilia A and B, respectively, in the absence of an inhibitor (see Complications below). Current rFVIII products include Recombinate, Kogenate FS, Helixate FS, Advate, and Xyntha, and rFIX products include Benefix and Rixubis. Recently, the FDA approved the use of rFVIII Fc fusion protein (Eloctate) and rFIX Fc fusion protein (Alprolix) for the treatment of hemophilia A and B, respectively. The Fc portion of IgG1 binds to the neonatal Fc receptor, delaying lysosomal degradation, and extending the half-life of rFVIII from 8 to 12 to 20 h and rFIX from 12 to 20 to 87 h [24, 25]. Other extended half-life factor products, including pegylated and albumin-fusion proteins, which are in various stages of clinical trials are expected to be available for clinical use in the near future.

All bleeds should be treated as soon as recognized to limit morbidity and chronic inflammation. All patients should have factor stored at home for home infusion as needed. Patients with hemophilia should refrain from all aspirin, antiplatelet, and nonsteroidal antiinflammatory containing drugs. Medications known to cause platelet dysfunction should be avoided. There is no strong evidence supporting treatment guidelines for acute bleeding and surgical prophylaxis in hemophilia, and standard practice is based on consensus expert opinion and varies among different hemophilia treatment centers. An overview of our hemophilia center's practice is presented in Table 6.2. As the optimal treatment with extended half-life products in the setting of surgery has not yet been established, and, as the cost would increase with more frequent use in the hospital setting, we reserve use of extended half-life products for prophylaxis in the outpatient setting, while continuing to recommend standard rFVIII and rFIX for surgery and use in the hospital. In an adult, 1 unit of FVIII per kg of body weight is expected to raise the FVIII level 2 %, and 1 unit of FIX per kg of body weight is expected to raise the FIX level 1 %; therefore, 50 and 100 units/kg of FVIII and FIX, respectively, are necessary to raise the factor level to 100 % [26]. The availability of safe and effective factor therapy dramatically changed the outlook for a generation of patients with hemophilia. The use of factor therapy as prophylaxis prior to the onset of joint disease has allowed many children with hemophilia to reach adulthood with minimal or no significant joint disease [27]. The goal of prophylaxis is to maintain factor levels above 1 %, which greatly diminishes the risk of spontaneous bleeding. Prophylaxis regimens used at our hemophilia center are detailed in Table 6.2. Adjunctive therapies include DDAVP for patients with mild hemophilia A, but it should only be used after an adequate response to treatment has been demonstrated. Antifibrinolytic therapy is effective for oral mucosa bleeding, but its use may be limited by nausea.

Table 6.2 Hemophilia management strategies[a]

	Hemophilia A	Hemophilia B
Acute bleed		
Minor (joint or soft tissue)	50 units/kg initially then 25 units/kg daily × 1–3 days	100 units/kg initially then 50 units/kg daily × 1–3 days
Major (abdominal, gastrointestinal, thoracic)	50 units/kg initially then 25 units/kg every 8 h × 3 doses then 25 units/kg every 12 h × 2 doses then 25 units/kg daily × 2 weeks	100 units/kg initially then 50 units/kg every 12 h × 2 doses then 50 units/kg daily × 2 weeks
CNS	50 units/kg initially then 25 units/kg every 8 h × 3 doses then 25 units/kg every 12 h × 2 doses then 25 units/kg daily × 3 weeks	100 units/kg initially then 50 units/kg every 12 h × 2 doses then 50 units/kg daily × 3 weeks
Bleeding prophylaxis	25 units/kg every Monday and Wednesday and 50 units/kg every Friday	50 units/kg every Monday and 100 units/kg every Thursday
Surgical prophylaxis		
Minor (biopsy, laparoscopic, arthroscopic)	50 units/kg immediately prior to surgery then 25 units/kg 8–12 h postoperatively then 25 units/kg daily × 1–5 days	100 units/kg immediately prior to surgery then 50 units/kg 12 h postoperatively then 50 units/kg daily × 1–5 days
Major (cardiac, CNS, orthopedic)	50 units/kg immediately prior to surgery then 25 units/kg every 8 h × 2 days then 25 units/kg every 12 h × 2 weeks then 25 units/kg daily × 1 week	100 units/kg immediately prior to surgery then 50 units/kg every 12 h × 2 weeks then 50 units/kg daily × 1 week
Dental	50 units/kg immediately prior to surgery then 25 units/kg 8–12 h postoperatively then 25 units/kg daily × 10 days (alternatively aminocaproic acid can be substituted)	100 units/kg immediately prior to surgery then 50 units/kg 12 h postoperatively then 50 units/kg daily × 10 days (alternatively aminocaproic acid can be substituted)

[a]Consistent with National Hemophilia Foundation Medical and Scientific Advisory Committee guidelines [50]

Complications

Chronic Hemophilic Arthropathy

Chronic hemophilic arthropathy is best treated through prevention with the regular use of factor infusions. Once present, chronic pain is best managed with acetaminophen or the judicious use of opioids in consultation with a pain medicine specialist. Physical therapy and orthotics can improve function of diseased joints significantly. Ultimately, orthopedic surgery, such as joint replacement or fusion, may be necessary if pain and functionality are refractory to more conservative management and having a significantly negative impact on quality of life.

Viral Infections

In the 1980s, a large percentage of patients with hemophilia receiving treatment with plasma-derived factor concentrates were infected with chronic hepatitis C virus (HCV) and human immunodeficiency virus (HIV). This was devastating to the hemophilia population resulting in significant morbidity and mortality over the course of the next several decades. However, HIV can now be managed as a chronic disease with the use of highly active antiretroviral therapy. Furthermore, chronic HCV is now curative in most patients receiving direct acting antiviral agents, such as sofosbuvir and ledipasvir (Harvoni). Most importantly, the risk of transmission of blood-borne viruses has been virtually eliminated in hemophilia patients with the use of recombinant factor products and a much safer blood supply.

Inhibitors

Inhibitor development is the most serious complication facing hemophilia patients today. An inhibitor is an IgG alloantibody directed against foreign infused FVIII, and rarely, FIX. Approximately 20–30 % of hemophilia A patients with severe disease will develop inhibitors, and 5–10 % of those with mild or moderate disease will be affected. Inhibitor formation is much less common in hemophilia B, affecting less than 5 % of patients [28]. At this time, it is impossible to predict who will develop an inhibitor, but certain factors have been shown to increase the risk, including disease severity, intensity of treatment, FVIII mutation, and family history of inhibitor development [29]. Inhibitor development typically occurs in the first 10–20 exposure days with over 95 % occurring within the first 50 exposure days [29]. Large deletion mutations are the FVIII mutations most commonly associated with inhibitor development [29]. While intron 22 mutations have been associated with inhibitor development, this is confounded by the fact that this is the most common mutation underlying hemophilia A. Nonsense mutations have been shown to be protective.

Inhibitors are suspected when patients bleed despite appropriate factor therapy. Diagnosis involves performing a mixing study, which will reveal a prolonged aPTT that does not correct in a 1:1 mix with normal plasma, confirmed in a Bethesda assay, which determines the inhibitor anti-FVIII titer. Low-responding inhibitors are associated with a anti-FVIII titer less than 5 Bethesda units (BU), no increase following rechallenge with rFVIII, and hemostasis with rFVIII. By contrast, the more common high-responding inhibitors are associated with a anti-FVIII titer greater than 5 BU, an increase following rechallenge with rFVIII exposure, and poor or no hemostatic response to infused rFVIII.

Treatment of bleeding in high-responding inhibitors requires the use of "bypass agents," i.e., agents such as recombinant FVIIa (rFVIIa) or FEIBA (Factor Eight Bypassing Activity), which bypass FVIII to promote clot formation for hemostasis. Recombinant FVIIa is given at a dose of 90 μg/kg every 2–3 h. FEIBA is given at a dose of 50–100 units/kg every 6–8 h. Both products carry a risk of thrombosis and no more than 20,000 units of FEIBA should be administered in a 24-h period. Low-titer inhibitors may resolve spontaneously with observation. Immune tolerance induction is necessary for high-titer inhibitor eradication and involves the use of high dose factor therapy, such as 200 units/kg on a daily basis up to 9–12 months.

Acquired Bleeding Disorders

Acquired bleeding disorders may result from a whole host of underlying pathologies, which can be broadly defined into two categories, coagulopathy and platelet disorders. The most common causes likely to be encountered in the ICU are discussed below.

Coagulopathy

Anticoagulants

Parental Anticoagulants

Unfractionated heparin (UFH) is an anionic, highly sulfated, mucopolysaccharide. It possesses anticoagulant activity by binding to antithrombin III (ATIII) and enhancing its ability to catalyze the inactivation of coagulation factors IIa, IXa, Xa, XIa, and XIIa. UFH can be administered intravenously or subcutaneously and has a half-life of 60–90 min. UFH binds to multiple plasma proteins, in addition to ATIII, and this phenomenon is responsible for the unpredictable nature of its anticoagulant effect; therefore, anticoagulation requires close monitoring using the aPTT or anti-Xa assay. A therapeutic aPTT is 1.5–2 times the normal aPTT value, or approximately 46–70 s, which corresponds to an anti-Xa level of 0.3–0.7 units/mL. Monitoring UFH using the anti-Xa assay is recommended when the aPTT is prolonged at baseline (i.e., in the presence of an underlying lupus anticoagulant), heparin resistance is present and requires the use of excessively large amounts of UFH to achieve a therapeutic aPTT (i.e., >35,000 units in a 24 h period), and in certain high risk bleeding situations. The major adverse effects of UFH are bleeding and heparin-induced thrombocytopenia. The incidence of major bleeding with therapeutic doses of UFH is approximately 3 %; however, this is likely higher in critically ill patients with multiple comorbidities [30]. Bleeding can be reversed with protamine sulfate, a cationic protein that binds to UFH forming an ionic complex that neutralizes its anticoagulant effects. One milligram of protamine will neutralize 100 units of UFH. Potential adverse effects include hypotension, bradycardia, or rarely anaphylaxis [31].

Another frequently used class of parental anticoagulants is low molecular weight heparins (LMWH). Enoxaparin is one of the most commonly used LMWHs in the

USA. Enoxaparin acts similarly to UFH exerting its anticoagulant effect by binding to and enhancing the activity of ATIII. Enoxaparin is administered subcutaneously with dosing based on weight. It has a half-life of 3–6 h. Enoxaparin has a reduced affinity for plasma proteins, so it exhibits a more predictable dose–response relationship and does not require monitoring of its anticoagulant effect except in certain situations, such as obesity, pregnancy, and renal dysfunction. Enoxaparin undergoes renal clearance and is contraindicated in severe renal insufficiency (creatinine clearance less than 30 mL/min). A therapeutic anti-Xa level is 0.6–1.0 units/mL. Adverse effects are bleeding and heparin-induced thrombocytopenia. If bleeding occurs, protamine is unable to completely neutralize the anticoagulant effect; however, it is still the recommended therapy. If enoxaparin was given the preceding 8 h, 1 mg of protamine should be given for each mg of enoxaparin given up to maximum of 50 mg of protamine. If bleeding continues a second dose of protamine can be given with 0.5 mg of protamine administered for each mg of enoxaparin [32].

Oral Anticoagulants

Vitamin K antagonists (VKAs) prevent activation of the vitamin K dependent coagulation factors II, VII, IX, and X through the inhibition of vitamin K oxide reductase, an enzyme necessary for cycling vitamin K to its reduced form. Vitamin K prevents the gamma carboxylation of glutamic acid residues on factors II, VII, IX, and X, which is necessary for their activation to promote procoagulant activity. VKAs require frequent monitoring to ensure an appropriate level of anticoagulation, by the use of the International Normalized Ratio (INR). Generally, the target INR is 2–3. There is significant variability in the anticoagulant effect with any given VKA dose. Further, the anticoagulant effect of VKAs is altered by numerous medications and changes in diet. The incidence of major bleeding with warfarin is 3–5 % per year [33]. Guidelines for the reversal of warfarin in patients with supratherapeutic INRs with and without bleeding are outlined in Table 6.3 [34].

For decades VKAs, such as warfarin, were the only oral option available for patients requiring anticoagulation; however, recently, we have seen the approval of

Table 6.3 Management of warfarin-induced supratherapeutic INR and bleeding

INR level	Management
INR 4-10	Omit next dose of warfarin Consider vitamin K 1–2.5 mg PO if bleeding risk is high Monitor INR and consider decreasing dose of warfarin
INR >10	Stop warfarin Given vitamin K 2.5–5 mg PO Monitor INR and resume warfarin at decrease dose when INR is therapeutic
Bleeding	Stop warfarin Given vitamin K 10 mg IV over 30 min If clinically significant or life-threatening bleeding then administer FFP 15–30 mL/kg or 4-factor PCC 25–50 IU/kg

Table 6.4 Target specific oral anticoagulants

	Dabigatran	Rivaroxaban	Apixaban
Target	Thrombin	Factor Xa	Factor Xa
Oral bioavailability	6 %	60 %	60 %
Time to peak affect	1–3 h	2–4 h	1–2 h
Half-life	8–15 h	7–11 h	12 h
Clearance	80 % Renal 20 % Biliary/fecal	66 % Renal 33 % Biliary/fecal	25 % Renal 75 % Biliary/fecal
Drug interactions	P-gp modulators	Strong CYP3A4 modulators P-gp modulators	Strong CYP3A4 modulators P-gp modulators
Drug monitoring	Exclude relevant anticoagulant effect—TCT Detect excessive anticoagulation—aPTT and TT Monitor drug activity—dilute TCT	Exclude relevant anticoagulant effect—anti-Xa[a] Detect excessive anticoagulation—PT and anti-Xa[a] Monitor drug activity—PT and anti-Xa[a]	Exclude relevant anticoagulant effect—anti-Xa[a] Detect excessive anticoagulation—anti-Xa[a] Monitor drug activity—anti-Xa[a]

CYP cytochrome P450, *P-gp* P-glycoprotein, *TCT* thrombin clotting time, *TT* thrombin time
[a]Anti-Xa assay using low molecular weight heparin standards can only be used to detect relevant anticoagulant effect. Monitoring drug activity requires the use drug-specific anti-Xa standards

several new oral anticoagulants, referred to as target specific oral anticoagulants (TSOACs), as alternatives to warfarin. TSOACs consist of direct thrombin inhibitors (dabigatran) and factor Xa inhibitors (rivaroxaban and apixaban). All are indicated for the prevention of stroke and systemic embolism in non-valvular atrial fibrillation and the treatment of acute and prevention of recurrent venous thromboembolism (VTE). Also, rivaroxaban and apixaban are indicated for the prevention of VTE following total hip and knee arthroplasty [35]. These therapies differ considerably from warfarin (Table 6.4) [36]. TSOACs have a rapid onset and short half-life. Metabolism and clearance is largely kidney-dependent and dose reductions are necessary with renal dysfunction to prevent hemorrhage. Drug interactions are limited to drugs that affect the P-glycoprotein and CYP3A4 systems (i.e., ketoconazole, ritonavir, rifampin, carbamazepine, etc.). Further, TSOACs exhibit predictable pharmacokinetic properties, obviating the need for drug monitoring; however, certain situations, such as major bleeding, emergency surgery, and renal failure, make it critical to be aware of the degree of anticoagulation present. Laboratory tests to measure anticoagulant activity and drug concentration with TSOACs vary in sensitivity and specificity. Recommended laboratory tests for detecting and excluding clinically significant anticoagulation are presented in Table 6.4 [37]. The use of drug concentrations to determine if a therapeutic anticoagulant effect is present is not recommended since therapeutic drug concentrations of TSOACs have not been established at this point. In contrast to warfarin, TSOACs have no specific antidote;

therefore, they are not readily reversible in the event of life-threatening hemorrhage or the need for emergency surgery. While no specific antidote exists to completely reverse TSOAC-induced anticoagulation, recommended strategies include the use of 4-factor Prothrombin Complex Concentrate, or PCC (Kcentra), activated PCC (FEIBA), or rFVIIa. Hemodialysis is useful for dabigatran removal. [38]. Results of early clinical trials evaluating the specific antidotes, idarucizumab and andexanet, for reversing direct thrombin and factor Xa inhibitor-induced anticoagulation, respectively, have been promising. Larger studies to confirm these findings are underway [39].

Disseminated Intravascular Coagulation

Activation of the coagulation cascade occurs following endothelial vascular disturbance. It is a tightly regulated process with each step being regulated by physiologic inhibitors, such as tissue factor pathway inhibitor, ATIII, and alpha-2 antiplasmin, which inhibit tissue factor, thrombin, and plasmin, respectively. In disseminated intravascular coagulation (DIC), there is an inciting stimulus, such as sepsis and trauma, resulting in sustained initiation of the coagulation cascade. This sustained activation overwhelms the inhibitory system leading to unopposed thrombin and plasmin production. The end result is pathologic thrombosis and fibrinolysis, or, in rare cases, severe hemorrhage.

DIC may be triggered by a variety of circumstances. The most common causes include sepsis, trauma, malignancy, and obstetric complications, such as abruptio placentae, placenta previa, and amniotic fluid embolism among others. DIC is clinically manifested as thrombosis, or, less often, bleeding, or a combination of thrombosis and bleeding associated with multiorgan dysfunction. Laboratory tests necessary for the diagnosis of DIC include platelet count, prothrombin time (PT), aPTT, fibrinogen, and markers of fibrin degradation, such as D-dimer or fibrin degradation products. Markers of microangiopathic hemolysis, such as lactate dehydrogenase and haptoglobin in combination with a hemoglobin and peripheral blood smear are often helpful. The International Society of Hemostasis and Thrombosis developed a scoring system with >90 % sensitivity and specificity for the diagnosis of overt DIC. It assigns points for degree of thrombocytopenia, PT prolongation, hypofibrinogenemia, and elevated markers of fibrin degradation. A score of 5 or greater is compatible with overt DIC [40].

The primary treatment of DIC is treating the underlying etiology. Transfusion of platelets and plasma should be reserved for patients with bleeding. It is not recommended to provide prophylactic transfusions for abnormal laboratory tests in the absence of clinically evident bleeding. Platelet transfusions should be administered for a platelet count less than 50,000/μL in the presence of bleeding. Plasma may be given in the form of fresh frozen plasma (FFP) for prolonged PT and aPTT or cryoprecipitate for hypofibrinogenemia. Large doses of FFP (starting dose of 15–30 mL/kg) are often necessary to improve coagulation parameters. Cryoprecipitate should be administered for a fibrinogen level less than 100 mg/dL with bleeding present. If thrombosis predominates, and the bleeding risk is not deemed too high, UFH should be considered. In the absence of clinical data supporting its effectiveness, ATIII concentrates are not currently recommended. ATIII concentrates may be necessary with UFH, if significant ATIII deficiency is present, due to heparin resistance. Lastly, if bleeding predominates, and is severe, antifibrinolytic agents, such as aminocaproic acid, should be given [41].

Liver Disease

The liver produces the majority of hemostatic proteins. As a consequence, liver disease can significantly alter the hemostatic system. Because the liver is responsible for the production of almost all procoagulant plasma proteins (recent evidence shows FVIII is primarily produced in vascular endothelial cells), liver disease may be associated with a bleeding diathesis; however, simultaneous decreases in anticoagulant and fibrinolytic proteins shifts results in a balanced hemostatic system in most individuals with liver disease [42, 43]. Exclusively assessing the risk of bleeding in patients with liver dysfunction using the PT and platelet count is misleading since neither are reflective of the prothrombotic changes that occur in liver disease. Changes that impair hemostasis include decreased production of factors II, V, VII, IX, X, XI, and XIII; fibrinogen; and thrombopoietin. Changes that promote hemostasis include decreased production of proteins C and S, ATIII, and plasminogen with simultaneous increased production of VWF and FVIII [44].

The hemostatic system in liver disease is easily disrupted and may result in hemorrhage and/or thrombosis. When hemorrhage occurs, it is not always related to hemostatic defects. One of the most common causes of bleeding in liver disease is esophageal varices, which are most often related to portal hypertension rather than a defect in the hemostatic system. Specific treatment of bleeding in liver disease should be selected based on the clinical scenario. If bleeding esophageal varices are present, then an interventional procedure, such as banding, should be performed. If bleeding is present in the setting of a significantly decreased platelet count or prolonged PT, corrective actions may consist of transfusion of platelets and FFP, respectively; however, correction of thrombocytopenia is often not possible due to splenomegaly and correction of prolonged PT may not be achieved due to inability to administer adequate dosing. The recommended dose of FFP is 15–20 mL/kg, but this is often not possible in liver disease due to the risk of transfusion associated circulatory overload. Other options include DDAVP and thrombopoietin receptor agonists; however, neither has proven to be effective in liver disease. Lastly, in the case of life-threatening refractory bleeding, rFVIIa may be used despite lack of data supporting its efficacy. The risk of thrombosis with rFVIIa in individuals with an otherwise normal coagulation system should be noted.

Trauma

Coagulopathy in trauma results from multiple factors [45]. First, trauma-related blood loss leads to the loss of coagulation factors. Volume resuscitation with asanguinous fluid and plasma-poor red blood cells dilutes the plasma concentration of coagulation factors. Furthermore, hypothermia and acidosis are often present, both of which reduce coagulation factor activity. Lastly, trauma may precipitate DIC resulting in coagulation factor consumption.

The treatment of the coagulopathy in trauma involves volume resuscitation to replace blood loss, body-warming efforts to reverse hypothermia, improvement of tissue oxygenation to minimize acidosis, and surgical management of trauma-related anatomical bleeding. Many hospitals employ a massive transfusion protocol to help instruct transfusion practices in life-threatening trauma. Administration of blood products is paramount in trauma-related blood loss, and the treatment of trauma-induced coagulopathy; however, asanguinous and plasma-poor red blood cell administration may worsen coagulopathy by diluting the plasma concentration of coagulation factors present. For massive transfusion (i.e., anticipated red blood cell transfusion of 10 or more units in 24 h), administration of fresh frozen plasma and red blood cell transfusions in a 1:1 ratio is widely practiced although a recently conducted randomized controlled trial showed no difference between 1:1 and 1:2 ratio transfusion practice in primary outcomes of 24 h and 30 days all-cause mortality [46]. In situations with refractory, uncontrolled, life threatening bleeding despite employing other measures above, rFVIIa may be given, but there is no high quality data supporting this practice.

Platelet disorders

Thrombocytopenia and platelet dysfunction are routinely present in critically ill patients and usually multifactorial in origin. While a complete overview of the many potential etiologies of thrombocytopenia and platelet dysfunction is beyond the scope of this chapter (Table 6.5), some of the more common causes encountered in the ICU are discussed below.

Thrombocytopenia

Medications

Numerous medications cause thrombocytopenia. The most common mechanisms include myelosuppression and immune-mediated destruction of platelets. Antibiotics are routinely prescribed in the ICU and are often associated with thrombocytopenia. Frequent culprits include sulfamethoxazole, vancomycin, linezolid,

Table 6.5 Causes of thrombocytopenia

Decreased production
Infections
CMV
EBV
HIV
Medications
Chemotherapy
Radiation therapy
Nutritional deficiencies
Vitamin B12 deficiency
Liver disease
Toxins
Intrinsic bone marrow disorders
Myelodysplastic syndrome
Malignancies
Leukemia
Lymphoma
Metastatic solid tumors
Increased destruction
Immune
Immune thrombocytopenia
Medications
Heparin-induced thrombocytopenia
Collagen vascular disorders
Antiphospholipid antibody syndrome
Posttransfusion purpura
Nonimmune
Thrombotic thrombocytopenia purpura
Hemolytic uremic syndrome
Disseminated intravascular coagulation
Sepsis
Mechanical valve
Artifact
Pseudothrombocytopenia
Splenomegaly
Congenital
MYH-9 related
Congenital amegakaryocytic thrombocytopenia
Thrombocytopenia with absent radius syndrome
Wiskott–Aldrich syndrome
Bernard–Soulier syndrome

and penicillins. Other common offenders include antiepileptic drugs, such as carbamazaepine and phenytoin; nonsteroidal antiinflammatory drugs; and antiplatelet agents, such as aspirin, clopidogrel, eptifibatide, and tirofiban. The ensuing thrombocytopenia may be profound with platelet counts of 20,000/μL or less, and often difficult to distinguish from immune thrombocytopenia (ITP). The onset of thrombocytopenia can occur anywhere from 1 day to more than 1 year after initiation of the offending medication; however, the median time to onset from initiating the drug is 14 days [47]. Treatment involves withdrawal of the offending agent. This is a difficult task in the ICU. Routinely, several medications known to cause thrombocytopenia are started simultaneously. Frequently, a trial-and-error method is necessary to determine the offending agent where potential culprit medications are stopped in succession. In the event that bleeding occurs, platelet transfusion is the recommended treatment. If an immune-mediated mechanism is suspected, steroids may be beneficial. In the setting of an immune-mediated thrombocytopenia, and rapid correction is necessary, intravenous immunoglobulin G (IVIG) may be given.

Infections

Another common cause of thrombocytopenia in the ICU is infection, including sepsis due to a variety of bacterial organisms, e.g., *Staphylococcus aureus*, *Pseudomonas aeruginosa*. In this setting, thrombocytopenia may be severe. Viral infections are often accompanied by thrombocytopenia, and include Epstein-Barr virus, cytomegalovirus, human immunodeficiency virus, and hepatitis B and hepatitis C virus. The mechanism of thrombocytopenia is often related to bone marrow suppression; however, immune-mediated mechanisms are sometimes responsible, too. Treatment is aimed at providing antimicrobial support as clinically indicated. If bleeding occurs, platelet transfusion is the recommended therapeutic course of action.

Disseminated Intravascular Coagulation

DIC is a common cause of thrombocytopenia in the ICU setting. Thrombocytopenia results from platelet activation, which is mediated by proinflammatory substances and thrombin. DIC is associated with a significant coagulopathy and is discussed in greater detail with the coagulopathies in section "Disseminated intravascular coagulation."

Liver Disease

Thrombocytopenia is commonly seen in liver disease. Splenomegaly, a result of portal hypertension in cirrhotic liver disease, sequesters platelets, and thrombopoietin production is reduced. Liver disease alters the production of several procoagulant and anticoagulant protein and is discussed in greater detail with the coagulopathies in section "Liver disease."

Platelet Dysfunction

Medications

Numerous medications alter platelet function and increase the risk of bleeding. Aspirin and nonsteroidal antiinflammatory drugs inhibit cyclooxygenase. Thienopyridines, such as clopidogrel and prasugrel, are P2Y12 receptor antagonists. Eptifibatide, tirofiban, and abciximab are glycoprotein IIb/IIIa receptor antagonists. All of these medications have mechanisms of action that reduce platelet activation or aggregation. Also, platelet dysfunction may arise from medications that alter the metabolism of cyclic adenosine/guanosine monophosphate, such as prostacyclin, nitroglycerin, and nitroprusside. Selective serotonin reuptake inhibitors reduce serotonin storage in platelets, which may result in platelet dysfunction. Several other medications, including penicillins and cephalosporins, affect platelet function but a complete review is beyond the scope of this chapter.

Hematologic Disorders

Paraproteinemias, such as multiple myeloma and monoclonal gammopathy, affect platelet function, which may be related to immunoglobulins binding to the surface of platelets [48]. Myeloproliferative neoplasms may affect platelet function, too, by affecting platelet secretion and aggregation.

Uremia

Uremia is responsible for multiple abnormalities in platelet function. Circulating metabolites are felt to be responsible for bleeding diathesis, though which of them is unclear [49]. Treatment consists of red blood cell transfusions, DDAVP, platelet transfusions, and hemodialysis.

Iatrogenic Bleeding

Iatrogenic bleeding may be related to invasive procedures, such as central venous placement or heart catheterization, and surgical procedures. If an anatomic source is identified, corrective steps should be taken. During this time, any coexisting laboratory abnormalities, such as thrombocytopenia or coagulopathy, should be corrected as necessary. Lastly, if bleeding is refractory to the above measures, and deemed life threatening, rFVIIa can be considered; however, there is no high quality evidence supporting its use in this situation.

References

1. Rodeghiero F, Castaman G, Dini E. Epidemiological investigation of the prevalence of von Willebrand's disease. Blood. 1987;69:454.
2. Nichols WL, Hultin MB, James AH, et al. The diagnosis, evaluation, and management of von Willebrand disease. National Heart, Lung, and Blood Institute. NIH Pub. No. 08-5832. 2007.
3. Lyons SE, Bruck ME, Bowie EJW. Impaired intracellular transport produced by a subset of type IIA von Willebrand disease mutations. J Biol Chem. 1992;267:4424.
4. Weiss HJ, Ball AP, Mannucci PM. Incidence of severe von Willebrand's disease. N Engl J Med. 1982;307:127.
5. Mancuso DJ, Tuley EA, Westfield LA, et al. Structure of the gene for human von Willebrand factor. J Biol Chem. 1989;264:19514.
6. Eikenboom JC, Matsushita T, Reitsma PH, et al. Dominant type 1 von Willebrand disease caused by mutated cysteine residues in the D3 domain of von Willebrand factor. Blood. 1996;88:2433–41.
7. Bonthron DT, Handin RI, Kauffman RJ, et al. Structure of pre-pro-von Willebrand factor and its expression in heterologous cells. Nature. 1986;324:270.
8. Franchini M, Mannucci PM. von Willebrand disease-associated angiodysplasia: a few answers, still many questions. Br J Hematol. 2013;161:177–82.
9. Rodeghiero F, Castaman G, Tosetto A. von Willebrand factor antigen is less sensitive than ristocetin cofactor for the diagnosis of type I von Willebrand disease—results based on a epidemiological investigation. Thromb Haemost. 1990;64:349.
10. Laffan M, Brown SA, Collins PW, et al. The diagnosis of von Willebrand disease: a guideline from the UK Haemophilia Centre Doctors' Organization. Haemophilia. 2004;10:199–217.
11. Bertholini DM, Butler CS. Severe hyponatraemia secondary to desmopressin therapy in von Willebrand's disease. Anaesth Intensive Care. 2000;28:199–201.
12. Federici AB, Mazurier C, Berntorp E, et al. Biologic response to desmopressin in patients with severe type 1 and type 2 von Willebrand disease. Results of a multicenter European study. Blood. 2004;103:2032.
13. Mannucci PM, Kempton C, Millar C, et al. Pharmacokinetics and safety of a novel recombinant human von Willebrand factor manufactured with a plasma-free method: a prospective clinical trial. Blood. 2013;122(5):648–57.
14. Brinkhous KM. A short history of hemophilia, with some comments on the word "hemophilia". In: Brinkhouse KM, Hemker HC, editors. Handbook of hemophilia. New York: Elsevier; 1975. p. 3.
15. Stonebraker JS, Bolton-Maggs PH, Soucie JM, et al. A study of variations in the reported haemophilia A prevalence around the world. Haemophilia. 2010;16(1):20–32.
16. Roberts HR. Contributions to the evolution of knowledge about hereditary hemorrhagic disorders. Cell Mol Life Sci. 2007;64:517.
17. Antonarakis SE, Youssoufian H, Kazazian H, et al. Molecular genetics of hemophilia in man factor VIII deficiency. Mol Biol Med. 1987;4:81.
18. Tuddenham EGD. FVIII. In: High KA, Roberts HR, editors. Molecular basis of thrombosis and hemostasis. New York: Marcel Dekker; 1995. p. 167.
19. Kurachi K, Davie EW. Isolation and characterization of a cDNA coding for factor IX. Proc Natl Acad Sci U S A. 1983;80:4200.
20. Payne AB, Miller CH, Kelly FM, et al. The CDC hemophilia A mutation project (CHAMP) mutation list: a new online resource. Hum Mutat. 2013;34(2):E2382–91.
21. Li T, Miller CH, Payne AB, et al. The CDC hemophilia B mutation project mutation list: a new online resource. Mol Genet Genomic Med. 2013;1(4):238–45.
22. Monroe DM, McCord DM, Huang MN, et al. Functional consequences of an arginine 180 to glutamine mutation in factor IX Hilo. Blood. 1989;73:1540.
23. Gilbert MS. Musculoskeletal complications of hemophilia: the joint. Hemophilia. 2000;6:34.
24. Eloctate™ [package insert]. Cambridge, MA: Biogen Idec Inc.; 2014.

25. Aprolix™ [package insert]. Cambridge, MA: Biogen Idec Inc.; 2014.
26. Björkman S, Berntorp E. Pharmacokinetics of coagulation factors: clinical relevance for patients with haemophilia. Clin Pharmacokinet. 2001;40:815–32.
27. Manco-Johnson MJ, Abshire TC, Shapiro AD, et al. Prophylaxis versus episodic treatment to prevent joint disease in boys with severe hemophilia. N Engl J Med. 2007;357:535–44.
28. Astermark J, Altisent C, Batorova A, European Haemophilia Therapy Standardization Board, et al. Non-genetic risk factors and the development of inhibitors in haemophilia: a comprehensive review and consensus report. Haemophilia. 2010;16:747–66.
29. Kempton CL, White GC. How we treat a hemophilia A patient with a factor VIII inhibitor. Blood. 2009;113:1–17.
30. Schulman S, Beyth RJ, Kearon C, et al. Hemorrhagic complications of anticoagulant and thrombolytic treatment: 9th ed: American College of Chest Physicians evidence-based clinical practice guidelines. Chest. 2008;133:257S–98.
31. Garcia DA, Baglin TP, Weitz JI, et al. Parenteral anticoagulants: antithrombotic therapy and prevention of thrombosis, 9th ed: American College of Chest Physicians evidence-based clinical practice guidelines. Chest. 2012;141:e24S–43.
32. Oden A, Fahlen M. Oral anticoagulation and risk of death: a medical record linkage study. Br Med J. 2002;325:1073–107.
33. Levi M, Eerenberg ES, Kampuisen PW. Anticoagulants. Old and new. Hamostaseologie. 2011;31:229–35.
34. Garcia DA, Crowther MA. Reversal of Warfarin. Circulation. 2012;125:2944–7.
35. Garcia DA. The target-specific oral anticoagulants: practical considerations. ASH Educ Program. 2014;2014(1):510–3.
36. Weitz JI, Gross PL. New oral anticoagulants: which one should my patient use? ASH Educ Program. 2012;2012:536–40.
37. Konkle BA. Monitoring target-specific oral anticoagulants. ASH Educ Program. 2014;2014(1):329–33.
38. Siegal DM, Garcia DA, Crowther MA. How I treat target-specific oral anticoagulant-associated bleeding. Blood. 2014;123(8):1152–8.
39. Greinacher A, Thiele T, Selleng K. Reversal of anticoagulants: an overview of current developments. Thromb Haemost. 2015;113:931–42.
40. Taylor FBJ, Toh CH, Hoots WK, et al. Towards definition, clinical and laboratory criteria, and a scoring system for disseminated intravascular coagulation. Thromb Haemost. 2001;86:1327.
41. Levi M, Toh CH, Thachil J, et al. Guidelines for the diagnosis and management of disseminated intravascular coagulation. Br J Haematol. 2009;145:24–33.
42. Lisman T, Porte RJ. Rebalanced hemostasis in patients with liver disease: evidence and clinical consequences. Blood. 2010;116:878–85.
43. Everett LA, Cleuren ACA, Khoriaty RN, et al. Murine coagulation factor VIII is synthesized in endothelial cell. Blood. 2014;123:3697–905.
44. Warnaar N, Lisman T, Porte RJ. The two tales of coagulation in liver transplantation. Curr Opin Organ Transplant. 2008;13:298–303.
45. Hess Jr B, Brohi K, Dutton RP, et al. The coagulopathy of trauma: a review of mechanisms. J Trauma. 2008;65:748–54.
46. Holcomb JB, Tilley BC, Baraniuk S, et al. Transfusion of plasma, platelets, and red blood cells in a 1:1:1 vs a 1:1:2 ratio and mortality in patients with severe trauma: the PROPPR randomized clinical trial. JAMA. 2015;313:471–82.
47. George JN, Raskob GE, Shah SR, et al. Drug-induced thrombocytopenia: a systematic review of published case reports. Ann Intern Med. 1998;129:886.
48. Zangari M, Elice F, Fink L, et al. Hemostatic dysfunction in paraproteinemias and amyloidosis. Semin Thromb Hemost. 2007;33:339–49.
49. Boccardo P, Remuzzi G, Galbusera M. Platelet dysfunction in renal failure. Semin Thromb Hemost. 2004;30(5):579–89.
50. National Hemophilia Foundation Medical and Scientific Advisory Council Recommendations. www.hemophilia.org. Accessed 23 Apr 2014.

Chapter 7
Acute Pulmonary Manifestations of Hematologic Malignancies

Andra Fee-Mulhearn and Patrick Nana-Sinkam

Pulmonary Infection

Pulmonary infections are a significant cause of mortality in patients with leukemia and lymphoma. While there is lack of data to support a precise incidence, studies suggest that approximately 42 % of patients with hematologic malignancies will be diagnosed with an infection during their disease course and most often it is a pulmonary infection [1, 2]. Another study indicates that pulmonary infiltrates develop in 30 % of neutropenic patients with acute leukemia during chemotherapy with a mortality of up to 50 % [3]. A recent study investigating the value of bronchoscopy in patients with hematologic malignancies found a bacterial organism as a pathogen in 41.3 % of patients, while fungi affected 23.8 % and viruses 28.6 % [4].

Hematologic malignancies directly cause a disruption in patient's immune systems due to the disease process. Additionally, the treatments for the disease disrupt the normal function of the immune system of the patient. This sets the stage for various infectious complications for these patients, especially pulmonary infections. Variable defects to specific immune mechanisms predispose patients to numerous pathogens.

A. Fee-Mulhearn, DO, MPH
Division of Pulmonary, Allergy, Critical Care and Sleep Medicine, The Ohio State University, Columbus, OH, USA

P. Nana-Sinkam, MD (✉)
Division of Pulmonary, Allergy, Critical Care and Sleep Medicine, The Ohio State University, Columbus, OH, USA

Division of Medical Oncology, The Ohio State University, Columbus, OH, USA

James Thoracic Oncology Center, The Ohio State University, Columbus, OH, USA

Faculty Advancement, Mentorship and Engagement, Center for FAME, The Ohio State University, Columbus, OH, USA
e-mail: Patrick.nana-sinkam@osumc.edu

J.S. Lee, M.P. Donahoe (eds.), *Hematologic Abnormalities and Acute Lung Syndromes*, Respiratory Medicine, DOI 10.1007/978-3-319-41912-1_7

Neutropenia as caused by leukemia, myelodysplastic syndrome, chemotherapy, or recent (within 30 days) hematopoietic stem cell transplantation, predisposes patients to gram-negative bacilli, gram positive cocci, and fungi [5]. Lymphomas, lymphoblastic leukemias, chemotherapy, administration of monoclonal antibodies, corticosteroid therapy, and hematopoietic stem cell transplant patients that are 30–100 days post procedure cause T cell defects. Patients with T cell defects are more susceptible to infections from *Nocardia, Mycobacterium*, viruses of which cytomegalovirus (CMV) is the most common, and fungi, particularly *Aspergillus* and *P jiroveci* [5].

The following sections detail predisposing factors, presentation, diagnosis, and treatment of the various organisms causing pulmonary infections in patients with hematologic malignancies.

Bacterial Infections

Neutropenia associated with hematologic malignancies from the disease process and treatment predisposes patients to bacterial pulmonary infections. Patients with hematologic malignancies are frequently evaluated within the health care system and as such given their immunocompromised state, have increased risk for nosocomial bacterial pulmonary infections. The most common health care associated pulmonary pathogen in patients with hematologic malignancy is *Pseudomonas* [6]. *Norcardia*, *Legionella*, *H. influenzae*, and *Enterobacter* are frequently isolated as causative agents of pneumonia as well [6].

Reviewing prior culture data of the patient being treated can help guide empiric antimicrobial coverage. As most commonly the pathogen is bacterial and often *Pseudomonas,* an anti-Pseudomonal antibiotic should be administered, such as Cefepime, Piperacillin/Tazobactam, or an anti-Pseudomonal carbapenem depending on the local antibiogram. Evaluation of the patient with diagnostic imaging is helpful. Chest radiography is usually the initial test of choice, but computed tomography (CT) is often more valuable at detecting earlier radiographic evidence of pneumonia [7]. Plain radiographs most commonly demonstrate airspace consolidation or no radiologic abnormality [8]. The most common finding on CT is segmental or lobar consolidation [8]; other findings include small airway plugging and branching centrilobular nodules (tree-in-bud appearance) [6].

Evaluation of the patient with respiratory symptoms should include laboratory, microbiology, and radiologic tests. Blood cultures are routinely drawn. Urine antigens for *Legionella* and *Streptococcus pneumonia* can also be evaluated. Quantitative and qualitative evaluation of bronchoalveolar lavage can often lead to a rapid diagnosis [7].

Bronchoscopy with bronchoalveolar lavage is considered the standard test to diagnose the cause of pulmonary infection [7]. Results from bronchoalveolar lavage changed management in 30.1 % of the cases studied in a sample of patients with chest radiographic infiltrates in the setting of a hematologic malignancy [4]. Given the common presence of comorbid factors, the clinician should consider whether or not the patient is suitable for bronchoscopy. For example, the risk of respiratory failure requiring mechanical ventilation in a patient that is requiring significant supplemental oxygen should be taken into consideration before proceeding to bronchoscopy.

Transbronchial lung biopsy (TBBx) at the time of bronchoscopy with BAL should also be considered. There are risks associated with TBBx that must be considered prior to performing the biopsy. Thrombocytopenia (platelets less than 50 K/μL) and neutropenic fever are quoted contraindications [9]. Pneumothorax and hemoptysis are complications that result in less than two percent of patients [10]. TBBx has a high sensitivity not only in clarifying neoplastic lung infiltrates but also with respect to toxic pneumonitis [9]. These etiologies appear to be more frequent than commonly estimated and are likely to go undiagnosed if TBBx is not applied. In contrast, infectious causes may be detected more reliably by BAL only, particularly with respect to the diagnosis of aspergillosis, when non-culture-based techniques are used [11] and combined with CT scans [12].

Fungal Infections

Fungal pathogens, most commonly *Aspergillus*, are a common cause of pneumonia in patients that become neutropenic following chemotherapy or HSCT [13]. *Aspergillus* galactomannan antigen testing has improved diagnosis of invasive pulmonary aspergillosis. There is concern for false positives with broad-spectrum beta lactam antibiotics, but a recent study indicated this is no longer a concern [14]. Radiographic imaging in patients with invasive aspergillosis is characterized as either angioinvasive or airway invasive [8]. Angioinvasive aspergillosis has a characteristic nodule surrounded by peripheral ground glass, commonly called a "halo-sign" (Fig. 7.1) [8]. This feature corresponds to a central area of consolidation of the fungal infection with surrounding areas of hemorrhagic infarction due to thrombosis [8]. Cavitation or air-crescent formation occurs at a late stage of infection [15]. Airway invasive aspergillosis has CT abnormalities in a peribronchial or peribronchiolar distribution of centrilobular nodules less than 0.5 cm in diameter or regions of consolidation as large as 5 cm in diameter [16].

Mucormycosis is typically indistinguishable from invasive aspergillosis, but more frequently has a "reverse halo sign," a round area of ground glass opacities surrounded by a crescent or complete ring of consolidation [17]. Pulmonary mucormycosis has a high mortality, often as high as 80 % [18]. Early recognition and treatment with lipid amphotericin B formulations and/or posaconazole can improve outcomes [19]. Patients with diabetes mellitus are predisposed to be infected with mucormycosis compared to those who do not have diabetes [20]. One study of infections in hematologic patients found that 56 % of the patients with mucormycosis were diabetic [20].

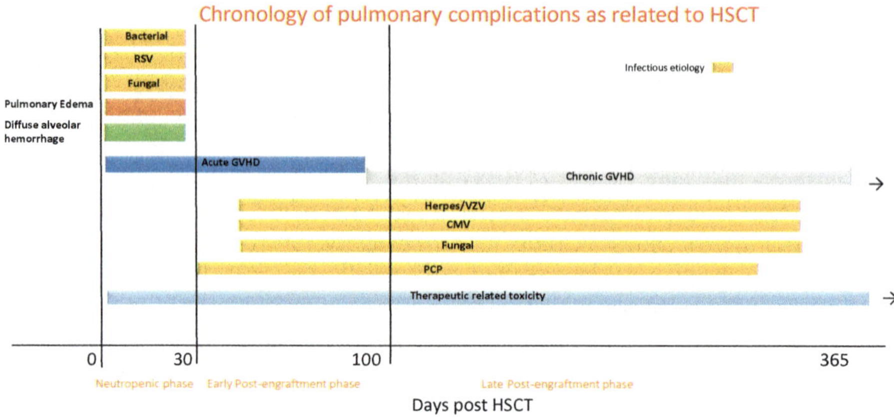

Fig. 7.1 Timing of pulmonary complications days after HSCT

Following HSCT, patients are typically placed on prophylactic trimethoprim/sulfamethoxazole to reduce infection from *Pneumocystis jiroveci*. Thirty to hundred days after HSCT, patients are frequently found to have *Pneumocystis jiroveci* induced pneumonia. In a study over 10 years at a single center, the diagnosis of *Pneumocystis jiroveci* was confirmed in a total of 154 patients negative for HIV [21]. The most common comorbid condition was a hematologic malignancy in 32.5 % of the cases [21]. Diffuse alveolar or interstitial opacities are often observed on plain radiographs [22]. On CT, a common pattern is widespread perihilar ground-glass opacities in a mosaic pattern, reflecting interspersion of areas of infected lung tissue with normal lung parenchyma [6].

Diagnosis of *Pneumocystis jiroveci* is most commonly obtained by polymerase chain reaction (PCR) of bronchoalveolar lavage fluid, fungal culture of bronchoalveolar lavage fluid, or transbronchial biopsy (TBLB) of infected lung tissue. Elevated LDH greater than 220 and beta-D-glucan serum testing can indicate likelihood of infection. PCR has a sensitivity of 72–100 % and specificity of 86.2 % in studies [23]. Bronchoscopic evaluation and subsequent evaluation of BAL represents the best approach to the identification of *Pneumocystis jiroveci*. Kim et al. demonstrated an incidence of *Pneumocystis jiroveci* in 17 % in patients who had a hematologic malignancy that underwent bronchoscopy with BAL and subsequent analysis with specific immunofluorescence staining and real time PCR [4].

Pneumonia from *Candida* spp. appears on imaging as any of the following: multiple patches of consolidation, cavitation and pulmonary nodules [9]. Empiric echinocandin coverage with narrowing of antibiotics after speciation is appropriate treatment. Similar to pneumonia caused by *P jiroveci*, pneumonia from *Candida* is seen less frequently with appropriate prophylactic treatment of patients with hematologic malignancies.

Viral Infections

With the utilization of molecular based diagnostic tools for viral pathogens, patients with hematologic malignancies that present with respiratory symptoms are increasingly screened for viral etiologies. CMV is the most common cause of viral pneumonia, yet morbidity is also caused by rhinoviruses, adenoviruses, influenza viruses, parainfluenza viruses, respiratory syncytial virus, and metapneumovirus [8]. Chest imaging of patients with viral pneumonia have similar appearances regardless of pathogen [24].

CMV pneumonia usually occurs in patients 31–100 days after HSCT. The most common radiographic findings are bilaterally distributed parenchymal opacities and innumerable nodules [8]. Prophylaxis with valganciclovir is the mainstay for patients after HSCT. Mortality rates of CMV pneumonia in patients after hematopoietic cell transplants are 50 %, but increase to 85 % if left untreated [25, 26]. Ganciclovir is the primary treatment for CMV pneumonia. CMV serum titers are often utilized to guide detection and management. The diagnosis can be made by analysis of the BAL fluid by specific immunofluorescence staining and real time PCR [4]. Identification of CMV is made by transbronchial lung biopsy or bronchoalveolar lavage (BAL) fluid (in the proper clinical setting) by a sensitive immunocytochemical method [27].

Noninfectious Acute Pulmonary Manifestations

The noninfectious pulmonary complications of hematologic malignancies carry significant morbidity and mortality as do the infectious complications. Noninfectious complications such as pulmonary hemorrhage and pulmonary edema can arise in any of the hematologic malignancies. Pulmonary leukostasis occurs in acute leukemia, most commonly in the myelomonocytic subtypes, and is a result of the disease process itself. Alternatively, there are therapies used in treatment of specific hematologic malignancies that can cause pulmonary complications. Hematopoietic stem cell transplantation (HSCT) can lead to infectious complications as mentioned above, but also noninfectious issues arise that affect the pulmonary system. Pulmonary complications can lead to life threatening illness in a patient with a hematologic malignancy. The specific associations with therapies should be well known to physicians treating these patients. Prompt recognition of the pulmonary complication and initiation of treatment is paramount for this patient population (Table 7.1).

Pulmonary Hemorrhage

Pulmonary hemorrhage is the most common noninfectious pulmonary complication of acute leukemia [28]. Pulmonary hemorrhage is associated with thrombocytopenia, infectious disease, and post HSCT. Diffuse alveolar hemorrhage is observed in

Table 7.1 Infectious acute pulmonary manifestations of acute hematologic malignancies

Pulmonary Infection	Clinical setting	Cause of immunosuppression	Common pathogens	Radiologic findings	Evaluation	Treatment
Bacterial pneumonia	Neutropenia	Leukemia, myelodysplastic syndrome, chemotherapy, recent (<30 days) HSCT	Gram-negative bacilli, gram-positive cocci	Segmental or lobar consolidation	Blood culture, sputum sample, analysis of BAL	Broad spectrum antibiotics, anti-*pseudomonal*, narrow on culture data
	T cell defect	Lymphomas, lymphoblastic leukemia, chemotherapy, monoclonal antibodies, corticosteroids, HSCT 30–100 days	*Nocardia, Mycobacterium*	Cavitation, lobar consolidation, nodules	AFB smears and culture, analysis of BAL	*Nocardia* Bactrim *Mycobacterium* pending speciation
	B cell defect	Lymphoma, leukemia, multiple myeloma, splenectomy	Encapsulated bacteria (*Streptococcus pneumonia, H. influenza*)	Segmental or lobar consolidation	Blood culture, sputum sample, analysis of BAL	Broad spectrum antibiotics, anti-*Pseudomonal*, narrow on culture data
Viral pneumonia	T cell defect	Lymphomas, lymphoblastic leukemia, chemotherapy, monoclonal antibodies, corticosteroids, HSCT 30–100 days	CMV Multiple other viruses	Ground-glass opacities, micronodules, airspace consolidation	Detection of CMV in BAL fluid or lung tissue samples, CMV serum PCR	CMV: Ganciclovir Supportive care

Pulmonary Infection	Clinical setting	Cause of immunosuppression	Common pathogens	Radiologic findings	Evaluation	Treatment
Fungal pneumonia	Neutropenia	Leukemia, myelodysplastic syndrome, chemotherapy, recent (<30 days) HSCT	*Candida, Aspergillus*	*Aspergillus*: "halo" sign, segmental or subsegmental pleura-based consolidation *Candida*: multiple microabscesses	*Aspergillus*: Galactomannan antigen test, analysis of BAL *Candida*: blood culture, analysis of BAL	Echinocandins in severe infections, narrow to Itraconazole or Voriconazole
	T cell defect	Lymphomas, lymphoblastic leukemia, chemotherapy, monoclonal antibodies, corticosteroids, HSCT 30–100 days	*Pneumocystis jiroveci Aspergillus* (as above)	Widespread perihilar ground-glass opacities	LDH, Detection of *P jiroveci* in BAL analysis, PCR	Bactrim

Table 7.2 Noninfectious acute pulmonary manifestations of patients with hematologic malignancies

Complication	Clinical setting	Radiologic findings	Evaluation	Treatment
Pulmonary hemorrhage	Thrombocytopenia, sudden onset of respiratory symptoms, rarely hemoptysis	Rapid progression of diffuse ground glass opacities and/or consolidation	Bronchoscopy, analysis of BAL	Augmentation with blood products, corticosteroids
Pulmonary edema	Multiple transfusions, cardiotoxic chemotherapy, renal impairment, large volume of intravenous fluids	Redistribution of blood flow toward the upper lobes, increased interstitial markings	Imaging, weights, strict measurement of intake and output	Fluid restriction (when able), diuretics
Leukostasis	Hyperleukocytosis (WBC > 100,000) and acute myelomonocytic leukemia (AML subtype M4)	Interstitial and/or alveolar opacities in varying degrees	Laboratory data, imaging, bone marrow bx	Leukapheresis, reduction in WBC

approximately 20 % of patients who have undergone HSCT and typically manifests within the first few weeks post-transplantation [8] (Table 7.2).

Hemoptysis is an uncommon initial presentation in patients with hematologic malignancy that have developed pulmonary hemorrhage. Rather, the clinical presentation consists typically of the sudden onset of progressive dyspnea, nonproductive cough, fever and hypoxia. Radiographic findings may appear to be out-of-proportion to the patient's relatively mild symptoms [29]. The radiographic changes progress rapidly to diffuse ground-glass opacities and patchy consolidation (Fig. 7.2) [29]. CT findings include widespread ground glass opacities, consolidation and reticulation or a crazy-paving pattern [30].

Bronchoscopic evaluation of the airway establishes the diagnosis of pulmonary hemorrhage. The BAL will demonstrate abnormally increased blood content that increases with subsequent aliquots of lavage. Microscopic evaluation of the BAL will show macrophages with hemosiderin content greater than 20 % without evidence of infection [31]. Importantly, infection can be a cause of pulmonary hemorrhage or hemoptysis. Therefore, careful examination of the BAL fluid for infectious organisms must be performed.

Treatment of pulmonary hemorrhage includes correcting coagulopathy, augmenting platelet counts with transfusion and supporting the patient during respiratory compromise.

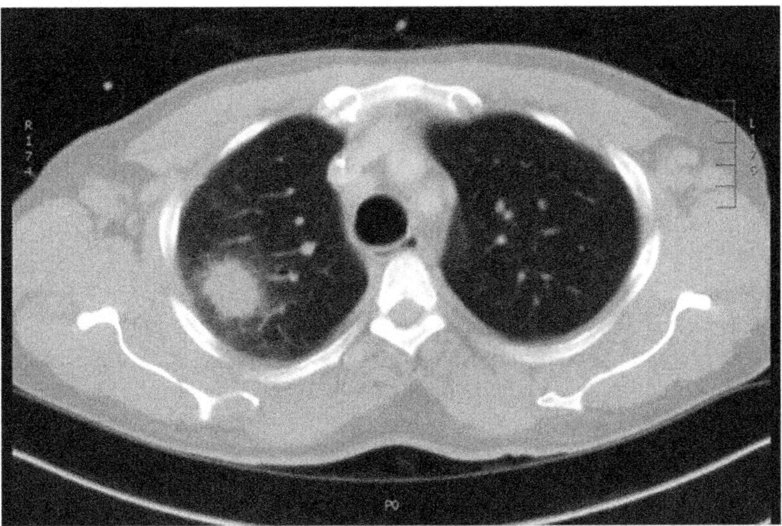

Fig. 7.2 Computed tomography slice demonstrating the classic halo sign associated with aspergillus infection in a 44-yo male with neutropenia. *Image courtesy of Mark King, MD. Division Chief Thoracic Imaging. The Ohio State University. Columbus, OH*

Pulmonary Edema

Patients with hematologic malignancies require intravenous administration of many medications including renal protective fluids during chemotherapy infusions. With the increased amount of volume introduced to the patient, pulmonary edema can develop. The etiology is multifactorial and includes increased hydrostatic pressure from high-volume infusions, multiple transfusions, parenteral nutrition, cardiotoxic effects of chemotherapy, renal impairment, and increased permeability of pulmonary vessels caused by a variety of other factors [32].

Radiographic evidence of pulmonary edema often includes cardiomegaly, redistribution of blood flow toward the upper lobes (cephalization), increased interstitial markings, Kerley B lines, and perihilar or peribronchial areas of ground glass opacities [8]. On CT, the same findings can indicate pulmonary edema with the addition of interlobular septal thickening [32].

Volume sparing strategies and diuresis are the mainstay of treatment for pulmonary edema. Supportive care for respiratory failure with noninvasive positive pressure ventilation can help reduce intubation and invasive mechanical ventilation. Early recognition and prompt treatment with diuretic agents improve outcomes.

Pulmonary Leukostasis

Patients with acute leukemia presenting with an initial hyperleukocytosis (white blood cell count of more than 100,000 per microliter) are at risk for pulmonary leukostasis. Leukemic cells accumulate in minor blood vessels in the lungs during pulmonary leukostasis. Other sites of accumulation include the heart, brain and testes. Patients typically present with cough, fever and dyspnea. In particular, patients with myelomonocytic subtypes of AML (M4/M5) are at increased risk that may be predicted by a specific surface marker [8]. The expression of CD56/NCAM, a surface marker used in routine immunophenotyping of AML, may help to predict severe and potentially fatal leukostasis in hyperleukocytic acute myelomonocytic leukemia [33]. Only the absolute count of CD56 positive blasts was a significant predictor of risk of severe leukostasis ($P=0.020$) [33]. This was not observed in AML without monocytic involvement (AML M1, M2, M3v) [33].

Chest radiographs in pulmonary leukostasis vary from normal to degrees of interstitial or alveolar opacification [34]. Chest CT findings of thickening of the bronchovascular bundles and prominence of peripheral pulmonary arteries correlate with the histopathologic findings [8] (Fig. 7.3).

Treatment with leukapheresis is often required in cases of life threatening pulmonary leukostasis [35]. Prompt reduction in the burden of leukocytes is often necessary.

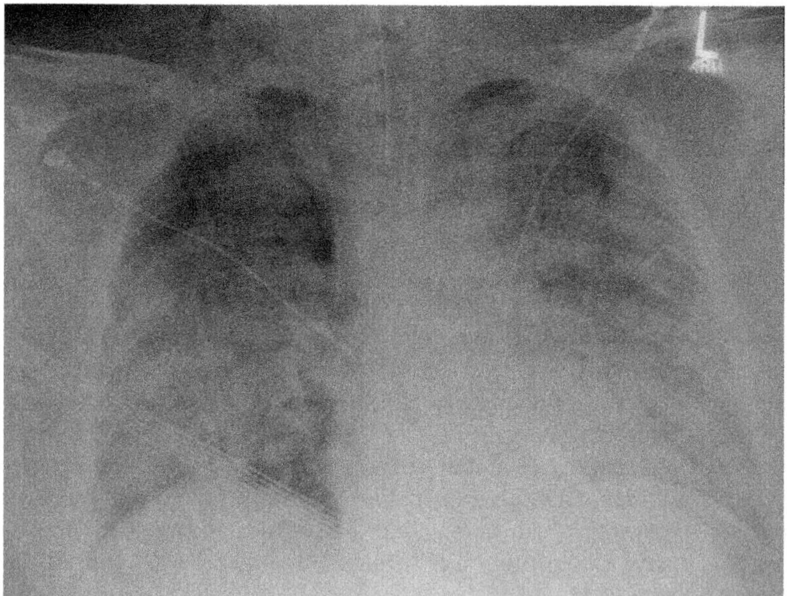

Fig. 7.3 Portable chest X-ray of a 30 yo male day 14 post HSCT with thrombocytopenia that developed pulmonary hemorrhage *Image courtesy of Mark King, MD. Division Chief Thoracic Imaging. The Ohio State University. Columbus, OH*

Hydroxyurea can also assist in reducing WBC count [36]. Both leukapheresis and hydroxyurea have limited data suggesting reduction in early mortality [37]. However, targeted low-dose chemotherapy has shown promise in reducing mortality in patients with pulmonary leukostasis [36].

Therapeutic Complications

Physicians prescribe regimens to help treat hematologic malignancies daily. Unfortunately, nearly all pharmaceuticals induce unwanted side effects. The following sections detail the pulmonary complications associated with treatments for hematologic malignancies. Therapies such as ATRA, tyrosine kinase, monoclonal antibodies, and HSCT help cure the disease but can cause life threatening pulmonary manifestations as a complication of treatment.

Retinoic Acid Syndrome

Retinoic acid syndrome is the result of a rare complication of treatment for acute promyelocytic leukemia (AML, M3). The agent used to differentiate blasts into mature granulocytes, ATRA or tretinoin acid is usually tolerated well. The prevalence of the syndrome ranges from 2 to 27 % [35]. Symptoms typically arise 10 days after initiation of treatment (range 2–21 days) [38]. Unexplained fever, respiratory distress, pulmonary opacities, weight gain and pleural effusion are all associated with retinoic acid syndrome [38]. A diagnosis of retinoic acid syndrome must include at least three of the following: fever, weight gain, respiratory distress, lung infiltrate, pleural or pericardial effusion, hypotension and renal failure [37].

Radiographic imaging is very similar to that of patients with pulmonary hemorrhage or edema. Prompt recognition of the syndrome with cessation of ATRA is essential. Treatment with corticosteroids after withdrawal of the offending agent can help reduce morbidity and mortality.

Effects of Tyrosine Kinase Inhibitors

Tyrosine kinase inhibitors (TKIs) are a class of pharmaceuticals used as targeted therapies for an increasing number of malignancies. Tyrosine kinases are enzymes responsible for the activation of many proteins by signal transduction cascades. The use of inhibitors of specific tyrosine kinase pathways has been applied to the treatment of renal cell carcinomas, gastrointestinal stromal tumors (GIST), and chronic leukemias [39].

Tyrosine Kinase Inhibitors of BCR-ABL: Imatinib, Dasatinib, and Nilotinib

Agents targeting BCR-ABL are utilized in chronic myeloid leukemia. The resultant rare pulmonary manifestations range from interstitial lung disease (ILD) to pleural effusions and precapillary pulmonary hypertension. The acute clinical manifestation is a pneumonitis that can present as significant dyspnea and hypoxia. The three main tyrosine kinase inhibitors that are FDA approved are imatinib, dasatinib, and nilotinib. Imatinib was shown to cause 27 cases of ILD among 5500 patients in a Japanese study [40]. Acute pneumonitis from TKIs has been reported between days 10 and 337 of therapy [41]. The acute pneumonitis differs from the ILD that can result years after treatment [41]. Acute pneumonitis often improves with removal of the offending tyrosine kinase inhibitor and initiation of corticosteroids.

Dasatinib is most frequently associated with pleural effusions occurring in 10–35 % of patients [40]. A more serious complication is severe precapillary pulmonary hypertension. There can be a delay in presentation of up to 34 months (8–48 months) [42]. The pathogenesis for this complication remains unclear. Some improvement does occur with removal of the agent, but hemodynamic recovery is usually incomplete [38].

Anti-lymphocyte Monoclonal Antibodies

Rituximab

Rituximab is a chimeric anti-CD20 monoclonal antibody that targets B-lymphocytes and is used to treat a variety of non-Hodgkin lymphomas (NHLs) as well as rheumatologic diseases, autoimmune hemolytic anemia, and idiopathic thrombocytopenic purpura (ITP) [39]. The most common and well-recognized pulmonary manifestation is bronchospasm during an acute infusion reaction that has been reported in nearly 10 % of patients [43]. The reaction including chills, fever, hypotension, and bronchospasm typically resolves shortly after stopping or decreasing the rate of infusion [43]. Fatal interstitial pneumonitis has been reported within weeks of starting rituximab [44]. A review of rituximab induced lung injury also identified both acute respiratory failure and diffuse alveolar hemorrhage as complications occurring within hours of administration of Rituximab [45].

Engraftment Syndrome

Engraftment syndrome occurs in the period of neutropenia following allogenic or autologous HSCT [8]. The clinical manifestations of fever, erythematous skin rash, and noncardiogenic pulmonary edema are indicative of the increased capillary permeability [46]. The median time to onset after transplantation is 11 days [46]. Chest radiographic findings are nonspecific and may include bilateral effusions and interstitial edema [8]. CT images often demonstrate bilateral ground-glass opacities, areas of airspace consolidation in the hilar or peribronchial regions and smooth thickening of the interlobular septa [8]. Treatment with corticosteroids typically results in rapid improvement [46].

Acute Graft Versus Host Disease (GVHD)

GVHD results from minor incompatibility differences between the donor and recipient in a HLA matched transplant and is thought to result from an immune reaction mediated by donor T-lymphocytes that recognize the recipient's tissue as a foreign body. In the early period (first 100 days) after BMT, acute GVHD develops in 25–75 % of patients and primarily affects the skin, liver, and gastrointestinal tract [47]. Pulmonary complications of acute GVHD are minimal [47]. The median time of onset of respiratory symptoms is approximately 5 months (range 1–13 months) [47]. The chest radiograph can be normal despite the presence of clinical symptoms and signs and abnormal pulmonary function tests. Chest radiography and computed tomography show that pulmonary infiltrates can vary from a few focal areas to diffuse bilateral disease. Pulmonary function tests demonstrate a reduction in vital capacity and forced expiratory volume in the first second, followed by marked decrease in forced expiratory volume in first second/vital capacity ratio suggestive of overt airway obstruction [47]. Histologically, pulmonary GVHD may manifest as diffuse alveolar damage, lymphocytic interstitial pneumonia, lymphocytic bronchitis, and bronchiolitis obliterans [47]. The majority of patients with GVHD respond to immunosuppressive treatment including high dose steroids (prednisolone 1–2 mg/kg) with a gradual taper over 3–12 months in those with sustained complete response [47]. In severe or steroid resistant cases, additional immunosuppressive drugs (cyclosporin A, azathioprine, or thalidomide) can be added [47]. In some patients, an initial favorable response is followed by a relapsing, remitting pattern, similar to other autoimmune diseases. A recent study suggested that the lung might be one of the target organs of acute GVHD and participation of T lymphocyte, macrophage and cytokines such as IFN-gamma and TNF-alpha contribute to the pathogenesis of acute GVHD-induced lung injury [48]. Acute GVHD-induced lung injury may progress to late-onset noninfectious lung injury [48].

Conclusion

Acute pulmonary complications of hematologic malignancies have various etiologies and treatments. The timing of the pulmonary illness in regard to the patient's treatment course, the history provided by the patient, the therapeutics used to treat the patient and the state of the patient's immune system are extremely helpful in determining the etiology and treatment of the pulmonary complication. Additionally, prompt use of diagnostic tools such as bronchoscopy with BAL or TBLB, serologic analysis, and chest imaging can aid in management. Anticipation of a pulmonary manifestation and quick reaction by the physician can reduce morbidity and mortality in these too often fatal pulmonary complications of hematologic malignancies.

References

1. Ewig S, Torres A, Riquelme R, et al. Pulmonary complications in patients with haematologic malignancies treated at a respiratory ICU. Eur Respir J. 1998;12:116–22.
2. Bugadaci M, Yanardag H, Ar M, et al. Pulmonary radiologic findings in patients with acute myeloid leukemia and their relation to chemotherapy and prognosis: a single center retrospective study. Turk J Hematol. 2012;29:217–22.
3. Ewig S, Glasmacher A, Ulrich B, et al. Pulmonary infiltrates in neutropenic patients with acute leukemia during chemotherapy: outcome and prognostic factors. Chest. 1998;114:444–51.
4. Kim SW, et al. Diagnostic value of bronchoscopy in patients with hematologic malignancy and pulmonary infiltrates. Ann Hematol. 2015;94:153–9.
5. Corti M, Palmero D, Eiguchi K. Respiratory infections in immunocompromised patients. Curr Opin Pulm Med. 2009;15(3):209–17.
6. Franquet T. High-resolution computed tomography of lung infections in non-AIDS immunocompromised patients. Eur Radiol. 2006;16(3):707–18.
7. Shorr AF, Susla GM, O'Grady NP. Pulmonary infiltrates in the non-HIV-infected immunocompromised patient: etiologies, diagnostic strategies, and outcomes. Chest. 2004;125(1):260–71.
8. Choi MH, Park SH, et al. Acute pulmonary complications in patients with hematologic malignancies. Radiographics 2014:1755–1768
9. Mulabecirovic A, et al. Pulmonary infiltrates in patients with haematologic malignancies: transbronchial lung biopsy increases the diagnostic yield with respect to neoplastic infiltrates and toxic pneumonitis. Ann Hematol. 2004;83:420–2.
10. Eapen GE, et al. Complications, consequences, and practice patterns of endobronchial ultrasound-guided transbronchial needle aspiration. Chest. 2013;143(4):1044–53.
11. Sanguinetti M, Posteraro B, Pagano L, et al. Comparison of real-time PCR, conventional PCR, and galactomannan antigen detection by enzyme-linked immunosorbent assay using bronchoalveolar lavage fluid samples from hematology patients for diagnosis of invasive pulmonary aspergillosis. J Clin Microbiol. 2003;41:3922–5.
12. Maschmeyer G, Beinert T, Buchheidt D, et al. Diagnosis and antimicrobial therapy of pulmonary infiltrates in febrile neutropenic patients. Ann Hematol. 2003;82:118–26.
13. Leung AN, Gosselin MV, Napper CH, et al. Pulmonary infections after bone marrow transplantation: clinical and radiographic findings. Radiology. 1999;210(3):699–710.
14. Otting KA, Stover KR, Cleary JD. Drug-laboratory interaction between beta-lactam antibiotics and the galactomannan antigen test used to detect mould infections. Braz J Infect Dis. 2014;18(5):544–7.
15. Kuhlman JE, Fishman EK, Sigelman SS. Invasive pulmonary aspergillosis in acute leukemia: characteristic findings on CT, the halo CT sign and role of CT in early diagnosis. Radiology. 1985;157(3):611–4.
16. Logan PM, Primack SL, Miller RR, Muller NL. Invasive aspergillosis of the airways: radiographic, CT and pathologic findings. Radiology. 1994;193(2):383–8.
17. Georgiadou SP, Sipsas NV, Marom EM, Konotoyiannis DP. The diagnostic value of halo and reversed halo sings for invasive mold infections in compromised hosts. Clin Infect Dis. 2011;52(9):1144–55.

18. Petrikkos G, Skiada A, Lortholary O, et al. Epidemiology and clinical manifestations of mucormycosis. Clin Infect Dis. 2012;54 Suppl 1:S23–34.
19. Kontoyiannis DP. Invasive mycoses: strategies for effective management. Am J Med. 2012;125(1 Suppl):S25–38.
20. Lee FYW, Mossad SB, Adal KA. Pulmonary mucormycosis: the last 30 years. Arch Intern Med. 1999;159(12):1301–9.
21. Tattevin P, et al. Incidence of Pneumocystis jiroveci pneumonia among groups at risk in HIV-negative patients. Am J Med. 2014;127(12):1242.e11–7.
22. Bollee G, Sarfati CM, Thiery G, et al. Clinical picture of Pneumocystis jiroveci pneumonia in cancer patients. Chest. 2007;132(4):1305–10.
23. Torres J, Lee CH, et al. Diagnosis of *Pneumocystis carinii (jiroveci)* pneumonia in human immunodeficiency virus-infected patients with polymerase chain reaction: a blinded comparison to standard methods. Clin Infect Dis. 2000;30:141–5.
24. Franquet T, Rodriguez S, Martino R, et al. Thin-section CT findings in hematopoietic stem cell transplantation recipients with respiratory virus pneumonia. Am J Roentgenol. 2006;187(4):1085–90.
25. Horger MS, Pfannenberg C, Einsele H, et al. Cytomegalovirus pneumonia after stem cell transplantation: correlation of CT findings with clinical outcome in 30 patients. Am J Roentgenol. 2006;187:636–43.
26. Vogel MN, Brodoefe H, Hierl T, et al. Differences and similarities of cytomegalovirus and Pneumocystis pneumonia in HIV negative immunocompromised patients thin section CT morphology in the early phase of the disease. Br J Radiol. 2007;80:516–23.
27. Florescu DF, Kalil AC. Cytomegalovirus infections in nonimmunocompromised and immunocompromised patients in the intensive care unit. Infect Disord Drug Targets. 2011;11:354–64.
28. Tenholder MF, Hooper RG. Pulmonary infiltrates in leukemia. Chest. 1980;78(3):468–73.
29. Witte RJ, Gurney JW, Robbins RA, et al. Diffuse pulmonary alveolar hemorrhage after bone marrow transplantation: radiographic findings in 39 patients. Am J Roentgenol. 1991;157(3):461–4.
30. Primark SL, Miller RR, Muller ND. Diffuse pulmonary hemorrhage: clinical, pathologic and imaging features. Am J Roentgenol. 1995;164(2):295–300.
31. Soubani AO, Miller KB, Hassoun PM. Pulmonary complications of bone marrow transplantation. Chest. 1996;109(4):1066–77.
32. Worthy SA, Flint JD, Muller NL. Pulmonary complications after bone marrow transplantation: high-resoluation CT and pathologic findings. Radiographics. 1997;17(6):1359–71.
33. Novotny JR, Nückel H, Dührsen U. Correlation between expression of CD56/NCAM and severe leukostasis in hyperleukocytic acute myelomonocytic leukaemia. Eur J Haematol. 2006;76(4):299–308.
34. Van Buchem MA, Wondergem JH, Kool LJ, et al. Pulmonary leukostasis: radiologic-pathologic study. Radiology. 1987;165(3):739–41.
35. Eisenstaedt RS, Berkman EM. Rapid cytoreduction in acute leukemia: management of cerebral leukostasis by cell pheresis. Transfusion. 1978;18(1):113–5.
36. Piro E, Carillio G, Levato L, Kropp M, Molica S. Reversal of leukostasis-related pulmonary distress syndrome after leukapheresis and low-dose chemotherapy in acute myeloid leukemia. J Clin Oncol. 2011;29(26):e725–6.
37. Porcu P, Danielson CF, Orazi A, et al. Therapeutic leukapheresis in hyperleucocytic leukemias: lack of correlation between degree of cytoreduction and early mortality rate. Br J Haematol. 1997;98:433–6.
38. De Botton S, Dombret H, Sanz M, et al. Incidence, clinical features and outomce oef all trans-retinoic acid syndrome in 413 cases of newly diagnosed acute promyelocytic leukemia. The European APL Group. Blood. 1998;92(8):2712–8.
39. Barber NA, Ganti AK. Pulmonary toxicities from targeted therapies: a review. Target Oncol. 2011;6(4):235–43.
40. Ohnishi K, Sakai F, Kudoh S, Ohno R. Twenty-seven cases of drug-induced interstitial disease associated with imatinib mesylate. Leukemia. 2006;20(6):1162–4.

41. Yokoyama T, Miyazawa K, Kurakawa E, et al. Interstitial pneumonia induced by imatinib mesylate: pathologic study demonstrates alveolar destruction and fibrosis with eosinophilic infiltration. Leukemia. 2004;18(3):645–6.
42. Montani D, Bergot E, Gunther S, et al. Pulmonary arterial hypertension in patients treated by dasatinib. Circulation. 2012;125(17):2128–37.
43. Lim KH, et al. Severe pulmonary adverse effects in lymphoma patients treated with cyclophosphamide, doxorubicin, vincristine, and prednisone (CHOP) regimen plus rituximab. Korean J Intern Med. 2010;25:86–92.
44. Kim KM, et al. Rituximab-CHOP induced interstitial pneumonitis in patients with disseminated extranodal marginal zone B cell lymphoma. Yonsei Med J. 2008;49:155–8.
45. Lioté H, et al. Rituximab-induced lung disease: a systematic literature review. Eur Respir J. 2010;35:681–7.
46. Spitzer TR. Engraftment syndrome following hematopoietic stem cell transplantation. Bone Marrow Transplant. 2001;27(9):893–8.
47. Khursid I, Anderson LC. Non-infectious pulmonary complications after bone marrow transplantation. Postgrad Med J. 2002;78:257–62.
48. Liu QF, et al. Association between acute graft versus host disease and lung injury after allogeneic haematopoietic stem cell transplantation. Hematology. 2009;14(2):63–72.

Chapter 8
Acute Pulmonary Complications of Bone Marrow and Stem Cell Transplantation

Guang-Shing Cheng and David K. Madtes

Introduction

In the past two decades, advances in the techniques of bone marrow and stem cell transplantation as well as infectious prophylaxis and supportive care have improved the outcomes of patients with hematologic malignancies and other conditions who undergo these procedures [1]. Yet the overall success of hematopoietic cell transplantation (HCT) as life-prolonging therapy remains limited by pulmonary complications, a significant and vexing source of morbidity and mortality. The purpose of this chapter is to provide an overview of the epidemiology and diagnostic considerations of acute pulmonary complications as well as an updated review of specific disease entities or clinical situations in which acute respiratory failure can occur in this unique population of patients. The complications discussed will focus primarily on what is observed in recipients of allogeneic HCT.

For the context of this chapter, the term *acute* will be used to describe pulmonary complications of high acuity that would require immediate medical attention in an acute care setting or result in acute respiratory failure. Traditionally, HCT-related pulmonary disease is considered in the context of the time frame after HCT. Complications that occur within the first 100 days are often categorized as early-onset; after the first 100 days is considered to be late-onset [2]. Early-onset complications tend to be acute in presentation and are directly related to lung injury from the transplantation procedure or infections associated with immune reconstitution status. Most episodes of acute respiratory failure occur in the early period, but acute respiratory failure can occur any time after HCT. After day 100, noninfectious pulmonary disease predominates in the spectrum of HCT-related complications as manifestations of late-onset lung injury or chronic graft-versus-host disease. Some

G.-S. Cheng, MD (✉) • D.K. Madtes, MD
Fred Hutchinson Cancer Research Center, University of Washington School of Medicine, Seattle, WA, USA
e-mail: gcheng2@fredhutch.org; dmadtes@fredhutch.org

J.S. Lee, M.P. Donahoe (eds.), *Hematologic Abnormalities and Acute Lung Syndromes*, Respiratory Medicine, DOI 10.1007/978-3-319-41912-1_8

patients experience acute respiratory failure as a consequence of these entities or from acute infections due to continued immunosuppression. There are several pulmonary syndromes that usually occur in the early post-HCT period, but can occasionally cause respiratory compromise in long-term survivors.

Outcomes of respiratory failure in a contemporary era of transplantation may be improving due to reduced incidence of severe lung injury and improvements in prophylaxis and supportive care [1]. Nonetheless, respiratory failure due to a variety of causes continues to account for the majority of the serious and fatal early complications after HCT.

Acute Respiratory Failure After HCT

Epidemiology of Acute Respiratory Failure

Approximately 15–25 % of HCT recipients require ICU admission. Respiratory failure is the most common indication, historically as well as in contemporary practice, affecting 60 % or more of HCT recipients in the ICU [3]. Acute respiratory failure occurs more frequently in allogeneic recipients compared with autologous recipients. Patients at highest risk for acute respiratory failure requiring mechanical ventilation include those who have a reduced pretransplant FEV_1 or have undergone myeloablative conditioning [4].

Overall, the prognosis of HCT recipients who experience respiratory failure and require mechanical support is poor. Rubenfeld and Crawford proposed an argument for withdrawal of ventilatory support based on a nested case-control study in which the combination of lung injury requiring mechanical ventilation, elevated liver function enzymes, renal dysfunction, and vasopressor support was 100 % predictive of death [5]. This message was tempered by the finding that overall survival of mechanically ventilated patients improved from 5 to 16 % in the last 5 years of their study, which took place between the years 1980 and 1992.

Since this influential article was published nearly 20 years ago, there have been significant advances in ICU care which have improved survival in critically ill patients [6]. A low tidal volume ventilation strategy, in which end-inspiratory plateau pressures are limited to reduce barotrauma and further lung injury, was shown to decrease the mortality from adult respiratory distress syndrome (ARDS) by 22 % as compared to conventional ventilatory settings [7]. Early goal-directed therapy for sepsis as well as an emphasis on prompt empiric antibiotic administration directly impact survival of patients with severe sepsis and circulatory shock [8]. Additional attention to supportive care measures such as aspiration precautions, reduction of sedation, and prevention of iatrogenic complications have likely contributed to improvement in ICU outcomes. HCT-specific factors such as nonmyeloablative conditioning regimens have become more widespread in use, reducing initial toxicities. The incidence of acute GVHD has declined due to prophylactic strategies, and infectious prophylaxis has decreased the incidence of severe early infectious complications [1].

Several recent studies have shown a modest improvement in outcomes of HCT recipients admitted to the ICU including those who require mechanical ventilation [9–11]. In a multicenter retrospective study in France, ICU hospital mortality decreased from 67 to 48 % from 1997–2003 to 2004–2011. Three month mortality of the subgroup requiring mechanical ventilation decreased from 84 to 70 % [11]. Although no longer considered futile, mechanical ventilation remains a significant independent risk factor for mortality in the ICU. Associated organ dysfunction, including shock and liver failure, also remain independent predictors of death [12].

Diagnostic Considerations

The differential diagnosis of acute respiratory failure after HCT is broad and depends on the timing of onset after HCT (Fig. 8.1) [2]. Early after HCT, direct noninfectious complications of the conditioning procedure including volume overload-related pulmonary edema or congestive heart failure and severe mucositis leading to aspiration pneumonitis should always be considered. Idiopathic pneumonia syndrome (IPS), pre-engraftment syndrome, diffuse alveolar hemorrhage (DAH), delayed pulmonary toxicity syndrome (DPTS), and acute fibrinous and organizing pneumonia (AFOP) represent forms of lung injury on a spectrum of histopathologic findings that are specific to the transplantation procedure. The etiology of infectious complications is related to the nature and degree of immunocompromise from the patient's engraftment status and pharmacologic immunosuppression.

These noninfectious etiologies must be distinguished from infectious complications in order to tailor antimicrobial therapy and to guide decisions to empirically augment immunosuppression. Computed tomography (CT) of the chest is mandatory in initial evaluation of respiratory failure, and radiographic patterns may suggest specific etiologies. The differential diagnosis of focal or diffuse infiltrates is broad, and further evaluation is usually undertaken.

Fiberoptic bronchoscopy with bronchoalveolar lavage (BAL) is a minimally invasive modality which is relied upon to make a specific diagnosis for new onset pulmonary infiltrates. The utility of bronchoscopy lies in exclusion of infection when clinical suspicion for a noninfectious etiology is high as much as it is to establish a specific infectious etiology [13]. The diagnostic yield of BAL has improved significantly for specific infectious diagnoses due to the advancements in diagnostic testing, including CMV rapid shell vial culture, aspergillus galactomannan, and respiratory viral PCR panel (Table 8.1) [14]. Two retrospective studies done in the era of routine anti-infective prophylaxis against fungus, CMV, and *Pneumocystis jirovecii*, report the yield of fiberoptic bronchoscopy for a specific diagnosis is 34–50 %, with a higher yield for allogeneic HCT [15, 16]. The majority of the diagnoses are achievable by BAL alone, with transbronchial biopsy adding additional specific information in <10 % of cases.

While aggressive diagnostic workup is appropriate for HCT patients, the impact of BAL on patient outcomes is difficult to ascertain [13]. Various factors including the

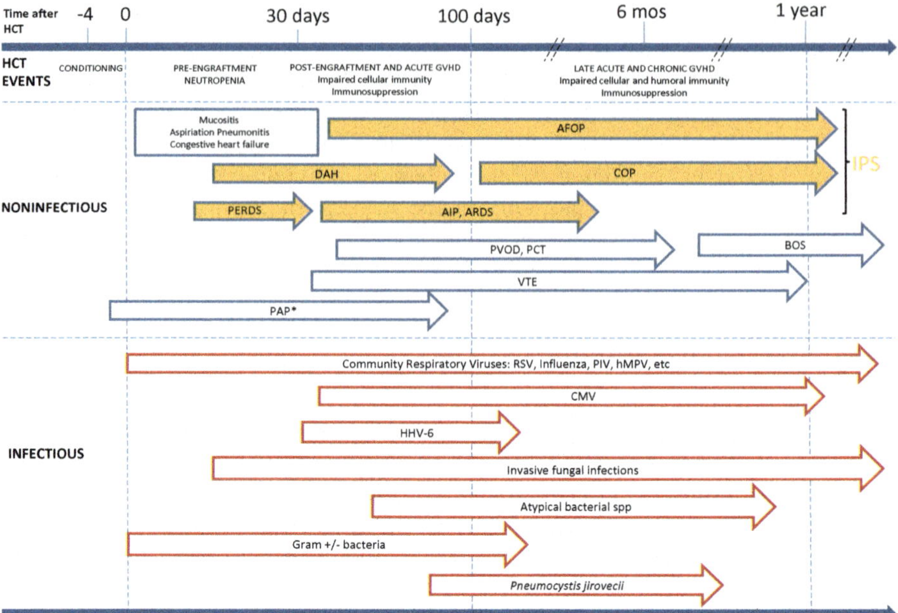

Fig. 8.1 Timeline of infectious and noninfectious pulmonary complications after allogeneic hematopoietic cell transplantation. *AFOP* acute fibrinous and organizing pneumonia, *AIP* acute interstitial pneumonitis, *ARDS* acute respiratory distress syndrome, *BOS* bronchiolitis obliterans syndrome, *COP* cryptogenic organizing pneumonia, *CMV* cytomegalovirus, *GVHD* graft-versus-host disease, *HHV-6* human herpesvirus-6, *HMPV* human metapneumovirus, *PAP* pulmonary alveolar proteinosis, *PCT* pulmonary cytolytic thrombi, *PIV* parainfluenza virus, *PVOD* pulmonary veno-occlusive disease, *PERDS* peri-engraftment respiratory distress syndrome, *VTE* venous thromboembolism, *RSV* respiratory syncytial virus. *PAP has been reported to occur >1 year post-HCT. Adapted from Ref. [13]

timing of procedure may influence the clinical outcome, as patients are often referred for BAL after persistence or progression of disease on empiric antibiotic therapy. A large retrospective study of 501 consecutive patients who underwent 598 BALs for the evaluation of new pulmonary infiltrates and suspected pneumonia during the first 100 days after HCT showed that the yield of BAL for clinically significant pathogens was 2.5-fold higher ($p<0.0001$) if performed within the first 4 days of presentation, compared to those performed late, and that the yield was highest when performed within 24 h of presentation. Mortality at 30 and 100 days following the BAL was significantly lower when a diagnosis of infection was confirmed by early BAL compared to late BAL, which was associated with multidrug-resistant and polymicrobial infections [17]. These findings suggest that BAL should be used in the early evaluation of HCT recipients with pulmonary infiltrates, as opposed to a conservative, expectant approach of bronchoscopy only after the failure of empiric therapy.

The use of bronchoscopy has largely supplanted surgical biopsy as means of diagnosing unknown lung disease in HCT patients. When treatment decisions depend on a definitive diagnosis of a noninfectious etiology and when empiric ther-

Table 8.1 Laboratory evaluation of bronchoalveolar lavage specimens for specific infectious agents

	Bacterial	Fungal	Viral	Parasitic
Pathologic exam	Wright-Giemsa Papanicolaou's Modified Jimenez stain (*Legionella*)	Silver stain (*Pneumocystis jirovecii*) Fungal hyphae Yeast forms	Viral inclusions (CMV)	Larval forms (*Strongyloides*)
Microbiology—stains	Gram stain Acid fast Modified acid fast	Wet mount KOH Calcofluor white stain		
Culture	Aerobic and anaerobic Chocolate yeast extract (*Legionella*) Acid-fast Nocardia Actinomycoses	Fungal	Routine viral culture Rapid centrifugation "shell vial" (CMV, RSV)	
Immunoassay	DFA (*Legionella*)	ELISA for galactomannan IFA/DFA (*Pneumocystis jirovecii*)	DFA (influenza) DFA (CMV)	Immunostain (*Toxoplasma*)
Molecular diagnostics: PCR	*Chlamydia* *Mycoplasma*	*Aspergillus* Pan-fungal (including *Mucorales* spp.	Herpesviruses: CMV, EBV, HSV, VZV, HHV-6 CRVs: RSV, influenza, PIV-3, hMPV, rhinovirus, bocavirus, adenovirus Coronavirus	*Toxoplasma*

apy is risky, surgical lung biopsy may be required to achieve a specific diagnosis, as is that case for pulmonary venoocclusive disease and pulmonary cytologic thrombi, for example. Surgical lung biopsy has the advantage of direct visualization of the biopsy site, as well as obtaining a large enough piece of tissue that allows for histologic examination and culture. Bleeding in the setting of thrombocytopenia can be controlled directly. In contemporary practice surgical lung biopsy is usually performed videoscopically (video assisted thoracic surgery, or VATS), which theoretically reduces the morbidity associated with thoracotomy. Lung biopsy in this population must be carefully considered, as the morbidity of surgery in the setting of neutropenia, thrombocytopenia and/or respiratory failure may be unacceptably high, particularly if the overall prognosis is poor and specific therapy is unlikely to alter the outcome. White and colleagues at Memorial Sloan Kettering Cancer Center reviewed 67 open lung biopsies in 63 patients with hematologic malignancies from 1996 to 1998, including 25 bone marrow transplant patients, and found that a specific diagnosis was found in 41 (62 %) of the biopsies. Focal lesions were much more likely than diffuse lesions to yield a specific diagnosis (79 % vs. 36 %), and neutropenic or mechanically ventilated patients had a low likelihood of having a specific diagnosis. The risk of complications was significant, affecting 13 % of the biopsies, including 1 death [18].

In contrast to classic reports in bone marrow transplant recipients prior to the era of CMV and fungal prophylaxis [19, 20], infectious etiologies are no longer the most common diagnoses at lung biopsy: inflammatory conditions were the most common specific diagnoses (23 %), followed by infection (21 %) and malignancy (18 %) [18]. The likelihood of an HCT recipient undergoing a surgical lung biopsy has continued to decline in the past two decades, and infectious etiologies at lung biopsy, particularly invasive aspergillosis, are significantly less likely than a noninfectious etiology, likely due to the introduction of broad spectrum triazole therapy against invasive fungal infection in the early 2000s [21]. A recent meta-analysis showed that the overall yield of a specific diagnosis was similar between BAL and surgery (53 % vs. 54 %), with a complication rate of 8 and 15 % for BAL and surgery, respectively. The proportion of noninfectious diagnosis exceeded the infectious diagnoses with surgical biopsy [22].

Noninfectious Etiologies

Lung Injury Syndromes, Early Onset

Idiopathic Pneumonia Syndrome

A spectrum of acute lung injuries can develop in the early posttransplantation period that fall under the category of the *idiopathic pneumonia syndrome* (IPS), and includes diffuse alveolar hemorrhage, peri-engraftment syndrome, delayed pulmonary toxicity syndrome and acute fibrinous and organizing pneumonia (Table 8.2). Broadly defined as widespread alveolar injury seen after HCT in the absence of active lower respiratory tract infection, cardiac dysfunction, acute renal failure, or iatrogenic fluid overload, IPS is thought to result from a variety of lung insults including toxic effects of the HCT conditioning regimen, immunologic cell-mediated injury, inflammatory cytokines, and occult pulmonary infections [2]. With the increasing use of new diagnostic methods such as multiplex PCR for respiratory viruses and the biomarker galactomannan for *Aspergillus* spp., the incidence of acute lung injury secondary to pulmonary infection has increased. Seo et al. have shown that approximately half of patients with IPS had pathogens detected in the BAL when these newer diagnostic methods were employed and that pathogen detection was associated with increased mortality. The most frequent pathogens were human herpes virus-6 (HHV-6), human rhinovirus (HRV), cytomegalovirus (CMV),

Table 8.2 The spectrum of clinical lung injury entities after HCT classified under IPS

Clinical entity	Timing of onset after HCT	Histology	Diagnostic considerations	Prognosis
Acute fibrinous organizing pneumonia (AFOP)	Early or late	Intra-alveolar fibrin, organizing pneumonia and type II pneumocyte hyperplasia		Poor
Acute interstitial pneumonia (AIP)	2–6 mos	Diffuse alveolar damage		Poor
Acute respiratory distress syndrome (ARDS)	2–6 mos	Diffuse alveolar damage		Poor
Cryptogenic organizing pneumonia (COP)	2–12 mos	Patchy plugs of granulation tissue and macrophages in distal airways and alveoli	Chest CT: Ground glass & linear opacities, upper lobe predominance	Favorable
Diffuse alveolar hemorrhage (DAH)	<1 mo–3 mos	Diffuse alveolar damage; intra-alveolar red blood cells and hemosiderin-laden macrophages	Progressively bloodier BAL fluid	Poor
Delayed pulmonary toxicity syndrome (DPTS)	1–6 mos	Type II pneumocyte hyperplasia, septal thickening, interstitial fibrosis, small vessel endothelial injury	Autologous transplants only	Favorable
Peri-engraftment respiratory distress syndrome (PERDS)	Within 5–7 days of neutrophil engraftment	Diffuse alveolar damage	Neutrophilic inflammation on BAL	Favorable

and *Aspergillus* spp. [23]. Of note, HHV-6, like CMV, is in the human β-herpesvirus family and latently infects 95 % of healthy adults. HHV-6 has been shown to reactivate frequently in critically ill patients, but its specific role in the pathogenesis of respiratory disease and outcomes in critical illness remains unknown [24].

IPS has been classified into specific entities based in large part on the presumed site of primary tissue injury. The primary anatomical sites of inflammation and dysfunction are divided into three subtypes: (1) pulmonary parenchymal, (2) vascular endothelial, and (3) airway epithelial [25]. Each subtype is further classified into distinct entities of noninfectious acute lung injury. While some IPS cases remain unclassified, this classification scheme may facilitate the development of therapeutic interventions that can be directed toward distinct subtypes of disease [25] (Table 8.2).

An association between IPS and acute GVHD has been reported, but the specific role of alloreactive donor T lymphocytes in the pathogenesis of IPS remains unclear. Although identified in the lungs of some patients with IPS, epithelial apoptosis, considered pathognomonic for acute GVHD, has not been consistently detected in allogeneic HCT recipients with acute lung dysfunction. There is no pathognomonic histologic finding that defines IPS [25], as the histology depends upon the anatomic site of injury. The diagnosis of IPS is rarely confirmed by tissue biopsy given the significant risks of open lung biopsy in this population and the low yield of lung tissue by transbronchial biopsy via fiberoptic bronchoscopy recovered from HCT patients with acute lung injury. The diagnosis of IPS is usually one of exclusion in the appropriate clinical context; BAL is often performed to exclude infection.

The cumulative incidence of IPS after allogeneic HCT ranges from 2.2 % following nonmyeloablative conditioning to 8.4 % following conventional, full-intensity radiation containing preparative regimens [26]. The median time of onset after allogeneic HCT is 19 days (range, 4–106 days) with mortality rates ranging from 60 to 80 % overall to greater than 95 % for patients requiring mechanical ventilation. Although IPS also develops after *autologous* HCT, the incidence is lower, the median time to onset is generally later (63 days; range 7–336 days), the response to corticosteroids is usually prompt and the prognosis is favorable compared with IPS in allogeneic HCT recipients.

Risk factors for IPS after allogeneic HCT include full-intensity conditioning with total body irradiation, acute GVHD, older recipient age, an underlying diagnosis of acute leukemia or myelodysplastic syndrome and the number of platelet transfusions administered [27]. Risk factors for IPS following autologous HCT include older patient age, severe oral mucositis, conditioning regimens using total body irradiation or carmustine (BCNU), chest irradiation within 2 weeks before transplant, female gender, and an underlying diagnosis of solid tumor [2, 25].

Current standard treatment strategies of IPS include broad-spectrum antibiotics and IV corticosteroids and supportive care with lung protective mechanical ventilation and venovenous ultrafiltration for those with respiratory failure. Response to corticosteroids (≤2 mg/kg/day) has shown mixed efficacy in allogeneic HCT recipients, which likely reflects the diversity of underlying causes responsible for the lung insult. Compared with lower doses, higher doses of corticosteroid therapy (>2 mg/kg/day) have not been shown to improve outcome but are associated with increased iatrogenic complications including fungal infection [26, 28]. Prophylaxis against filamentous fungal infection with voriconazole or micafungin is recommended during treatment with corticosteroids (≥0.5 mg/kg/day) because fungal pneumonia was identified in 16 % (4/25) of IPS patients at the time of autopsy in a single-center study.

Preclinical and clinical studies suggest that neutralization of *tumor necrosis factor* (TNF)-α may be a useful therapeutic strategy for IPS. In a multicenter, Phase II single-arm, open-label study by Yanik and colleagues in pediatric HCT recipients, treatment with etanercept (0.4 mg/kg/dose twice weekly for 8 doses)

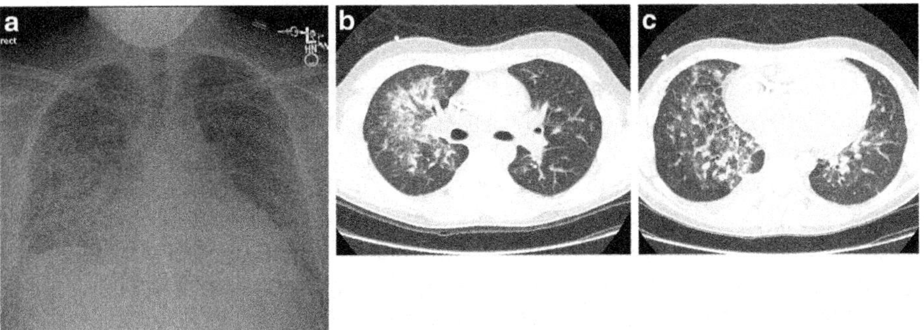

Fig. 8.2 DAH in a patient 23 days following an allogeneic stem cell transplant with new onset hemoptysis and respiratory insufficiency. DAH was diagnosed by bronchoscopy which showed progressively bloodier lavage fluid. (**a**) Chest radiograph shows patchy consolidation. (**b**, **c**) Chest CT shows diffuse ground glass opacities with areas of denser consolidation within a peribronchial vascular distribution

plus corticosteroids (2 mg/kg/day) resulted in a complete response in 71 % (20 of 28) of patients and was associated with a high overall survival compared with historical controls [29]. In a randomized, double-blind, placebo-controlled trial of corticosteroids (2 mg/kg/day) with etanercept (0.4 mg/kg/dose twice weekly for 8 doses) or placebo for the treatment of IPS, the use of corticosteroids was associated with higher response rates (defined as alive with complete discontinuation of supplemental oxygen support at days 28 and 54 after initiation of therapy) and overall survival compared to historical controls, but the addition of etanercept did not lead to further increases in response [30]. This study was truncated early and the small sample size precluded a definitive conclusion regarding the benefit of etanercept therapy.

Diffuse alveolar hemorrhage (DAH), also called *acute pulmonary hemorrhage* or *hemorrhagic alveolitis,* is a common subset of IPS that generally develops in the immediate post-transplant period and is characterized by progressive dyspnea, cough, and hypoxemia with or without fever and diffuse bilateral pulmonary infiltrates (Fig. 8.2). The cumulative incidence of DAH is 5–12 % of HCT patients with a median time of onset of 19 days (range, 5–34 days) in allogeneic recipients and 12 days (range, 0–40 days) in autologous patients. The diagnosis is based on progressively bloodier return of BAL fluid. Treatment of DAH consists of aggressive platelet support to maintain a platelet count greater than or equal to 100,000 and high-dose systemic corticosteroids (2 mg/kg/day to 1 g/m^2/day). The addition of aminocaproic acid or recombinant factor VII may further improve outcomes. Despite these interventions, the mortality from DAH ranges from 60 to 100 % with death usually due to multiorgan failure within 3 weeks of diagnosis [2].

Peri-engraftment respiratory distress syndrome (PERDS) develops within 5–7 days of engraftment and accounts for 33 % of IPS cases after allogeneic HCT. Although the clinical presentation of PERDS after HCT is similar to other subsets of IPS, lung dysfunction is more responsive to corticosteroids and the prognosis is better [31].

The incidence of *delayed pulmonary toxicity syndrome* (DPTS) is 29–64 % in autologous HCT recipients receiving chemotherapy with regimens containing BCNU, cyclophosphamide, and cisplatin. The median time of onset is 45 days (range, 21–149 days), and treatment with corticosteroids (1 mg/kg/day) results in resolution in up to 92 % of cases [32].

Acute fibrinous and organizing pneumonia (AFOP) is an infrequently observed subset of IPS that is histologically characterized by the presence of intra-alveolar fibrin that form fibrin "balls" within the alveolar spaces, organizing pneumonia composed of intraluminal loose connective tissue within alveolar ducts and bronchioles in association with the fibrin and type II pneumocyte hyperplasia, typically in a patchy distribution. AFOP has been associated with a variety of disease states, including HCT [33], infections, rheumatologic diseases as well as environmental and drug exposures. The presenting symptoms may include fever, cough, dyspnea, hemoptysis, malaise, arthralgias, and chest, pleural, or abdominal pain. Two distinct clinical courses have been reported: (1) an acute and fulminant course typically leading to respiratory failure and death and (2) a less severe, subacute course. The radiographic findings of patients with an acute presentation and rapid decline are similar to those of diffuse alveolar damage including diffuse but basilar predominant consolidation and ground glass opacities. The radiographic features of patients with subacute AFOP are indistinguishable from those of organizing pneumonia with both focal and diffuse parenchymal abnormalities. Although no specific therapy exists, case reports describe response to corticosteroids [34] and immunosuppressant therapy [35].

Lung Injury Syndromes, Late Onset

Cryptogenic Organizing Pneumonia

Cryptogenic organizing pneumonia (COP), originally given the term *bronchiolitis obliterans organizing pneumonia* (BOOP), was first described by Epler in 1985 as a distinct clinicopathologic entity that can affect the general population. As a histologic entity, organizing pneumonia (OP) may be associated with bacterial and viral infections, but most OP in the general population is idiopathic, hence the term cryptogenic organizing pneumonia (COP). In HCT recipients, the histology is characterized by patchy plugs of granulation tissue occupying distal terminal airways, alveolar ducts and alveolar sacs, widened alveolar septa and mononuclear cell infiltration, and accumulation of foamy macrophages within alveoli (Fig. 8.3) [36]. In the context of noninfectious pulmonary entities after HCT, COP may be considered a late-onset manifestation on one end of the spectrum of lung injury syndromes, of which IPS occupies the early onset, acute end of the spectrum [37].

In an analysis of 49 biopsy-proven cases of COP after allogeneic HCT, there was a significant association with the presence of acute or chronic graft-versus-host disease (GVHD) by multivariate analysis. Of note, the severity of the GVHD, acute or

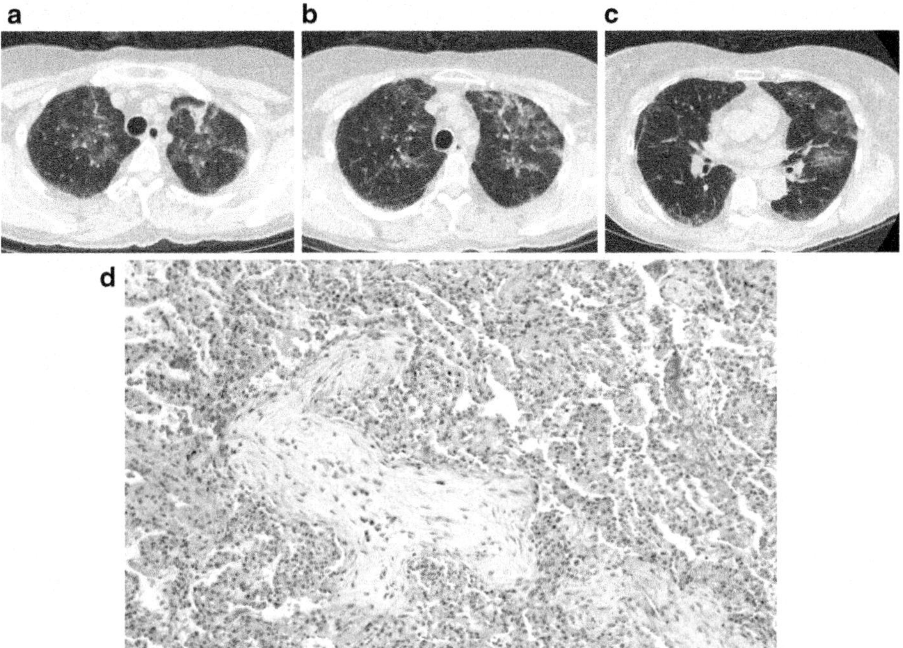

Fig. 8.3 COP after HCT. (**a**–**c**) Serial Chest CT images in the same individual showing upper lobe predominant reticular linear and ground glass opacities. (**d**) Example of COP on lung biopsy showing patchy plugs of granulation tissue within distal small airways and alveolar spaces with macrophages and inflammatory infiltrate. Courtesy of Drs. Robert Hackman and David Myerson

chronic, was significantly greater in patients with COP compared with controls, and 22 % of the cases were diagnosed in the setting of corticosteroid taper for GVHD [36]. The association with severe acute GVHD and extensive chronic GVHD in survivors beyond day 100 was also shown in a large retrospective study of 193 HCT recipients from a Japanese registry of 9550 allogeneic HCT recipients. Other risk factors that were shown to be associated with COP included donor HLA disparity, female-to-male HCT, related peripheral blood stem cell transplantation and radiation as part of a myeloablative conditioning regimen [38]. Although an alloimmune mechanism may be postulated from the reported association with GVHD, there is currently no direct evidence of a donor T-cell-mediated immune response against lung tissue in this entity.

The clinical presentation of COP after HCT is similar to that in other clinical settings: fever, cough, and progressive dyspnea arising in a subacute to acute tempo. The median time of onset in allogeneic HCT recipients is approximately 3 months after transplant, although many cases are diagnosed after day 100 and in long-term survivors up to several years after transplant. Since the presentation may be subacute and insidious, many patients are diagnosed in the outpatient setting, but the disease can progress to acute respiratory failure necessitating ventilator support. In the aforementioned case series, the median time to diagnosis was 108 days after

HCT (range 5–2819 days), after a median symptom duration of 13 days. Pulmonary function testing may reveal a new restrictive defect (43 %), obstructive defect (11 %), mixed restrictive and obstructive defect (8 %), or normal physiology (38 %). Sixty-four percent had a new diffusing capacity deficit [36]. The radiographic hallmark of COP on chest CT is ground glass opacities, with linear opacities in an upper lobe, often bilateral, distribution (Fig. 8.3). Features of biopsy-proven COP on chest CT include ground glass opacities (94 %), consolidation (50 %), and linear opacities (50 %) with an upper lobe predominance (63 %) [39]. These linear opacities are usually not described in COP that occurs in non-HCT settings. Because the radiographic findings as well as the clinical presentation may mimic infectious pneumonia, bronchoscopy with lavage is recommended to exclude infectious etiologies. In cases in which a clinical diagnosis is still unclear, a histologic diagnosis by surgical lung biopsy may be warranted.

The mainstay of treatment for COP after HCT is corticosteroids, usually initiated at a dose of 0.5–1.0 mg/kg/day, depending on the severity. If the patient has severe disease or is in acute respiratory failure, administration of pulse steroids with 1–2 g initial dosing is justified. Recent recommendations suggest treating with corticosteroids starting at 0.75 mg/kg/day until symptomatic or radiographic improvement is noted then tapering slowly over a minimum of 4–6 months [40]. Although there is little more than anecdotal evidence for the use of macrolides in this population, chronic clarithromycin or azithromycin may be added as an adjunctive immunomodulatory agent in patients who have difficulty tapering or tolerating corticosteroids [41].

Overall, prognosis for COP after HCT is good, with a majority of cases resolving or stabilizing with corticosteroids. Relapse is common, particularly when corticosteroid taper is accelerated. A small, but significant proportion of patients will progress in spite of therapy and ultimately succumb to respiratory failure. In refractory cases, it is hypothesized that the interstitial inflammation sets up a process of progressive interstitial fibrosis, evidenced by progressive interstitial changes on computed tomography. It is not known what factors contribute to progression, or which individuals are at risk for progression. As more patients survive past day 100 after allogeneic HCT, there is a sense amongst transplant physicians that COP is increasing in frequency, but the true incidence is difficult to ascertain given the relative rarity of the condition and histologic confirmation by lung biopsy is now rarely undertaken. Investigation into this entity and its impact on HCT outcomes and non-relapse mortality is warranted.

Bronchiolitis Obliterans Syndrome

Bronchiolitis obliterans syndrome (BOS) is a late-onset and chronic pulmonary problem, but it is considered here because acute respiratory failure can occur in the setting of rapid airflow decline and infectious complications. BOS is characterized by new onset irreversible airflow obstruction in the setting of prior or active chronic graft-versus-host disease and usually occurs within the first 2 years after

HCT. Although the pathogenesis of BOS is unknown, it is likely a form of lung injury caused by an alloimmune response to the airway epithelium. An aberrant repair response results in the obliteration of small airways with fibrous material, which leads to the physiologic correlate of airways obstruction [42]. The clinical manifestations of BOS are usually insidious, but there is a phenotype of rapidly progressive airflow obstruction which can lead to primary respiratory failure [43]. Even when patients with BOS are stabilized, morbidity and mortality from BOS are high, and result mainly from infectious pneumonia or progressive chronic respiratory failure [42].

Drug-Induced Pneumonitis

Individual components of some conditioning regimens used in HCT are associated with pulmonary toxicity. Carmustine (or bischloroethylnitrosourea, BCNU), used as a single agent or in combination prior to autologous HCT for solid tumor and hematologic malignancies, is associated with acute onset pneumonitis with an incidence of 4–59 %. Prior mediastinal radiation therapy, BCNU dose greater than 1000 mg and age less than 54 were independent risk factors for developing pneumonitis after autologous HCT for lymphoma [44]. The mechanism of BCNU-associated pulmonary toxicity has not been entirely elucidated but is thought to include oxidative stress, glutathione dysfunction and immune-mediated lung injury [45].

Cyclophosphamide is another agent used in combination with total body radiation or other chemotherapy agents in preparative regimens for autologous and allogeneic HCT that is associated with pulmonary toxicity thought to be related to increased reactive oxygen species generation and depletion of glutathione stores [46].

A spectrum of drug-induced lung diseases has been reported after transplantation in association with immunosuppressive therapies. Implicated immunosuppressive agents and their patterns of pulmonary toxicity are listed in Table 8.3. Noncardiogenic pulmonary edema and ARDS have been reported in association with intravenous and oral cyclosporine after bone marrow transplantation that resolves when the medication is discontinued and is postulated to be an idiosyncratic reaction [2].

The mammalian target of rapamycin (mTOR) inhibitor, sirolimus, binds to rapamycin-FK binding protein-12 to inhibit T and B lymphocyte proliferation for induction and long term maintenance of immunosuppression. In HCT, it is used for acute GVHD prophylaxis in the early post-HCT period [47], and then as primary immunosuppression in active chronic GVHD. Pulmonary toxicities are rare but do occur with sirolimus in this context, and may be severe and fatal [48, 49]. The clinical presentation of sirolimus–induced lung injury is well described in the solid organ transplantation population, and includes cough (96 %), fatigue (83 %), fever (67 %), dyspnea (33 %), and hemoptysis (8 %). Physical exam is noted for hypoxemia (50 %) and inspiratory crackles (50 %). Radiographic findings on CT scan include patchy bilateral asymmetrical peripheral consolidations (COP-like pattern) (79 %), reticular and ground glass opacities (17 %) and lobar consolidation (4 %)

Table 8.3 Pulmonary toxicity of immunosuppressant agents

Immunosuppressant	Pulmonary toxicity
Monoclonal antibodies	
Muromanab-CD3 (OKT3)	Capillary leak (noncardiogenic pulmonary edema), ARDS
Basiliximab-CD25 (anti-IL2 receptor) antibody	Capillary leak (noncardiogenic pulmonary edema)
Alemtuzumab anti-CD52 antibody	Diffuse alveolar hemorrhage
Rituximab anti-CD-20 antibody	ARDS, diffuse alveolar hemorrhage interstitial pneumonitis, cryptogenic organizing pneumonia, pulmonary fibrosis, hypersensitivity pneumonitis
Calcineurin inhibitors	
Cyclosporine	Capillary leak (noncardiogenic pulmonary edema), ARDS
Tacrolimus	Cryptogenic organizing pneumonia
mTOR inhibitors	
Sirolimus	Organizing pneumonia, diffuse alveolar hemorrhage, ARDS, pulmonary alveolar proteinosis
Everolimus	Interstitial pneumonitis, diffuse alveolar hemorrhage, ARDS
Mycophenolate mofetil	Pulmonary edema, ARDS, pulmonary fibrosis, bronchiectasis
Azathioprine	Cryptogenic organizing pneumonia, diffuse alveolar hemorrhage, interstitial pneumonitis,laryngeal edema, vasculitis

[50]. BAL reveals lymphocytic or eosinophilic alveolitis in up to 92 % of cases. The predominant histologic patterns are organizing pneumonia, pulmonary hemorrhage, diffuse alveolar damage, and in a minority of cases, pulmonary alveolar proteinosis. The mainstay of treatment is discontinuation of the drug with or without corticosteroids (1 mg/kg/day), which results in complete resolution of symptoms within 2–4 months. Less severe cases can be managed by a reduction in the sirolimus dose with close monitoring of serum levels, however, relapses have been reported with this approach [2].

Pulmonary Alveolar Proteinosis

Pulmonary alveolar proteinosis (PAP) is a rare disease characterized by the accumulation of surfactant lipids and protein in alveolar spaces resulting in gas exchange impairment. Primary, or autoimmune PAP, is due to the presence of autoantibodies against GM-CSF, which is a critical regulator of surfactant homeostasis. Secondary PAP comprises 7–10 % of PAP cases, and occurs primarily in the setting of hematologic malignancies or unusual infections (e.g., *Pneumocystis jirovecii* or *Nocardia* spp). The underlying defect is thought to be due to qualitative and quantitative macrophage dysfunction, as by definition, there are no autoantibodies against GM-CSF, which distinguishes it from primary PAP [51]. In the context of HCT, secondary

PAP is extremely rare but has been shown in autopsy series as a cause of undiagnosed premortem noninfectious pulmonary disease. PAP has been reported following autologous HCT, cord blood transplantation and cord blood transplantation in association with parainfluenza virus 3 [52]. There are cases of PAP which have resolved after chemotherapy or HCT for the underlying leukemia, presumably due to correction of the quantitative defect of macrophages present in marrow-infiltrating disease processes. Patients with PAP are at risk for infections, which may also confound the presentation and diagnosis in HCT recipients.

As with primary PAP, secondary PAP may be mild and self-limited or may progress to respiratory failure. Patients with secondary PAP present with progressive exertional dyspnea and nonproductive cough, a restrictive pattern and severely reduced diffusing capacity on pulmonary function tests. Computed tomography of the chest shows diffuse or patchy ground glass opacities, interlobular thickening, and subpleural sparing, or a "crazy paving" pattern, although this is more typical of primary PAP. Bronchoscopy reveals a milky, opaque lavage fluid containing large and foamy alveolar macrophages that stains positive with periodic acid-Schiff and is diagnostic in the appropriate clinical setting. The BAL may not reveal PAS+ material, as described in a recent case report [52], in which case surgical biopsy showing PAS+ material in architecturally preserved alveolar spaces may be required to confirm the diagnosis. Therapy of secondary PAP is directed at the underlying condition, i.e., treatment of infection or malignancy, in addition to supportive care. Corticosteroids are generally ineffective for this condition, and the mainstay of treatment is whole lung lavage. Exogenous GM-CSF for PAP after HCT is not effective, and the course of the disease may be self-limited.

Pulmonary Vascular Disease

Venous thromboembolism (VTE) is an under-recognized complication of HCT. In a retrospective study of 1514 HCT recipients, the incidence of symptomatic VTE within the first 180 days post transplantation was 4.6 % including 0.7 % incidence of non-catheter-associated lower extremity DVT and 0.6 % incidence of pulmonary emboli [53]. The median time after HCT admission to the development of non-catheter-associated lower extremity DVT and pulmonary embolism was 63 and 66 days, respectively. Risk factors for the development of VTE were prior VTE and GVHD. Thrombocytopenia was only partially protective against the development of VTE [53]. The safety and efficacy of thromboprophylaxis in HCT patients remains uncertain. In patients with thrombocytopenia, anticoagulant therapy for documented VTE should be accompanied by platelet transfusions to maintain a platelet count of 50×10^9/L or greater to reduce the risk of bleeding complications [2].

Pulmonary veno-occlusive disease (PVOD) is a rare, late-onset complication after HCT that presents with the insidious onset of fatigue and exertional dyspnea within 3–4 months after transplant. The physical examination typically shows hypoxemia and resting tachycardia consistent with pulmonary hypertension. Right heart catheterization demonstrates elevated pulmonary artery pressures with normal pulmonary capillary wedge pressure, and angiography is used to exclude pulmonary emboli as the etiology for the pulmonary hypertension. The diagnosis of PVOD is strongly supported by the triad of pulmonary artery hypertension, radiographic evidence of pulmonary edema, and normal pulmonary artery occlusion pressures; however, lung biopsy confirms the diagnosis by the presence of extensive and diffuse intimal proliferation and fibrosis of pulmonary venules [54]. Treatment consists of high-dose corticosteroids (methylprednisolone 2 mg/kg/day) with anecdotal success, but the overall prognosis of PVOD after HCT remains poor [55].

Pulmonary cytolytic thrombus (PCT) is seen exclusively in allogeneic HCT recipients and almost always in children. The incidence of PCT has been reported to range from 1.2 to 4 % with a median onset at 3 months (range 1.3–11.3 months) after transplant. Clinical manifestations include fever, cough, and respiratory distress, and CT findings range from small, peripheral nodules to diffuse opacities. Diagnosis requires lung biopsy with histology characterized by vascular occlusions in distal pulmonary vessels, entrapment of leukocytes, endothelial disruption, and infarction of adjacent tissue. In a single-center, retrospective study, grades II to IV acute and chronic GVHD were independent risk factors for developing PCT. Treatment for PCT consists of systemic corticosteroids (prednisone 1–2 mg/kg/day) until pulmonary symptoms resolve (typically within 2 weeks) followed by a steroid taper over 2–4 weeks. The strong association with acute and chronic GVHD, as well as the response to corticosteroid therapy, suggests that PCT is a manifestation of alloreactive lung injury. The prognosis with PCT is favorable, and there have been no reported deaths attributable to this entity [56, 57].

Infectious Etiologies

The profound alterations in immune status associated with bone marrow and stem cell transplantation renders this population vulnerable to severe opportunistic and community-acquired pneumonias that can precipitate acute respiratory failure (Fig. 8.1). In the first month after HCT, neutropenia and immune suppression from management of acute early GVHD contribute to the infection risk predominantly due to bacterial pneumonia from nosocomial gram-positive and gram-negative organisms, herpes simplex virus, and *Candida* species. The early post-engraftment phase from 1 to 6 month post-HCT is characterized by impaired cellular immunity, continued immune suppression for GVHD, and interruptions in prophylaxis; opportunistic viral and fungal infections predominate. In the late post-engraftment phase, when immunosuppressive therapy is decreased in most patients, pulmonary infections are due more commonly to community-acquired organisms than opportunistic pathogens [2].

Because HCT recipients are particularly vulnerable to uncommon pathogens and suffer severe manifestations of common pathogens, much of what has been learned about these particular agents comes from the experience in this population. In this section we focus our review on the most important viral and fungal pathogens affecting HCT recipients in the contemporary era.

Cytomegalovirus

Although specific antiviral therapy and preemptive treatment strategies have reduced the impact of cytomegalovirus (CMV) pneumonia in the early posttransplant period, CMV remains the most important opportunistic viral pathogen and cause of acute respiratory disease and mortality in HCT recipients. Prior to the implementation of CMV prophylaxis in the late 1990s, the incidence of CMV pneumonia was 10–30 % after allogeneic HCT and 1–6 % in autologous recipients. The use of ganciclovir for prophylaxis in the early posttransplant period has decreased the overall incidence to 5–8 % and has increased the proportion of disease occurring in the late transplant period (>100 days) [58]. Risk factors for developing late onset disease include CMV antigenemia in the first 3 months, delayed lymphocyte engraftment, low CD4 counts, and acute graft-versus-host disease [59]. In a single center retrospective review of 421 cases of CMV pneumonia over a 25 year span, the overall survival of HCT recipients after CMV pneumonia onset was approximately 30 %; treatment with IV ganciclovir or foscarnet was associated with decreased overall mortality of patients with CMV pneumonia over time. Not surprisingly, coinfection with other lung pathogens was associated with increased overall mortality. Lymphopenia and the use of mechanical ventilation at the time of CMV onset were independently associated with an increased risk of 6-month CMV-attributable mortality [60].

The diagnosis of CMV pneumonia requires evidence of the virus by culture, cytology, immunohistochemistry, polymerase chain reaction (PCR), or direct fluorescent antibody methods in BAL fluid or lung biopsy, in conjunction with bilateral infiltrates on chest imaging. The use of rapid detection of CMV by shell vial culture is a highly sensitive method of detecting CMV that has improved the utility of bronchoscopy in making the diagnosis [14]. Quantitative PCR from the BAL may have higher sensitivity for CMV and is now used by many centers; however, lack of an appropriate cutoff for the viral load limits the interpretation of positive results. The presence of intranuclear inclusions on lung biopsy confirms the presence of CMV pneumonia, but lung biopsy is now rarely required to achieve diagnosis. The majority of patients with CMV pneumonia will have evidence of CMV reactivation in the blood [58].

First line antiviral therapy for CMV disease is IV ganciclovir, a nucleoside analog that inhibits DNA synthesis, with an induction phase of 7–21 days followed by at least 2 weeks of maintenance therapy. The major side effect of ganciclovir is neutropenia which limits its use in the pre-engraftment phase. High-dose intravenous pooled immunoglobulin or CMV-specific immunoglobulin administered as an adjunct to IV ganciclovir has been the standard of care for many years based on early open label trials, but recent analyses show no effect on attributable mortality [60]. Foscarnet, which inhibits CMV viral polymerase, is second line therapy in patients with known resistance to ganciclovir. Its major side effect is nephrotoxicity. Third line therapy is cidofovir, a competitive inhibitor of DNA polymerase, which has significant renal and hematologic toxicities [58].

Antiviral prophylaxis with gancyclovir has been shown in clinical trials to reduce the burden of disease early after transplant at the cost of prolonged neutropenia and increased bacterial and fungal infections as well as selection of ganciclovir-resistant strains of CMV. Most institutions use a preemptive strategy in which only those patients who show evidence of CMV reactivation in the blood by antigenemia or viral load on weekly screening are treated with ganciclovir to decrease the risk of CMV pneumonia [58].

Community Respiratory Viruses

Community respiratory viruses (CRV) cause considerable morbidity and mortality in the immunocompromised population when upper respiratory tract illness progresses to lower tract disease and acute respiratory failure. Risk factors for progression to pneumonia in HCT recipients include infection early after transplantation, allogeneic HCT, myeloablative conditioning, GVHD, and lymphopenia [61]. The majority of clinically relevant CRV can be diagnosed with nasal washing, nasopharyngeal swabs, or BAL by rapid antigen detection or RT-PCR methods. There are few specific antiviral agents with efficacy against CRV and management is primarily supportive. HCT recipients may shed virus for prolonged periods of time [62].

CRVs include influenza, respiratory syncytial virus (RSV), and parainfluenza serotypes-1 and 2, which have their peak primarily in the winter months, and parainfluenza serotype-3 and adenovirus, which occur year round. Patterns of influenza infection in HCT recipients reflect the seasonal occurrence in the community, with an incidence of seasonal influenza infection after HCT of 1–4 % and a mortality rate of 15–28 % in the setting of pneumonia [61]. Due to the prevalence of resistance to the M2 inhibitors (amantadine and rimantadine), neuraminidase inhibitors (oseltamavir and zanamivir) are used in the immunosuppressed host with suspected or documented influenza [63].

Parainfluenza virus is a major cause of laryngotracheobronchitis in children; parainfluenza serotype-3 (PIV-3) is the most frequently found in immunocompromised patients. Almost half of HCT recipients with PIV infection progress to lower respiratory tract infection with a mortality rate of 17 % [64]. Although sometimes used, ribarivin and IVIG have not been shown to be efficacious in treating PIV pneumonia. DAS181 is a novel sialidase fusion protein currently being tested in clinical trials for treating PIV disease in severely immunocompromised individuals [63].

Newly discovered respiratory viruses of clinical significance that have emerged within the past decade include human metapneumovirus (HMPV), human bocavirus, and new coronaviruses. HMPV was first reported in 2001 and has an associated mortality of 33–40 % for lower respiratory tract disease [61] HMPV has been detected in HCT recipients with fulminant respiratory failure initially attributed to IPS [65].

Respiratory syncytial virus (RSV) is one of the leading causes of viral pneumonia in HCT recipients, affecting 24–31 % of HCT recipients with a documented respiratory viral infection [62]. Usually presenting as an upper respiratory tract infection with rhinorrhea, sinus congestion and a sore throat, RSV infection can progress to bronchiolitis, pneumonitis, and pneumonia. Patients who have not yet engrafted are at highest risk for progression to lower tract disease, and once pneumonia is established, mortality is 43 % [62]. Risk factors for mortality include hypoxemia, steroids at the time of diagnosis, or mechanical ventilation [66]. In survivors of HCT, lower respiratory tract infection with RSV in the first 100 day is associated with increased risk of developing airflow decline (OR 3.6) [67], which may be recognized as BOS. Uncontrolled studies suggest that treatment of RSV lower respiratory tract infection with aerosolized ribavirin and RSV-Ig can reduce mortality to <20 % if initiated before the onset of respiratory failure [62]. The novel compound GS-5806, an RSV entry inhibitor, reduces the viral load and severity of clinical disease in healthy adult volunteers and is currently in phase II clinical trials to treat RSV in HCT recipients [68].

Invasive Fungal Disease

The epidemiology of invasive fungal infection (IFI) continues to evolve with advances in detection, prophylaxis and treatment. When recently revised definitions for proven and probable invasive fungal disease [69] are applied, the incidence of all IFI is 14 % in allogeneic HCT recipients. Aspergillosis accounts for 50 % of the IFI, followed by candidiasis and mucormycosis [70]. Widespread use of voriconazole may be contributing to emergence of mold infections with decreased susceptibility to voriconazole, including *Mucorales* spp. [71].

Manifestations of *Aspergillus* in the HCT population include airway colonization, tracheobronchitis, pneumonia, sinusitis or disseminated disease. Symptoms of pulmonary invasive aspergillosis (IA) include dyspnea, fever, productive cough, chest pain and hemoptysis; patients may also be asymptomatic [2]. After recovery from neutropenia, 64 % of allogeneic HCT recipients with invasive filamentous fungal infection presented with dyspnea but only 32 % were febrile [72]. Mortality at 3 months from the time of IA diagnosis ranges from 53.8 % of autologous recipients to 84.6 % for unrelated donor recipients and does not differ for those with early-versus late-onset infections [73, 74].

The gold standard for the diagnosis of IA is biopsy with culture in the setting of compatible clinical and radiographic features; however biopsy is now rarely performed to confirm IA. Galactomannan, a fungal polysaccharide specific to *Aspergillus* spp, is a widely used biomarker for the detection of IA from both the serum and BAL fluid. The serum galactomannan assay has a sensitivity and specificity of 82 and 86 %, respectively, for the detection of IA in HCT recipients [75]. Galactomannan testing of BAL has a sensitivity of 60–82 % and a specificity of 95 %. PCR-based methods for the detection of *Aspergillus* are not yet standardized for clinical use although published studies indicate that BAL analysis using quantitative RT-PCR has a sensitivity of 67–77 % and specificity of 90–100 % [76].

The approach to treatment of IA should involve reducing the level of immunosuppression to the extent possible in addition to the use of an antifungal agent with appropriate efficacy and minimal toxicity profile. It is important to recognize that all clinically relevant azole antimicrobials inhibit cytochrome P450 isoenzyme activity to varying degrees resulting in increased serum concentrations of cyclosporine, tacrolimus, sirolimus and everolimus that could lead to neurotoxicity and/or nephrotoxicity. These medications must be dose-adjusted when the patient requires azole treatment for IFI [2]. Voriconazole, a broad-spectrum triazole derivative that became available in 2002, is the agent of choice for the treatment of IA based on its superior efficacy and survival benefit in comparison to amphotericin [77]. Liposomal amphotericin B is an alternative in patients who are azole intolerant. Echinocandins (caspofungin, micafungin, anidulafungin) are also an option for the treatment of IA and have very low potential for drug interactions although tacrolimus levels may be reduced. Surgical resection for focally invasive disease that is refractory to medical therapy can be considered in neutropenic patients. Inhaled liposomal amphotericin B, in addition to systemic antifungals, can be used for the treatment of fungal tracheobronchitis [2].

Mucormycosis is an aggressive infection with high mortality associated with prolonged neutropenia. It accounts for 8 % of IFI in HCT recipients, most often as a late complication (>3 months after transplantation) with pulmonary involvement in over half of cases. The overall mortality rate among HCT recipients is at least 75 % [78]. First line therapy is liposomal amphotericin B for at least 6–8 weeks and extensive early surgical debridement. A combination of liposomal amphotericin and an echinocandin may be considered in cases that are refractory to first line therapy. Isavuconazole is a promising new extended spectrum triazole with excellent oral bioavailability and a low side effect profile, which may have utility as primary therapy against invasive mucormycosis and other IFI [79].

Key Points

- Acute respiratory disease is a significant contributor to the morbidity and mortality of hematopoietic cell transplantation.
- The differential diagnosis of pulmonary disease depends on the time frame after HCT and the patient's immune status.
- A spectrum of noninfectious acute lung injuries that develop in the early post-transplantation period falls under the category of the *idiopathic pneumonia syndrome* (IPS). Late-onset lung injury usually manifests as cryptogenic organizing pneumonia.
- Other noninfectious pulmonary complications include pulmonary alveolar proteinosis, pulmonary vascular disease, and drug toxicities.
- The epidemiology of acute lung injury and classic infectious etiologies of acute respiratory disease in this population has changed since the advent of improved supportive care, diagnostic detection, and treatments.

References

1. Gooley TA, Chien JW, Pergam SA, Hingorani S, Sorror ML, Boeckh M, et al. Reduced mortality after allogeneic hematopoietic-cell transplantation. N Engl J Med. 2010;363(22): 2091–101.
2. Madtes DK. Pulmonary complications of stem cell and solid organ transplantation. In: Broaddus VC, editor. Murray and Nadel's textbook of respiratory medicine, vol. 2. 6th ed. Philadelphia, PA: Saunders; 2016. p. 1612–23.e8.
3. Afessa B, Azoulay E. Critical care of the hematopoietic stem cell transplant recipient. Crit Care Clin. 2010;26(1):133–50.
4. Ho VT, Weller E, Lee SJ, Alyea EP, Antin JH, Soiffer RJ. Prognostic factors for early severe pulmonary complications after hematopoietic stem cell transplantation. Biol Blood Marrow Transplant. 2001;7(4):223–9.
5. Rubenfeld GD, Crawford SW. Withdrawing life support from mechanically ventilated recipients of bone marrow transplants: a case for evidence-based guidelines. Ann Intern Med. 1996;125(8):625–33.
6. Naeem N, Reed MD, Creger RJ, Youngner SJ, Lazarus HM. Transfer of the hematopoietic stem cell transplant patient to the intensive care unit: does it really matter? Bone Marrow Transplant. 2006;37(2):119–33.
7. The Acute Respiratory Distress Syndrome Network. Ventilation with lower tidal volumes as compared with traditional tidal volumes for acute lung injury and the acute respiratory distress syndrome. N Engl J Med. 2000;342(18):1301–8.
8. Rivers E, Nguyen B, Havstad S, Ressler J, Muzzin A, Knoblich B, et al. Early goal-directed therapy in the treatment of severe sepsis and septic shock. N Engl J Med. 2001;345(19):1368–77.
9. Soubani AO, Kseibi E, Bander JJ, Klein JL, Khanchandani G, Ahmed HP, et al. Outcome and prognostic factors of hematopoietic stem cell transplantation recipients admitted to a medical ICU. Chest. 2004;126(5):1604–11.
10. Kew AK, Couban S, Patrick W, Thompson K, White D. Outcome of hematopoietic stem cell transplant recipients admitted to the intensive care unit. Biol Blood Marrow Transplant. 2006;12(3):301–5.
11. Lengline E, Chevret S, Moreau AS, Pene F, Blot F, Bourhis JH, et al. Changes in intensive care for allogeneic hematopoietic stem cell transplant recipients. Bone Marrow Transplant. 2015;50(6):840–5.
12. Pene F, Aubron C, Azoulay E, Blot F, Thiery G, Raynard B, et al. Outcome of critically ill allogeneic hematopoietic stem-cell transplantation recipients: a reappraisal of indications for organ failure supports. J Clin Oncol. 2006;24(4):643–9.
13. Harris B, Lowy FD, Stover DE, Arcasoy SM. Diagnostic bronchoscopy in solid-organ and hematopoietic stem cell transplantation. Ann Am Thorac Soc. 2013;10(1):39–49.
14. Crawford SW, Bowden RA, Hackman RC, Gleaves CA, Meyers JD, Clark JG. Rapid detection of cytomegalovirus pulmonary infection by bronchoalveolar lavage and centrifugation culture. Ann Intern Med. 1988;108(2):180–5.
15. Patel NR, Lee PS, Kim JH, Weinhouse GL, Koziel H. The influence of diagnostic bronchoscopy on clinical outcomes comparing adult autologous and allogeneic bone marrow transplant patients. Chest. 2005;127(4):1388–96.
16. Hofmeister CC, Czerlanis C, Forsythe S, Stiff PJ. Retrospective utility of bronchoscopy after hematopoietic stem cell transplant. Bone Marrow Transplant. 2006;38(10):693–8.
17. Shannon VR, Andersson BS, Lei X, Champlin RE, Kontoyiannis DP. Utility of early versus late fiberoptic bronchoscopy in the evaluation of new pulmonary infiltrates following hematopoietic stem cell transplantation. Bone Marrow Transplant. 2010;45(4):647–55.
18. White DA, Wong PW, Downey R. The utility of open lung biopsy in patients with hematologic malignancies. Am J Respir Crit Care Med. 2000;161(3 Pt 1):723–9.

19. Crawford SW, Hackman RC, Clark JG. Open lung biopsy diagnosis of diffuse pulmonary infiltrates after marrow transplantation. Chest. 1988;94(5):949–53.
20. Crawford SW, Hackman RC, Clark JG. Biopsy diagnosis and clinical outcome of persistent focal pulmonary lesions after marrow transplantation. Transplantation. 1989;48(2):266–71.
21. Cheng GS, Stednick Z, Madtes DK, McDonald G, Boeckh M, Pergam SA. Changing trends in the use of surgical biopsy for diagnosis of pulmonary disease in hematopoietic cell transplant recipients. 2013 BMT Tandem Meetings; Salt Lake City, UT. Biol Blood Marrow Transplant. 2013;19:S297.
22. Chellapandian D, Lehrnbecher T, Phillips B, Fisher BT, Zaoutis TE, Steinbach WJ, et al. Bronchoalveolar lavage and lung biopsy in patients with cancer and hematopoietic stem-cell transplantation recipients: a systematic review and meta-analysis. J Clin Oncol. 2015;33(5):501–9.
23. Seo S, Renaud C, Kuypers JM, Chiu CY, Huang ML, Samayoa E, et al. Idiopathic pneumonia syndrome after hematopoietic cell transplantation: evidence of occult infectious etiologies. Blood. 2015;125(24):3789–97.
24. Razonable RR, Fanning C, Brown RA, Espy MJ, Rivero A, Wilson J, et al. Selective reactivation of human herpesvirus 6 variant a occurs in critically ill immunocompetent hosts. J Infect Dis. 2002;185(1):110–3.
25. Panoskaltsis-Mortari A, Griese M, Madtes DK, Belperio JA, Haddad IY, Folz RJ, et al. An official American Thoracic Society research statement: noninfectious lung injury after hematopoietic stem cell transplantation: idiopathic pneumonia syndrome. Am J Respir Crit Care Med. 2011;183(9):1262–79.
26. Fukuda T, Hackman RC, Guthrie KA, Sandmaier BM, Boeckh M, Maris MB, et al. Risks and outcomes of idiopathic pneumonia syndrome after nonmyeloablative and conventional conditioning regimens for allogeneic hematopoietic stem cell transplantation. Blood. 2003;102(8):2777–85.
27. Vande Vusse LK, Madtes DK, Guthrie KA, Gernsheimer TB, Curtis JR, Watkins TR. The association between red blood cell and platelet transfusion and subsequently developing idiopathic pneumonia syndrome after hematopoietic stem cell transplantation. Transfusion. 2014;54(4):1071–80.
28. Marr KA. Fungal infections in hematopoietic stem cell transplant recipients. Med Mycol. 2008;46(4):293–302.
29. Yanik GA, Grupp SA, Pulsipher MA, Levine JE, Schultz KR, Wall DA, et al. TNF-receptor inhibitor therapy for the treatment of children with idiopathic pneumonia syndrome. A joint Pediatric Blood and Marrow Transplant Consortium and Children's Oncology Group Study (ASCT0521). Biol Blood Marrow Transplant. 2015;21(1):67–73.
30. Yanik GA, Horowitz MM, Weisdorf DJ, Logan BR, Ho VT, Soiffer RJ, et al. Randomized, double-blind, placebo-controlled trial of soluble tumor necrosis factor receptor: enbrel (etanercept) for the treatment of idiopathic pneumonia syndrome after allogeneic stem cell transplantation: blood and marrow transplant clinical trials network protocol. Biol Blood Marrow Transplant. 2014;20(6):858–64.
31. Gorak E, Geller N, Srinivasan R, Espinoza-Delgado I, Donohue T, Barrett AJ, et al. Engraftment syndrome after nonmyeloablative allogeneic hematopoietic stem cell transplantation: incidence and effects on survival. Biol Blood Marrow Transplant. 2005;11(7):542–50.
32. Wilczynski SW, Erasmus JJ, Petros WP, Vredenburgh JJ, Folz RJ. Delayed pulmonary toxicity syndrome following high-dose chemotherapy and bone marrow transplantation for breast cancer. Am J Respir Crit Care Med. 1998;157(2):565–73.
33. Lee SM, Park JJ, Sung SH, Kim Y, Lee KE, Mun YC, et al. Acute fibrinous and organizing pneumonia following hematopoietic stem cell transplantation. Korean J Intern Med. 2009;24(2):156–9.
34. Beasley MB, Franks TJ, Galvin JR, Gochuico B, Travis WD. Acute fibrinous and organizing pneumonia: a histological pattern of lung injury and possible variant of diffuse alveolar damage. Arch Pathol Lab Med. 2002;126(9):1064–70.

35. Bhatti S, Hakeem A, Torrealba J, McMahon JP, Meyer KC. Severe acute fibrinous and organizing pneumonia (AFOP) causing ventilatory failure: successful treatment with mycophenolate mofetil and corticosteroids. Respir Med. 2009;103(11):1764–7.
36. Freudenberger TD, Madtes DK, Curtis JR, Cummings P, Storer BE, Hackman RC. Association between acute and chronic graft-versus-host disease and bronchiolitis obliterans organizing pneumonia in recipients of hematopoietic stem cell transplants. Blood. 2003;102(10):3822–8.
37. Yanik G, Kitko C. Management of noninfectious lung injury following hematopoietic cell transplantation. Curr Opin Oncol. 2013;25(2):187–94.
38. Nakasone H, Onizuka M, Suzuki N, Fujii N, Taniguchi S, Kakihana K, et al. Pre-transplant risk factors for cryptogenic organizing pneumonia/bronchiolitis obliterans organizing pneumonia after hematopoietic cell transplantation. Bone Marrow Transplant. 2013;48(10):1317–23.
39. Pipavath SN, Chung JH, Chien JW, Godwin JD. Organizing pneumonia in recipients of hematopoietic stem cell transplantation: CT features in 16 patients. J Comput Assist Tomogr. 2012;36(4):431–6.
40. Cottin V, Cordier JF. Cryptogenic organizing pneumonia. Semin Respir Crit Care Med. 2012;33(5):462–75.
41. Stover DE, Mangino D. Macrolides: a treatment alternative for bronchiolitis obliterans organizing pneumonia? Chest. 2005;128(5):3611–7.
42. Au BK, Au MA, Chien JW. Bronchiolitis obliterans syndrome epidemiology after allogeneic hematopoietic cell transplantation. Biol Blood Marrow Transplant. 2011;17(7):1072–8.
43. Clark JG, Crawford SW, Madtes DK, Sullivan KM. Obstructive lung disease after allogeneic marrow transplantation. Clinical presentation and course. Ann Intern Med. 1989;111(5):368–76.
44. Lane AA, Armand P, Feng Y, Neuberg DS, Abramson JS, Brown JR, et al. Risk factors for development of pneumonitis after high-dose chemotherapy with cyclophosphamide, BCNU and etoposide followed by autologous stem cell transplant. Leuk Lymphoma. 2012;53(6):1130–6.
45. Abushamaa AM, Sporn TA, Folz RJ. Oxidative stress and inflammation contribute to lung toxicity after a common breast cancer chemotherapy regimen. Am J Physiol Lung Cell Mol Physiol. 2002;283(2):L336–45.
46. Malik SW, Myers JL, DeRemee RA, Specks U. Lung toxicity associated with cyclophosphamide use. Two distinct patterns. Am J Respir Crit Care Med. 1996;154(6 Pt 1):1851–6.
47. Cutler C, Logan B, Nakamura R, Johnston L, Choi S, Porter D, et al. Tacrolimus/sirolimus vs tacrolimus/methotrexate as GVHD prophylaxis after matched, related donor allogeneic HCT. Blood. 2014;124(8):1372–7.
48. Garrod AS, Goyal RK, Weiner DJ. Sirolimus-induced interstitial lung disease following pediatric stem cell transplantation. Pediatr Transplant. 2015;19(3):E75–7.
49. Patel AV, Hahn T, Bogner PN, Loud PA, Brown K, Paplham P, et al. Fatal diffuse alveolar hemorrhage associated with sirolimus after allogeneic hematopoietic cell transplantation. Bone Marrow Transplant. 2010;45(8):1363–4.
50. Champion L, Stern M, Israel-Biet D, Mamzer-Bruneel MF, Peraldi MN, Kreis H, et al. Brief communication: sirolimus-associated pneumonitis: 24 cases in renal transplant recipients. Ann Intern Med. 2006;144(7):505–9.
51. Trapnell BC, Whitsett JA, Nakata K. Pulmonary alveolar proteinosis. N Engl J Med. 2003;349(26):2527–39.
52. Pidala J, Khalil F, Fernandez H. Pulmonary alveolar proteinosis following allogeneic hematopoietic cell transplantation. Bone Marrow Transplant. 2011;46(11):1480–3.
53. Gerber DE, Segal JB, Levy MY, Kane J, Jones RJ, Streiff MB. The incidence of and risk factors for venous thromboembolism (VTE) and bleeding among 1514 patients undergoing hematopoietic stem cell transplantation: implications for VTE prevention. Blood. 2008;112(3):504–10.
54. Mandel J, Mark EJ, Hales CA. Pulmonary veno-occlusive disease. Am J Respir Crit Care Med. 2000;162(5):1964–73.
55. Hackman RC, Madtes DK, Petersen FB, Clark JG. Pulmonary venoocclusive disease following bone marrow transplantation. Transplantation. 1989;47(6):989–92.

56. Woodard JP, Gulbahce E, Shreve M, Steiner M, Peters C, Hite S, et al. Pulmonary cytolytic thrombi: a newly recognized complication of stem cell transplantation. Bone Marrow Transplant. 2000;25(3):293–300.
57. Peters A, Manivel JC, Dolan M, Gulbahce HE, Baker KS, Verneris MR. Pulmonary cytolytic thrombi after allogeneic hematopoietic cell transplantation: a further histologic description. Biol Blood Marrow Transplant. 2005;11(6):484–5.
58. Travi G, Pergam SA. Cytomegalovirus pneumonia in hematopoietic stem cell recipients. J Intensive Care Med. 2014;29(4):200–12.
59. Boeckh M, Leisenring W, Riddell SR, Bowden RA, Huang ML, Myerson D, et al. Late cytomegalovirus disease and mortality in recipients of allogeneic hematopoietic stem cell transplants: importance of viral load and T-cell immunity. Blood. 2003;101(2):407–14.
60. Erard V, Guthrie KA, Seo S, Smith J, Huang M, Chien J, et al. Reduced mortality of cytomegalovirus pneumonia after hematopoietic cell transplantation due to antiviral therapy and changes in transplantation practices. Clin Infect Dis. 2015;61(1):31–9.
61. Renaud C, Campbell AP. Changing epidemiology of respiratory viral infections in hematopoietic cell transplant recipients and solid organ transplant recipients. Curr Opin Infect Dis. 2011;24(4):333–43.
62. Kim YJ, Boeckh M, Englund JA. Community respiratory virus infections in immunocompromised patients: hematopoietic stem cell and solid organ transplant recipients, and individuals with human immunodeficiency virus infection. Semin Respir Crit Care Med. 2007;28(2):222–42.
63. Chemaly RF, Shah DP, Boeckh MJ. Management of respiratory viral infections in hematopoietic cell transplant recipients and patients with hematologic malignancies. Clin Infect Dis. 2014;59 Suppl 5:S344–51.
64. Chemaly RF, Hanmod SS, Rathod DB, Ghantoji SS, Jiang Y, Doshi A, et al. The characteristics and outcomes of parainfluenza virus infections in 200 patients with leukemia or recipients of hematopoietic stem cell transplantation. Blood. 2012;119(12):2738–45. quiz 969.
65. Englund JA, Boeckh M, Kuypers J, Nichols WG, Hackman RC, Morrow RA, et al. Brief communication: fatal human metapneumovirus infection in stem-cell transplant recipients. Ann Intern Med. 2006;144(5):344–9.
66. Renaud C, Xie H, Seo S, Kuypers J, Cent A, Corey L, et al. Mortality rates of human metapneumovirus and respiratory syncytial virus lower respiratory tract infections in hematopoietic cell transplantation recipients. Biol Blood Marrow Transplant. 2013;19(8):1220–6.
67. Erard V, Chien JW, Kim HW, Nichols WG, Flowers ME, Martin PJ, et al. Airflow decline after myeloablative allogeneic hematopoietic cell transplantation: the role of community respiratory viruses. J Infect Dis. 2006;193(12):1619–25.
68. DeVincenzo JP, Whitley RJ, Mackman RL, Scaglioni-Weinlich C, Harrison L, Farrell E, et al. Oral GS-5806 activity in a respiratory syncytial virus challenge study. N Engl J Med. 2014;371(8):711–22.
69. De Pauw B, Walsh TJ, Donnelly JP, Stevens DA, Edwards JE, Calandra T, et al. Revised definitions of invasive fungal disease from the European Organization for Research and Treatment of Cancer/Invasive Fungal Infections Cooperative Group and the National Institute of Allergy and Infectious Diseases Mycoses Study Group (EORTC/MSG) Consensus Group. Clin Infect Dis. 2008;46(12):1813–21.
70. Corzo-Leon DE, Satlin MJ, Soave R, Shore TB, Schuetz AN, Jacobs SE, et al. Epidemiology and outcomes of invasive fungal infections in allogeneic haematopoietic stem cell transplant recipients in the era of antifungal prophylaxis: a single-centre study with focus on emerging pathogens. Mycoses. 2015;58(6):325–36.
71. Ziakas PD, Kourbeti IS, Mylonakis E. Systemic antifungal prophylaxis after hematopoietic stem cell transplantation: a meta-analysis. Clin Ther. 2014;36(2):292–306 e1.
72. Shaukat A, Bakri F, Young P, Hahn T, Ball D, Baer MR, et al. Invasive filamentous fungal infections in allogeneic hematopoietic stem cell transplant recipients after recovery from neutropenia: clinical, radiologic, and pathologic characteristics. Mycopathologia. 2005;159(2):181–8.
73. Morgan J, Wannemuehler KA, Marr KA, Hadley S, Kontoyiannis DP, Walsh TJ, et al. Incidence of invasive aspergillosis following hematopoietic stem cell and solid organ transplantation:

interim results of a prospective multicenter surveillance program. Med Mycol. 2005;43 Suppl 1:S49–58.
74. Singh N, Paterson DL. Aspergillus infections in transplant recipients. Clin Microbiol Rev. 2005;18(1):44–69.
75. Pfeiffer CD, Fine JP, Safdar N. Diagnosis of invasive aspergillosis using a galactomannan assay: a meta-analysis. Clin Infect Dis. 2006;42(10):1417–27.
76. Wengenack NL, Binnicker MJ. Fungal molecular diagnostics. Clin Chest Med. 2009;30(2):391–408. viii.
77. Herbrecht R, Denning DW, Patterson TF, Bennett JE, Greene RE, Oestmann JW, et al. Voriconazole versus amphotericin B for primary therapy of invasive aspergillosis. N Engl J Med. 2002;347(6):408–15.
78. Lanternier F, Sun HY, Ribaud P, Singh N, Kontoyiannis DP, Lortholary O. Mucormycosis in organ and stem cell transplant recipients. Clin Infect Dis. 2012;54(11):1629–36.
79. Miceli MH, Kauffman CA. Isavuconazole: a new broad-spectrum triazole antifungal agent. Clin Infect Dis. 2015;61(10):1558–65.

Part III
Transfusion-Related Complications

Chapter 9
Storage Lesion: Evolving Concepts and Controversies

Stefanie Forest, Francesca Rapido, and Eldad A. Hod

Storage of Red Blood Cell Components

An estimated 92 million packed red blood cell (RBC) units are collected worldwide each year making RBC transfusions the most common procedure requiring informed consent performed during hospitalization [1]. These RBC transfusions are a vital part of medical treatment and are essential for the management of inherited disorders such as thalassemia and sickle cell disease, acute blood loss from trauma or surgery, and for patients undergoing chemotherapy or stem cell transplants [2]. Nearly, thirty percent of critical care service admissions receive RBC transfusions, and those transfused receive an average of 5 units of RBCs during their stay in the intensive care unit [3].

The first successful human blood transfusion was performed in the seventeenth century by James Blundell [4]. Blood transfusions were performed with direct artery to vein anastomosis or indirect syringe or flask techniques; however, these methods required the blood donor and recipient to be side by side [5]. The discovery of the first RBC storage solution by Rous and Turner [6] allowed stable storage of RBCs by anticoagulating the blood with citrate and providing nutrients to RBCs with glucose, so that the donor and recipient could be separated by both space and time for the transfusion procedure. The discovery of this storage solution set the

S. Forest, MD, PhD • E.A. Hod, MD (✉)
Department of Pathology and Cell Biology at Columbia University Medical Center,
New York Presbyterian Hospital, New York, NY 10032, USA
e-mail: eldad.hod@gmail.com

F. Rapido, MD
Department of Pathology and Cell Biology at Columbia University Medical Center,
New York Presbyterian Hospital, New York, NY 10032, USA

Department of Medical Surgical Pathophysiology and Organ Transplantation,
Università degli Studi di Milano, Milan, Italy

J.S. Lee, M.P. Donahoe (eds.), *Hematologic Abnormalities and Acute Lung Syndromes*, Respiratory Medicine, DOI 10.1007/978-3-319-41912-1_9

Table 9.1 RBC additive solutions currently in routine use around the world [10]

	Licensed RBC additive solutions						
Constituents (mM)	SAGM	AS-1	AS-3	AS-5	AS-7	MAP	PAGGSM
NaCl	150	154	70	150		85	72
$NaHCO_3$					26		
Na_2HPO_4					12		16
NaH_2PO_4			23			6	8
Citric acid			2			1	
Na-citrate			23			5	
Adenine	1.25	2	2	2.2	2	1.5	1.4
Guanosine							1.4
Glucose	45	111	55	45	80	40	47
Mannitol	30	41		45.5	55	80	55
pH	5.7	5.5	5.8	5.5	8.5	5.7	5.7
FDA licensed	No	Yes	Yes	Yes	Yes	No	No
Approved shelf life (d)	42	42	42	42	42[a]	42	49

[a]Approved in Europe for 56 days of storage

stage for Captain Oswald Hope Robertson (who worked in Rous's laboratory in 1915–1916) to build the world's first blood bank in France during World War I. Dr. Oswald recognized the utility of storing blood products to improve availability of blood to soldiers suffering wartime trauma. He utilized the Rous–Turner solution and stored bottles on ice for up to 26 days [5]. These wartime transfusions were lifesaving and provided the proof-of-principle that blood products could be stored for future use.

Today, RBC units are stored to allow for inventory management that insures that needed blood types are readily available. Donated RBCs destined for transfusion are prepared from whole blood collected into a solution containing citrate, phosphate, and dextrose (CPD or CP2D) or from apheresis collection into CP2D or into anticoagulant citrate dextrose solution A (ACD-A). To allow for longer-term storage, additional nutrients are provided to the RBCs in the form of additive solutions (AS), and the RBCs stored at 1–6 °C [5]. Several additive solutions have been developed (see Table 9.1). The first additive solution developed was SAG (saline, adenine and glucose) in the late 1970s [7]. The addition of mannitol to SAG solution, to produce SAGM, reduced hemolysis and allowed storage for an additional week, up to 6 weeks of refrigerated storage [5]. SAGM is now the standard additive solution with two variants approved for use in the USA, AS-1 and AS-5, which have different concentrations of the same constituents. Sodium chloride is necessary for proper tonicity. Adenine provides a source for ATP, the energy unit of the cell. Glucose (dextrose) provides nutrients for the RBCs. Finally, mannitol is a free radical scavenger and membrane stabilizer, which reduces hemolysis and allows for a longer shelf-life of packed RBC units. AS-3 is composed of SAG with citrate and phosphate. Phosphate also provides a component source for ATP generation and the citrate serves a protective function for the membrane by balancing the osmotic pressures in RBCs [5]. A newer isotonic additive solution, phosphate–adenine–glucose–

guanosine–saline–mannitol (PAGGS-M), allows for maximal storage up to 49 days compared to the hypertonic additive solutions; however, this is not Food and Drug Administration (FDA)-approved [8]. The most recently FDA-approved additive solution is AS-7, an alkaline RBC storage solution designed to improve RBC metabolism during storage by increasing the range and capacity of pH buffering [9].

The FDA and foreign counterparts allow for RBCs to be stored for a maximum of 42 days (49 days for PAGGS-M and 56 days for AS-7 in Europe) [11]; however, no clinical study assessing the clinical safety of this somewhat arbitrary decision was ever conducted. The expiration date of RBC units are mainly based on post transfusion recovery studies, which measure the quantity of chromium radiolabeled RBCs remaining in the peripheral circulation 24 h after a dose of autologous RBCs is reinfused into healthy subjects on the last day of storage [12]. Hemolysis levels in the bag are also taken into consideration [13]. Earlier FDA standards in the 1970s set 70 % as an acceptable 24-h post transfusion RBC recovery. This level was decided for concern that any lower recovery could result in hemoglobinuria which would be confused with an immunologic reaction to incompatible RBCs [12]. The FDA standards were arbitrarily updated in 1985 to a minimum mean recovery of 75 % of radiolabeled RBCs at 24 h [12]. Additionally, in the USA and Europe, hemolysis must be less than 1.0 and 0.8 %, respectively, at the end of storage (with 95 % confidence that at least 95 % of the population meets or exceeds the specification) [13].

Blood banking has come a long way since the first blood banks during World War I. The development of additive solutions allowed for longer storage of RBC units [5]. Due to the challenges of providing RBCs with a limited supply, there is pressure to increase the shelf life of RBC units. However this must be balanced with the RBC storage lesion that results from prolonged refrigerator storage of RBCs. The storage lesion is "a series of biochemical and biomechanical changes in the RBC and storage media during ex vivo preservation that reduce RBC survival and function" [14]. The storage lesion has been studied for decades. The potential contributors to the storage lesion include changes in RBC morphology and deformability, reductions in 2,3-DPG, ATP, pH, reduced glutathione, membrane expression of CD47, as well as membrane loss and increased formation of microvesicles, oxidation of cellular lipids and proteins, phosphatidylserine exposure, supernatant lipid accumulation and desialylation of RBCs (see Fig. 9.1). The underlying mechanisms of these contributors to the storage lesion will be further described below.

Potential Contributors to the RBC Storage Lesion

RBC Morphology and Deformability

During storage, red blood cells undergo a predictable morphologic change that can be visualized by electron microscopy (see Fig. 9.2). Some of these shape changes are reversible following transfusion, while some changes are irreversible. RBCs undergo a transition from the normal biconcave disk shape to reversibly deformed

Fig. 9.1 Features of the RBC storage lesion. The biochemical and biomechanical changes occur in the storage media or RBC additive solution, RBC membrane, and RBC. Hemoglobin (Hb), phosphatidylserine (PS)

Additive Solution	
↑Microvesicles	↓pH
↑Lipid Accumulation	
↑Free Hb/Heme/Iron	
↑K +	
↑Lactate	
↑Histamine	
RBC Membrane	
↑Echinocytes	↓Membrane Deformability
↑Spheroechinocytes	↓CD47
↑Lipid peroxidation	↓Sialic acid
↑Protein oxidation	
↑PS exposure	
RBC Cytosol	
↑Lactate	↓2,3-DPG
↑NADPH	↓ATP
	↓Glutathione
	↓Glutathione-peroxidase

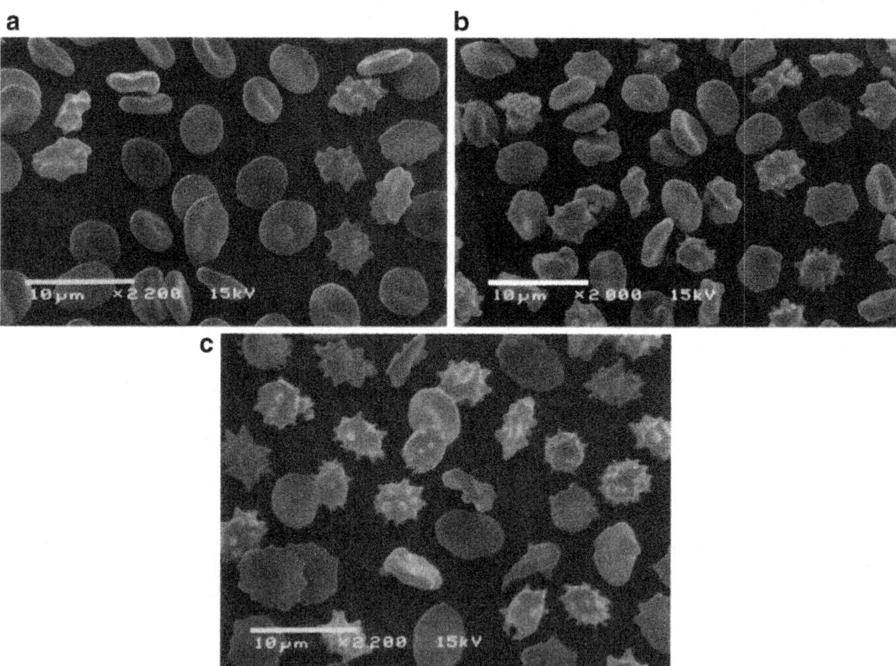

Fig. 9.2 Scanning electron microscopic image of RBCs during storage. (**a**) On the 5th day of storage, discocytes predominate and only a few irreversibly changed RBC can be seen. (**b**) On the 14th day of storage, numerous echinocytes and spheroechinocytes are observed. (**c**) By the 42nd day of storage, spheroechinocytes and degenerated forms predominate among the irreversibly changed RBCs. (Reproduced from Berezina et al. 2002)

echinocytes, which have projections extending from the surface resembling a spiked ball. Eventually, the changes become irreversible as the RBCs become spheroechinocytic. During the first week of storage, discocytes predominate. By day 21 of storage, nearly half of the RBCs are abnormally echinocytically shaped, and by day 42 over 76 % of RBCs are abnormally shaped with a substantial percentage of irreversibly changed spheroechinocytes [15]. These morphologic transitions are accompanied by a decrease in RBC membrane deformability [15, 16]. The relationship between abnormally shaped RBC and RBC deformability is unclear. However, at early stages of storage, normal appearing biconcave disks exhibited reduced deformability [17] suggesting that changes in membrane deformability may precede the alterations in cell shape. Using a microbead sorting device to recapitulate the splenic microcirculation, older stored RBCs were shown to have a significant increase in elongation index and retention rate. This suggests that older stored RBCs are less deformable and are more likely to be retained and destroyed by the spleen [18]. The full implications of the changes in morphologic and rheological properties of RBCs during storage remain to be fully determined.

2,3-Diphosphoglycerate (DPG)

2,3-DPG is the major allosteric modifier of oxygen affinity and causes a right shift in the oxygen-hemoglobin dissociation curve thereby enhancing off loading of oxygen. A decrease in RBC levels of 2,3 DPG has been observed with RBC storage with nearly undetectable levels by 2–3 weeks of storage [19]. This change impairs oxygen release to tissues following transfusion; however, RBC 2,3-DPG levels regenerate relatively quickly and levels have been shown to increase by 25–30, 50, and 100 % by 1 h, 24 h, and 3 days following transfusion, respectively [20]. In addition to decreased 2,3-DPG levels, metabolomics studies suggest decreases in ATP, pH, and reduced glutathione levels accompanied by increases in oxidized glutathione, lactate, NADPH, and oxidation of membrane proteins and lipids during prolonged storage [16, 21].

Adenosine Triphosphate (ATP), pH, Lactate

Multiple studies observe a decrease in pH, a decrease in ATP, and an increase in lactate during storage [16, 21, 22]. Experimental ATP depletion results in morphologic changes in RBCs from their normal discoid shape to a crenated one and then eventually to smooth spheres after 6 h. These changes are similar to those observed during RBC storage. Furthermore, restoration of RBC ATP levels results in return of their normal biconcave disk shape [23]. This demonstrates the importance of ATP in normal RBC morphology. However, although parallels can be drawn between these experiments involving rapid ATP depletion and then restoration, the depletion of ATP in RBCs during storage is a much more gradual process. Higher ATP levels in stored blood from different storage media has little effect on the viability of RBCs when transfused, suggesting that higher ATP levels may not be critical for RBC survival [24]. Additionally, despite ATP restoration to normal levels, a number of irreversible spherocytes are still present [14].

Glutathione and NADPH

Oxidation occurs in RBCs due to transported oxygen and the reactive iron present in hemoglobin [25]. Oxidizing radicals such as superoxide anions, hydrogen peroxide, and hydroxyl radicals are generated during RBC storage [26]. In stored RBCs these oxidizing radicals modify both lipids and proteins, damaging RBC membrane integrity. Antioxidants are available to counteract the destructive effects of this oxidation. The primary antioxidant defense system in stored RBCs is reduced glutathione and glutathione peroxidase. During storage, there is a significant decline in both reduced glutathione and glutathione peroxidase levels with a concomitant rise in oxidized glutathione [21, 26]. These changes are indicators of oxidative stress during storage.

Metabolomics studies of RBCs during refrigerated storage reveal a shift towards the oxidative phase of the pentose phosphate pathway [27]. This shift is likely a response to the increase in oxidative stress and accumulation of reactive oxygen species observed during storage. Thus, NADPH levels increase during storage in line with the switch towards the pentose phosphate pathway [21]. This potentially allows the RBC to maintain oxidation–reduction balance and protect itself against oxidative injury [28].

Oxidation of Cellular Lipids and Proteins

The generation of oxidizing radicals results in oxidative damage to the RBC membrane lipids and proteins. There is both a loss of membrane lipids as well as increase in lipid peroxidation with RBC storage [21, 26]. Peroxidation of RBC membrane phospholipids results in the formation of malondialdehyde, a highly reactive molecule that interacts with RBC membrane phospholipids and proteins and impairs their function. Malondialdehyde has been observed to increase progressively during storage [21, 26]. Oxidative damage also modifies membrane proteins of RBCs. Oxidation further induces aggregation of proteins, introducing carbonyl groups to specific residues of polypeptide chains. During RBC storage, carbonylation of band 4.1 protein, an important cytoskeletal protein, increases significantly [26]. Additionally, protein aggregation of band 3 and a shift of small and large band 3 oligomers to large aggregates is observed [29]. Band 3, the anion exchanger 1, is a membrane receptor and transporter protein with a number of important roles including maintenance of the oxygen transport system, docking site for glycolytic enzymes, and structural protein in the cytoskeletal network [30].

Glycolytic enzymes form complexes with band 3 on the RBC membrane. When glycolytic enzymes are bound to band 3 their function is inhibited, when they are released and free in the cytoplasm, their activity is restored. During blood bank storage, in response to oxidative stress, these glycolytic enzymes are increasingly bound to band 3 and thus inhibited. Thus, this may explain the mechanism for the shift towards the oxidative phase of the pentose phosphate pathway, resulting in increased production of NADPH [31]. Finally, band 3 aggregation occurs both in vitro in the storage lesion as well as in vivo associated with aging RBCs in circulation and potentially serves as a membrane neoantigen for IgG to bind and mediate phagocytosis by Kupffer cells [30].

Membrane Loss and Microvesicles

Stored RBCs undergo membrane oxidation, damage, and exocytosis to form microvesicles (50–100 nm), which contain a substantial amount of hemoglobin. Some studies demonstrate that a small proportion of microvesicles are already evident at 4 days, but the percentage of microvesicles in packed RBC units increases dramatically with storage duration [32]. These microvesicles are prothrombotic, proinflammatory, and immunogenic and therefore are a potential source of adverse post-transfusion effects [33].

Supernatant Lipid Accumulation

During RBC storage, both nonpolar lipids and lysophosphatidylcholines accumulate in the supernatant. These lipids can prime polymorphonuclear cells and mediate acute lung injury in vivo [34]. The nature of the lipids responsible for this effect is different for leukoreduced and non-leukoreduced RBC units. Leukoreduced RBCs contain mostly the nonpolar lipids with arachidonic acid and 5-, 12-, 15-hydroxyeicostetraenoic acid (HETE) responsible for the priming activity; non-leukoreduced units also accumulate lysophosphatidylcholines, which can also mediate this potentially deleterious effect [34].

Phosphatidylserine

The RBC plasma membrane, like other cell membranes, is composed of a phospholipid bilayer. This bilayer demonstrates a distinct asymmetry with choline-containing lipids, phosphatidylcholine and sphingomyelin, predominately in the outer leaflet, while the aminophospholipids, phosphatidylethanolamine and phosphatidylserine (PS) are located mainly in the inner leaflet of erythrocytes [35]. This asymmetric distribution is tightly regulated by the enzymes flippase and scramblase. Flippase is an ATP-dependent aminophospholipid translocase that transports PS from the outer to inner leaflet; conversely, phospholipid scramblase is responsible for the transport of PS from the outer to inner leaflet. The maintenance of the phospholipid asymmetry is essential for cell survival. Specifically, PS exposure is an apoptotic signal and enhances pro-coagulant activity as it serves as a negatively charged surface for the coagulation cascade. RBC storage results in an increase in PS exposure in some [35], but not all studies [16]. However, although PS exposure may not occur during cold storage in vitro [16], it is difficult to assess whether stored RBCs are more prone to expose PS on their external membrane surface once transfused. Furthermore, flippase activity declines with storage. Flippase activity is modulated by ATP levels and intracellular pH; notably, both ATP levels and pH decline with RBC storage. Flippase activity can be restored to those seen in freshly isolated RBCs through experimental manipulation restoring ATP levels and pH [35]. These findings suggest that incubation in a high pH rejuvenation solution of inosine, phosphate, pyruvate, and adenine can rejuvenate stored RBCs and improve post-transfusion recovery [36].

Desialylation of RBCs

Exposure of the penultimate β-galactosyl residues as a result of desialylation of membrane glycoconjugates has been demonstrated to promote phagocytosis of senescent RBCs in circulation [37]. During storage of non-leukoreduced RBC units, RBCs are desialylated leading to exposure of terminal β-galactosyl residues. However, leukoreduction of RBC units dramatically reduces this desialylation. This finding, along with the accumulation of lysophosphatidylcholines in non-leukoreduced RBC units, which could potentially mediate acute lung injury [34], demonstrate some of the benefits of leukoreducing RBC units.

Decreased Membrane Expression of CD47

CD47, or integrin associated protein, is a transmembrane protein found on RBCs. It has been shown to have an important role as a self-recognition marker, acting as a "don't eat me" signal, and thus protects circulating RBCs from destruction by macrophages [38]. CD47 interacts with signal regulatory protein alpha (SIRPα) receptors found on macrophages, which causes inhibition of macrophage activation and thus survival of circulating RBCs [39]. CD47 antigen expression decreases on RBCs during storage, potentially enhancing their phagocytosis by macrophages. Additionally, with the loss of CD47 from the RBC surface, an increase in CD47 is observed in the supernatant of the RBC units. This extracellular CD47 may mediate a deleterious effect on the host during transfusion by binding and interfering with signal transduction pathways [38].

Clinical Consequences of Transfusion of Stored RBCs

RBC Hemolysis

Controversy exists as to whether transfusion of older, stored RBCs has negative clinical implications. Furthermore, the mechanism(s) responsible for adverse effects has yet to be determined. It is well-accepted that with increasing storage there is decreasing recovery of RBCs following transfusion leading to the FDA criteria that on average >75 % of RBCs remain in the circulation 24-h following transfusion. Thus, up to 25 % of transfused RBCs can be cleared from the circulation. Two leading hypotheses regarding the adverse effects of the storage lesion relate to hemolysis and differ in terms of the relative contribution of intravascular versus extravascular hemolysis. Hemolysis is defined as the destruction or removal of old or damaged RBCs from the circulation [40]. Certain types of damage result in intravascular hemolysis, in which the RBCs are destroyed within the circulation, releasing free hemoglobin and the remaining RBC contents. Extravascular hemolysis occurs by phagocytosis in the monocyte–macrophage system of organs such as the liver and spleen, which are considered the primary site of RBC removal from the circulation [41, 42]. Finally, to the extent that clinically relevant adverse effects of transfusion exist, it is likely that a combination of intravascular and extravascular hemolysis, along with other elements of the storage lesion described above, is responsible for these effects (Fig. 9.3).

Intravascular Hemolysis

Transfusion of older, stored RBCs is associated with increased plasma free hemoglobin and pulmonary artery pressure in recipients [43]. During intravascular hemolysis, the toxic compounds, hemoglobin and heme, are released into the circulation. Because of the toxicity of these compounds, mammals are equipped with efficient but saturable systems to clear them from the circulation. Haptoglobin and hemopexin are the most important scavenger systems.

Haptoglobin is an acute-phase reactant. When intravascular destruction of RBCs occurs, the released hemoglobin binds to haptoglobin. The resulting hemoglobin-haptoglobin complex is rapidly removed via receptor-mediated endocytosis and degraded in the liver, leading to a reduction in plasma haptoglobin. Once the haptoglobin scavenging capacity has been exceeded, the remaining free hemoglobin may form methemoglobin, which releases free heme, at the expense of endothelial NO (see Fig. 9.3). Hemopexin, another acute phase protein, binds heme and is then rapidly cleared from the circulation by receptor-mediated endocytosis. Thus, the combination of haptoglobin and hemopexin can reduce heme toxicity during intravascular hemolysis. However, once these systems are saturated, free heme can lead to adverse consequences as described below.

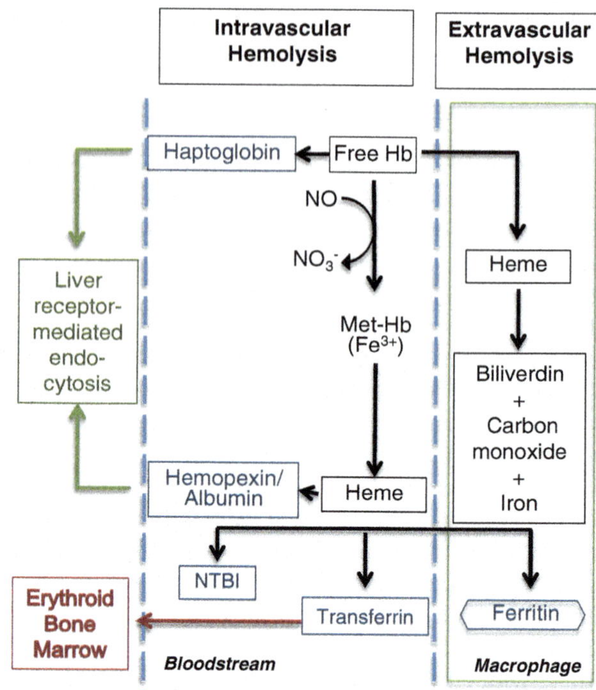

Intravascular Hemolysis

- Endothelial dysfunction
- Systemic vasoconstriction
- ROS generation
- Activation of platelets and hemostatic system
- Macrophage and neutrophil localization within the lung
- Neutrophil extracellular traps

Extravascular Hemolysis

- Innate immune activation
- Cytokine production
- Proliferation of pathogens
- Endothelial activation

Fig. 9.3 Intravascular and extravascular hemolytic pathways. Intravascular hemolysis results in the formation of free hemoglobin (Hb) and heme, which bind haptoglobin and hemopexin, respectively, and are delivered to the liver for degradation. Extravascular hemolysis occurs within reticuloendothelial macrophages. The breakdown of free Hb results in the production of iron, carbon monoxide, and biliverdin. Outside of the macrophages, free iron binds transferrin to be safely transported in the bloodstream. If these systems are saturated, non-transferrin-bound iron (NTBI) is produced and nitric oxide (NO) is consumed. The production of NTBI, free hemoglobin (Hb), and heme can lead to the listed consequences, contributing to organ dysfunction and tissue ischemia

Effects of Free Hemoglobin/Heme in the Circulation

A number of mechanisms have been postulated to mediate endothelial and lung injury from the release of molecules that are typically compartmentalized within RBCs.

Increasing studies are characterizing the pathogenic properties of these intracellular molecules released into the plasma, collectively referring to them as erythrocyte danger-associated molecular pattern molecules (eDAMPs) [44–47]. Free heme can act as an eDAMP serving as a pro-inflammatory ligand of innate immune receptors (e.g., TLR4) and can cause endothelial dysfunction by several mechanisms: increasing adhesion molecule expression and endothelial activation, promoting inflammatory cell recruitment and platelet aggregation, causing nitric oxide consumption and vasoconstriction, and/or oxidizing low-density lipoprotein [48–51]. Additionally, heme is a source of iron. Iron, both in the ferrous (Fe^{2+}) and in the ferric (Fe^{3+}) oxidation states, can participate in the Fenton reaction to produce highly toxic hydroxyl radicals [52, 53]. Finally, heme can amplify the hemolytic process, since it intercalates into RBC membranes favoring cell rupture [54]. In light of the properties of the RBC contents and the saturability of the scavenger systems, RBC hemolysis has been postulated to lead to vascular dysfunction, injury, and inflammation [55].

Imbalance Between Nitric Oxide and Reactive Oxygen Species

Circulating free hemoglobin interacts with NO in a fast and irreversible way via the NO deoxygenation reaction and iron nitrosylation reactions [56]. In addition, microvesicles containing hemoglobin can react with NO much faster than the hemoglobin contained in RBCs; these microvesicles may be the major source of NO-scavenging following transfusion [47]. Therefore, during intravascular hemolysis, a small amount of cell free plasma hemoglobin can impair NO signaling, leading to endothelial dysfunction and systemic vasoconstriction. In addition, RBCs contain significant concentrations of the enzyme arginase 1, which can metabolize L-arginine to ornithine. During hemolysis, this enzyme is released, reducing the availability of L-arginine, which is required for NO synthesis by the endothelial NO synthase enzyme.

In addition to impairment in NO synthesis and function, reactive oxygen species (ROS) generation from heme/hemoglobin also occurs during hemolysis. Extracellular hemoglobin auto-oxidizes to methemoglobin and participates in a catalytic pseudoperoxidase cycle producing ROS. Heme is responsible for the production of ROS because it contains iron, able, as mentioned before, to generate toxic ROS through the Fenton reaction. In addition to direct ROS production, heme can contribute to ROS generation by other distinct signaling pathways [53].

Platelet and Hemostatic Activation

In vitro experiments demonstrate that NO inhibits both platelet aggregation and endothelial adhesion molecule expression. Thus, the acute reduction in NO bioavailability by free hemoglobin can lead to the activation of platelets and the hemostatic system [57, 58]. Furthermore, NO may affect coagulation by inhibiting Factor XIII, enhancing clot stability and reducing clot dissolution [59]. Finally, RBCs contain high levels of ADP, the release of which during hemolysis can activate platelets via the P2Y receptors [54].

Heme and ATP-Mediated Activation of the Innate Immune System

Plasma free hemoglobin and heme affects endothelial function by causing macrophage and neutrophil localization within the lung parenchyma and activating the endothelium to generate pro-inflammatory effects. Heme, in particular, induces neutrophil migration to the lung and the release of DNA neutrophil extracellular traps (NETs) [60–62]. NETs recruit RBCs, activate platelets and promote fibrin deposition, contributing to the development of inflammation and thrombosis. Intravascular hemolysis also leads to ATP release, which can activate inflammatory pathways leading to sterile inflammation. Finally, heme has been shown to be an extracellular cell-signaling molecule and a causal factor in the development of vascular inflammation and vaso-occlusion [63]. In fact, recent studies suggest that heme binds macrophage and endothelial cell toll-like receptor (TLR)-4, stimulating parallel pro-inflammatory and pro-thrombotic pathways involving Weibel–Palade Body degranulation and nuclear factor-kappa B (NF-kB) activation [49, 50]. Together, these can trigger rapid pro-inflammatory, pro-thrombotic, and vasoconstrictive responses in the vasculature.

Extravascular Hemolysis

Although some RBCs hemolyze in the bag during storage (up to 1 and 0.8 % in the USA and Europe, respectively), on average, up to 25 % of the RBCs can be cleared from the circulation following transfusion. A majority of the RBCs cleared in vivo following transfusion are cleared by extravascular hemolysis in the monocyte–macrophage system of the reticuloendothelial system [64]. Furthermore, a majority of the storage-damaged RBCs that are cleared from the circulation are cleared very rapidly within the first hour of transfusion [65]. In a normal, healthy adult, approximately 1 mL of RBCs reach the end of their natural life span and are cleared each hour. This results in approximately 1 mg of iron recycled to the bone marrow with production of 1 mL of new RBCs every hour. After transfusion of 1 unit of stored RBCs, up to 25 % of the RBCs are cleared within 24 h, and most of this clearance takes place during the first hour [65]. As one unit of RBC contains about 250 mg iron, this translates into a rate of delivery of heme-iron to reticuloendothelial macrophages that is increased by as much as 60-fold after transfusion of even a single unit of packed RBCs. The delivered iron is either stored intracellularly or returned to the plasma to be bound by transferrin and transported to the erythroid marrow and other tissues for reuse. However, the rate of release of iron into the circulation can surpass the rate of uptake by transferrin producing circulating non-transferrin-bound iron [64, 66].

The full implications of the increased extravascular hemolysis remain to be determined. However, animal studies using mice [67] and dogs [68] suggest that there is a pro-inflammatory response following transfusion of older, stored RBCs.

This can exacerbate an underlying systemic inflammatory response syndrome (SIRS) [67] and can increase alloimmunogenicity to RBC antigens [69]. Furthermore, increased circulating iron, especially non-transferrin-bound iron, enhances proliferation of certain pathogens [64, 70, 71]. Thus, it would be expected that studies comparing the outcomes of patients receiving fresher or older RBC transfusions would yield differences in clinical outcome favoring the use of fresher RBCs.

Clinical Studies of Fresh Versus Old RBC Transfusions

Multiple observational studies have suggested an association between worse clinical outcomes (including increases in sepsis, pneumonia, multiorgan failure, myocardial infarction, acute renal failure, thrombosis, and mortality) and transfusion of RBC stored for longer durations [72]. However, these important studies have significant flaws, mainly owing to the difficulty in disentangling the contribution of the age of the RBCs from the increased underlying disease severity in patients receiving more, and therefore older units of RBCs. Thus, the conclusions are subject to much controversy and a number of randomized, controlled trials have been completed or are in progress to address these limitations.

The Age of Red Blood Cells in Premature Infants (ARIPI) study [73] randomized very low-birth-weight neonates to fresh blood stored for 7 days or less (mean 5.1 days) compared with standard issue RBC units (mean 14.6 days). There was no difference in the primary composite outcome, which included various neonatal morbidities and mortality. Similarly, in the Age of Transfused Blood in Critically Ill Adults (ABLE) study [74], there was no difference in the mortality of critically ill adults when randomized to fresh (mean 6.1 days) compared to standard issue (mean 22.0 days) RBC transfusions. Although these studies reported negative findings, it must be noted that the standard issue group did not receive many units near the FDA-approved outdate and these studies were not designed to answer the question of whether the use of RBCs stored for very prolonged periods (e.g., 35–42 days) results in harm [74]. Finally, in the Red Cell Storage Duration Study (RECESS) [75], patients undergoing complex cardiac surgery were randomly assigned to receive leukocyte-reduced RBCs stored for 10 days or less (mean 7.8 days) or for 21 days or more (mean 28.3 days) for all intraoperative and postoperative transfusions. Again, there was no difference in the primary outcome of the change in Multiple Organ Dysfunction Score observed between the groups suggesting that the current storage standards are acceptable for patients undergoing complex cardiac surgery. It is debatable whether this conclusion should be generalized to other populations. Of note, patients undergoing cardiopulmonary bypass (96% of the RECESS study population) exhibit signs of hemolysis from damage induced by the bypass pump [76]. Thus, these patients have a higher baseline level of hemolysis than other patient populations and to the extent that hemolysis is responsible for the adverse effects of stored RBC transfusions, the additional contribution of RBC transfusion to the damage already induced by the pump may not be clinically significant. Thus, despite the reports of these randomized controlled studies, the issue of whether prolonged storage of RBCs prior to transfusion results in harm is still controversial.

Summary

The clinical implications of the RBC storage lesion remain controversial. There are several well-studied biochemical and biomechanical changes that occur and alter the RBCs as well as the storage media in which the RBCs are preserved during prolonged refrigerated storage. Once transfused, RBCs that are stored longer undergo increased hemolysis. At the very least, hemolyzed RBCs cannot deliver oxygen to tissues. Furthermore, several observational studies suggest that patients receiving older RBCs have worse outcomes. The hemolysis associated with transfusion of stored RBCs may be responsible for these adverse effects. Randomized controlled trials examining the benefits of fresher RBC transfusions demonstrate no significant difference in clinical outcomes. However, these studies do not examine whether RBCs stored for very prolonged periods (i.e., 35–42 days) result in harm. Thus, controversy still remains regarding the clinical significance of the RBC storage lesion.

References

1. Pfuntner A, Wier LM, Stocks C. Most Frequent Conditions in U.S. Hospitals, 2011: Statistical Brief #162. Healthcare Cost and Utilization Project (HCUP) Statistical Briefs. Rockville, MD; 2013.
2. Klein HG. Should blood be an essential medicine? N Engl J Med. 2013;368(3):199–201.
3. Shehata N, Forster A, Lawrence N, Rothwell DM, Fergusson D, Tinmouth A, et al. Changing trends in blood transfusion: an analysis of 244,013 hospitalizations. Transfusion. 2014;54(10 Pt 2):2631–9.
4. Klein HG, Spahn DR, Carson JL. Red blood cell transfusion in clinical practice. Lancet. 2007;370(9585):415–26.
5. Hess JR. An update on solutions for red cell storage. Vox Sang. 2006;91(1):13–9.
6. Rous P, Turner JR. The preservation of living red blood cells in vitro: II. The transfusion of kept cells. J Exp Med. 1916;23(2):239–48.
7. Hogman CF, Hedlund K, Zetterstrom H. Clinical usefulness of red cells preserved in protein-poor mediums. N Engl J Med. 1978;299(25):1377–82.
8. Zehnder L, Schulzki T, Goede JS, Hayes J, Reinhart WH. Erythrocyte storage in hypertonic (SAGM) or isotonic (PAGGSM) conservation medium: influence on cell properties. Vox Sang. 2008;95(4):280–7.
9. Cancelas JA, Dumont LJ, Maes LA, Rugg N, Herschel L, Whitley PH, et al. Additive solution-7 reduces the red blood cell cold storage lesion. Transfusion. 2015;55(3):491–8.
10. Sparrow RL. Time to revisit red blood cell additive solutions and storage conditions: a role for "omics" analyses. Blood Transfus. 2012;10 Suppl 2:s7–11.
11. Flegel WA, Natanson C, Klein HG. Does prolonged storage of red blood cells cause harm? Br J Haematol. 2014;165(1):3–16.

12. Dumont LJ, AuBuchon JP. Evaluation of proposed FDA criteria for the evaluation of radiolabeled red cell recovery trials. Transfusion. 2008;48(6):1053–60.
13. Hess JR, Sparrow RL, van der Meer PF, Acker JP, Cardigan RA, Devine DV. Red blood cell hemolysis during blood bank storage: using national quality management data to answer basic scientific questions. Transfusion. 2009;49(12):2599–603.
14. Tinmouth A, Fergusson D, Yee IC, Hébert PC, Investigators A, The Canadian Critical Care Trials Group. Clinical consequences of red cell storage in the critically ill. Transfusion. 2006;46(11):2014–27.
15. Berezina TL, Zaets SB, Morgan C, Spillert CR, Kamiyama M, Spolarics Z, et al. Influence of storage on red blood cell rheological properties. J Surg Res. 2002;102(1):6–12.
16. Bennett-Guerrero E, Veldman TH, Doctor A, Telen MJ, Ortel TL, Reid TS, et al. Evolution of adverse changes in stored RBCs. Proc Natl Acad Sci. 2007;104(43):17063–8.
17. La Celle PL. Alteration of deformability of the erythrocyte membrane in stored blood. Transfusion. 1969;9(5):238–45.
18. Deplaine G, Safeukui I, Jeddi F, Lacoste F, Brousse V, Perrot S, et al. The sensing of poorly deformable red blood cells by the human spleen can be mimicked in vitro. Blood. 2011;117(8):e88–95.
19. Raat NJ, Verhoeven AJ, Mik EG, Gouwerok CW, Verhaar R, Goedhart PT, et al. The effect of storage time of human red cells on intestinal microcirculatory oxygenation in a rat isovolemic exchange model. Crit Care Med. 2005;33(1):39–45. discussion 238-9.
20. Lion N, Crettaz D, Rubin O, Tissot J-D. Stored red blood cells: a changing universe waiting for its map(s). J Proteomics. 2010;73(3):374–85.
21. D'Alessandro A, D'Amici GM, Vaglio S, Zolla L. Time-course investigation of SAGM-stored leukocyte-filtered red blood cell concentrates: from metabolism to proteomics. Haematologica. 2012;97(1):107–15.
22. D'Alessandro A, Nemkov T, Kelher M, West FB, Schwindt RK, Banerjee A, et al. Routine storage of red blood cell (RBC) units in additive solution-3: a comprehensive investigation of the RBC metabolome. Transfusion. 2014.
23. Nakao M, Nakao T, Yamazoe S. Adenosine triphosphate and maintenance of shape of the human red cells. Nature. 1960;187:945–6.
24. Wood L, Beutler E. The viability of human blood stored in phosphate adenine media. Transfusion. 1967;7(6):401–8.
25. Whillier S, Raftos JE, Sparrow RL, Kuchel PW. The effects of long-term storage of human red blood cells on the glutathione synthesis rate and steady-state concentration. Transfusion. 2011;51(7):1450–9.
26. Dumaswala UJ, Zhuo L, Jacobsen DW, Jain SK, Sukalski KA. Protein and lipid oxidation of banked human erythrocytes: role of glutathione. Free Radic Biol Med. 1999;27(9–10):1041–9.
27. Gevi F, D'Alessandro A, Rinalducci S, Zolla L. Alterations of red blood cell metabolome during cold liquid storage of erythrocyte concentrates in CPD-SAGM. J Proteomics. 2012;76 Spec No.:168–80.
28. Ralser M, Wamelink MM, Kowald A, Gerisch B, Heeren G, Struys EA, et al. Dynamic rerouting of the carbohydrate flux is key to counteracting oxidative stress. J Biol. 2007;6(4):10.
29. Karon BS, Hoyer JD, Stubbs JR, Thomas DD. Changes in Band 3 oligomeric state precede cell membrane phospholipid loss during blood bank storage of red blood cells. Transfusion. 2009;49(7):1435–42.
30. D'Alessandro A, Liumbruno G, Grazzini G, Zolla L. Red blood cell storage: the story so far. Blood Transfus. 2010;8(2):82–8.
31. Rinalducci S, Marrocco C, Zolla L. Thiol-based regulation of glyceraldehyde-3-phosphate dehydrogenase in blood bank-stored red blood cells: a strategy to counteract oxidative stress. Transfusion. 2015;55(3):499–506.
32. Donadee C, Raat NJ, Kanias T, Tejero J, Lee JS, Kelley EE, et al. Nitric oxide scavenging by red blood cell microparticles and cell-free hemoglobin as a mechanism for the red cell storage lesion. Circulation. 2011;124(4):465–76.
33. D'Alessandro A, Kriebardis AG, Rinalducci S, Antonelou MH, Hansen KC, Papassideri IS, et al. An update on red blood cell storage lesions, as gleaned through biochemistry and omics technologies. Transfusion. 2015;55(1):205–19.

34. Silliman CC, Moore EE, Kelher MR, Khan SY, Gellar L, Elzi DJ. Identification of lipids that accumulate during the routine storage of prestorage leukoreduced red blood cells and cause acute lung injury. Transfusion. 2011;51(12):2549–54.
35. Verhoeven AJ, Hilarius PM, Dekkers DWC, Lagerberg JWM, De Korte D. Prolonged storage of red blood cells affects aminophospholipid translocase activity. Vox Sang. 2006;91(3):244–51.
36. Szymanski IO, Teno RA, Lockwood WB, Hudgens R, Johnson GS. Effect of rejuvenation and frozen storage on 42-day-old AS-1 RBCs. Transfusion. 2001;41(4):550–5.
37. Bratosin D, Estaquier J, Petit F, Arnoult D, Quatannens B, Tissier JP, et al. Programmed cell death in mature erythrocytes: a model for investigating death effector pathways operating in the absence of mitochondria. Cell Death Differ. 2001;8(12):1143–56.
38. Anniss AM, Sparrow RL. Expression of CD47 (integrin-associated protein) decreases on red blood cells during storage. Transfus Apher Sci. 2002;27(3):233–8.
39. Oldenborg PA, Zheleznyak A, Fang YF, Lagenaur CF, Gresham HD, Lindberg FP. Role of CD47 as a marker of self on red blood cells. Science. 2000;288(5473):2051–4.
40. DhaliwalG,CornettPA,TierneyJrLM.Hemolyticanemia.AmFamPhysician.2004;69(11):2599–606.
41. Cazzola M, Beguin Y. New tools for clinical evaluation of erythron function in man. Br J Haematol. 1992;80(3):278–84.
42. Bossi D, Giardina B. Red cell physiology. Mol Aspects Med. 1996;17(2):117–28.
43. Berra L, Pinciroli R, Stowell CP, Wang L, Yu B, Fernandez BO, et al. Autologous transfusion of stored red blood cells increases pulmonary artery pressure. Am J Respir Crit Care Med. 2014;190(7):800–7.
44. Chiabrando D, Vinchi F, Fiorito V, Mercurio S, Tolosano E. Heme in pathophysiology: a matter of scavenging, metabolism and trafficking across cell membranes. Front Pharmacol. 2014;5:61.
45. Matzinger P. Tolerance, danger, and the extended family. Annu Rev Immunol. 1994;12:991–1045.
46. Matzinger P. The danger model: a renewed sense of self. Science. 2002;296(5566):301–5.
47. Jeney V, Balla G, Balla J. Red blood cell, hemoglobin and heme in the progression of atherosclerosis. Front Physiol. 2014;5:379.
48. Belcher JD, Nath KA, Vercellotti GM. Vasculotoxic and proinflammatory effects of plasma heme: cell signaling and cytoprotective responses. ISRN Oxidative Med. 2013;2013. pii: 831596.
49. Belcher JD, Nguyen J, Chen CS, et al. Plasma hemoglobin and heme trigger Weibel Palade body exocytosis and vaso-occlusion in transgenic sickle mice. Blood. 2011;118(21):896.
50. Palsson-McDermott EM, O'Neill LA. Signal transduction by the lipopolysaccharide receptor, toll-like receptor-4. Immunology. 2004;113(2):153–62.
51. Valentijn KM, Sadler JE, Valentijn JA, Voorberg J, Eikenboom J. Functional architecture of Weibel-Palade bodies. Blood. 2011;117(19):5033–43.
52. Prousek J. Fenton chemistry in biology and medicine. Pure Appl Chem. 2007;79(12):13.
53. Goldstein S, Meyerstein D, Czapski G. The Fenton reagents. Free Radic Biol Med. 1993;15(4):435–45.
54. Dutra FF, Bozza MT. Heme on innate immunity and inflammation. Front Pharmacol. 2014;5:115.
55. Potoka KP, Gladwin MT. Vasculopathy and pulmonary hypertension in sickle cell disease. Am J Physiol Lung Cell Mol Physiol. 2015;308(4):L314–24.
56. Rother RP, Bell L, Hillmen P, Gladwin MT. The clinical sequelae of intravascular hemolysis and extracellular plasma hemoglobin: a novel mechanism of human disease. JAMA. 2005;293(13):1653–62.
57. Hu W, Jin R, Zhang J, You T, Peng Z, Ge X, et al. The critical roles of platelet activation and reduced NO bioavailability in fatal pulmonary arterial hypertension in a murine hemolysis model. Blood. 2010;116(9):1613–22.
58. Patel RP, McAndrew J, Sellak H, White CR, Jo H, Freeman BA, et al. Biological aspects of reactive nitrogen species. Biochim Biophys Acta. 1999;1411(2–3):385–400.

59. Gries A, Bode C, Peter K, Herr A, Bohrer H, Motsch J, et al. Inhaled nitric oxide inhibits human platelet aggregation, P-selectin expression, and fibrinogen binding in vitro and in vivo. Circulation. 1998;97(15):1481–7.
60. Chen G, Zhang D, Fuchs TA, Manwani D, Wagner DD, Frenette PS. Heme-induced neutrophil extracellular traps contribute to the pathogenesis of sickle cell disease. Blood. 2014;123(24):3818–27.
61. Graca-Souza AV, Arruda MA, de Freitas MS, Barja-Fidalgo C, Oliveira PL. Neutrophil activation by heme: implications for inflammatory processes. Blood. 2002;99(11):4160–5.
62. Porto BN, Alves LS, Fernandez PL, Dutra TP, Figueiredo RT, Graca-Souza AV, et al. Heme induces neutrophil migration and reactive oxygen species generation through signaling pathways characteristic of chemotactic receptors. J Biol Chem. 2007;282(33):24430–6.
63. Belcher JD, Chen C, Nguyen J, Milbauer L, Abdulla F, Alayash AI, et al. Heme triggers TLR4 signaling leading to endothelial cell activation and vaso-occlusion in murine sickle cell disease. Blood. 2014;123(3):377–90.
64. Hod EA, Brittenham GM, Billote GB, Francis RO, Ginzburg YZ, Hendrickson JE, et al. Transfusion of human volunteers with older, stored red blood cells produces extravascular hemolysis and circulating non-transferrin-bound iron. Blood. 2011;118(25):6675–82.
65. Luten M, Roerdinkholder-Stoelwinder B, Schaap NP, de Grip WJ, Bos HJ, Bosman GJ. Survival of red blood cells after transfusion: a comparison between red cells concentrates of different storage periods. Transfusion. 2008;48(7):1478–85.
66. Stark MJ, Keir AK, Andersen CC. Does non-transferrin bound iron contribute to transfusion related immune-modulation in preterms? Arch Dis Child Fetal Neonatal Ed. 2013;98(5):F424–9.
67. Hod EA, Zhang N, Sokol SA, Wojczyk BS, Francis RO, Ansaldi D, et al. Transfusion of red blood cells after prolonged storage produces harmful effects that are mediated by iron and inflammation. Blood. 2010;115(21):4284–92.
68. Callan MB, Patel RT, Rux AH, Bandyopadhyay S, Sireci AN, O'Donnell PA, et al. Transfusion of 28-day-old leucoreduced or non-leucoreduced stored red blood cells induces an inflammatory response in healthy dogs. Vox Sang. 2013;105(4):319–27.
69. Hendrickson JE, Hod EA, Spitalnik SL, Hillyer CD, Zimring JC. Storage of murine red blood cells enhances alloantibody responses to an erythroid-specific model antigen. Transfusion. 2010;50(3):642–8.
70. Prestia K, Bandyopadhyay S, Slate A, Francis RO, Francis KP, Spitalnik SL, et al. Transfusion of stored blood impairs host defenses against Gram-negative pathogens in mice. Transfusion. 2014;54(11):2842–51.
71. Solomon SB, Wang D, Sun J, Kanias T, Feng J, Helms CC, et al. Mortality increases after massive exchange transfusion with older stored blood in canines with experimental pneumonia. Blood. 2013;121(9):1663–72.
72. Wang D, Sun J, Solomon SB, Klein HG, Natanson C. Transfusion of older stored blood and risk of death: a meta-analysis. Transfusion. 2012;52(6):1184–95.
73. Fergusson DA, Hebert P, Hogan DL, LeBel L, Rouvinez-Bouali N, Smyth JA, et al. Effect of fresh red blood cell transfusions on clinical outcomes in premature, very low-birth-weight infants: the ARIPI randomized trial. JAMA. 2012;308(14):1443–51.
74. Lacroix J, Hebert PC, Fergusson DA, Tinmouth A, Cook DJ, Marshall JC, et al. Age of transfused blood in critically ill adults. N Engl J Med. 2015;372(15):1410–8.
75. Steiner ME, Ness PM, Assmann SF, Triulzi DJ, Sloan SR, Delaney M, et al. Effects of red-cell storage duration on patients undergoing cardiac surgery. N Engl J Med. 2015;372(15):1419–29.
76. Vermeulen Windsant IC, Hanssen SJ, Buurman WA, Jacobs MJ. Cardiovascular surgery and organ damage: time to reconsider the role of hemolysis. J Thorac Cardiovasc Surg. 2011;142(1):1–11.

Chapter 10
Transfusion and Acute Respiratory Distress Syndrome: Pathogenesis and Potential Mechanisms

Nicole P. Juffermans and Alexander P. Vlaar

Introduction

The association between blood transfusion and lung injury or its more severe form acute respiratory distress syndrome (ARDS) has been noted already since the early seventies. Since then, it is a consistent finding in multiple clinical trials in different patient populations. In the association between transfusion and lung injury, both patient- and transfusion-related risk factors play a role. Identification of these risk factors has shed some light on the pathogenesis of lung injury following transfusion, although many questions remain.

In terms of patient factors, it has become more and more clear that the association between transfusion and ARDS is more prevalent in the critically ill, in trauma and other surgical patients [1], the epidemiology of which is discussed in Chap. 11. In terms of mechanisms, it can be argued that the relation between transfusion and ARDS reflects the fact that transfusion is merely a confounder in the occurrence of lung injury, as patients who have lung injury are more ill, with a concomitant more profound anemia and subsequent more frequent exposure to transfusion. However, recent data strongly suggests that there is a causal relationship between transfusion and lung injury, with clear proof of principal in either experimental settings [2–7] or using experimental methods of measuring lung edema in the clinical setting [8]. Increasingly, patient-related risk factors are recognized as the most relevant risk factors for the development of lung injury following transfusion [9].

In terms of transfusion-related risk factors, plasma containing blood products are the blood products most frequently involved in the occurrence of lung injury, and are also associated with fatal pulmonary reactions. Antibodies in the blood product directed at cognate antigens in the recipient have been implicated, but these

N.P. Juffermans, MD, PhD (✉) • A.P. Vlaar, MD, PhD
Laboratory of Experimental Intensive Care and Anesthesiology, Department of Intensive Care Medicine, Academic Medical Center, Amsterdam, The Netherlands
e-mail: n.p.juffermans@amc.uva.nl

J.S. Lee, M.P. Donahoe (eds.), *Hematologic Abnormalities and Acute Lung Syndromes*, Respiratory Medicine, DOI 10.1007/978-3-319-41912-1_10

Table 10.1 Definition of transfusion-related acute lung injury

TRALI
– Acute onset within 6 h after a blood transfusion
– PaO_2/FiO_2 <300 mmHg
– Bilateral infiltrative changes on the chest X-ray
– No sign of hydrostatic pulmonary edema (PAOP <18 mmHg or CVP <15 mmHg)
– No other risk factor for ALI present
Possible TRALI
– Other risk factor for ALI present
Delayed TRALI
– Onset of TRALI between 6 and 72 h after a blood transfusion

PAOP pulmonary arterial occlusion pressure, *CVP* central venous pressure, *ALI* acute lung injury

antibodies are not a prerequisite for the development of lung injury, nor do they explain all cases of lung injury. Currently, there is a surge of research aimed at identifying other causative factors in the blood product.

Lung injury immediately following transfusion is a well-known syndrome, termed transfusion-related acute lung injury (TRALI, Table 10.1). However, the association between transfusion and ARDS has also repeatedly been observed outside the context of a clear temporal relationship, in particular in the critically ill. Characteristically, another risk factor for lung injury is often present in these patients with a delayed reaction. Obviously, causality is more difficult to prove in this setting.

In this chapter, we summarize available knowledge on the pathogenesis and potential mechanisms of the relation between transfusion and ARDS, highlighting both the role of the recipient as well as of the blood product. We describe both TRALI as well as the association between transfusion and ARDS which does not fulfill TRALI criteria, with the aim to integrate pathophysiology in an explanatory model.

Transfusion and ARDS in Clear Temporal Relationship: TRALI

Transfusion-related acute lung injury (TRALI) is a subcategory of acute lung injury/acute respiratory distress syndrome (ALI/ARDS). According to a consensus definition, TRALI is defined as the occurrence of ALI within 6 h of transfusion of a blood product [10]. Any cell- or plasma-containing blood product can elicit a TRALI reaction and even small volumes can trigger the reaction. When other risk factors for ALI are concurrently present, one speaks of possible TRALI (Table 10.1).

Clinically, TRALI is indistinguishable from ALI due to other causes, characterized by pulmonary edema resulting in bilateral infiltrates on chest radiograph, with decreased oxygenation and subsequent dyspnea and tachypnea. Other clinical features are nonspecific and can include fever or hypothermia, hypotension as well as hypertension. Also laboratory testing in TRALI is not specific. The most prevalent symptom is a transient leukopenia, which occurs in 35–75 % [11], mostly occurring in patients after transfusion with an antibody containing blood product, which are thought to be due to neutrophil-specific antibodies. Also transient thrombocytopenia occurs.

Pathogenesis of TRALI: Two-Hit Mechanism

TRALI is mediated by the interaction of neutrophils with pulmonary endothelial cells. TRALI is thought to occur as a result of two independent hits. The first hit is the clinical condition of the patient at the time of the transfusion. An inflammatory reaction due to any cause attracts neutrophils to the pulmonary compartment. Primed neutrophils, trapped in the lung's microvasculature, are functionally hyperactive. The second hit is the transfusion, which further activates the primed neutrophils in the lung vasculature of the recipient, resulting in endothelial damage, with ensuing pulmonary edema and extravasation of neutrophils. The second hit can be divided in antibody and non-antibody-mediated TRALI. There is near universal agreement that passive infusion of human neutrophil antibodies (HNA) or human leukocyte antibodies (HLA) directed against the recipients antigens can result in TRALI, called antibody-mediated TRALI. This is detailed below. However, many TRALI cases are reported in which no specific anti-neutrophil antibodies are detected [12, 13]. Also, the majority of recipients do not develop TRALI after infusion of antibodies, even when cognate antigen is present [14, 15]. Also, observational studies report associations between prolonged storage of blood products and ARDS in the critically ill [16, 17], although this was not confirmed in a recent randomized trial [18]. Thereby, there is also a non-antibody-mediated pathway in TRALI. The causative factor is presently not known. Data on the role of bioactive lipids (lysophosphatidylcholines, lysoPCs) or other neutrophil priming agents which have accumulated during blood storage are summarized below.

Pathogenesis of TRALI: Importance of Host Factors in the First Hit

The First Hit

Recent data point towards an important role for host factors in TRALI pathogenesis. In a study on risk factors for TRALI in a cohort of critically ill adults [19] as well as in critically ill children [20], around 90 % of the patients that confirmed to the diagnostic criteria for TRALI, also had a risk factor for ALI prior to onset of TRALI (possible TRALI). In the multivariate analysis, patient related risk factors were more important for the onset of TRALI than transfusion related risk factors, suggesting that development of a TRALI reaction depends more on host factors then on factors in the blood product. Of note, in a cohort of general TRALI patients as well as in cardiac surgery patients with TRALI, systemic levels of IL-6 and IL-8 were found to be elevated prior to the development of TRALI compared to controls [21, 22].

Specific Patient Risk Factors

These are summarized in Fig. 10.1. The presence of mechanical ventilation predisposes to acquiring TRALI. This was shown in experimental models [23]. Also, the application of high peak airway pressures increases the risk for TRALI in patients [21]. Thereby, it seems likely that mechanical stretch of the lungs can prime pulmonary neutrophils. Given that an inflammatory condition can be a first hit, it is unsurprising that sepsis has repeatedly been shown to be an important risk factor for TRALI [17, 21]. Also specific surgical procedures seem a risk factor. The high incidence of TRALI in cardiac surgery is associated with duration of cardiopulmonary bypass, suggesting that this device may contribute to neutrophil priming. Also thoracic, vascular and transplant surgeries carry a high rate of perioperative TRALI, with an incidence of 2–3 %. Interestingly, obstetric and gynecologic surgeries are not risk factors [24]. Conditions in which patients typically receive multiple transfusions are also risk factors for TRALI, including hematologic malignancy, bleeding

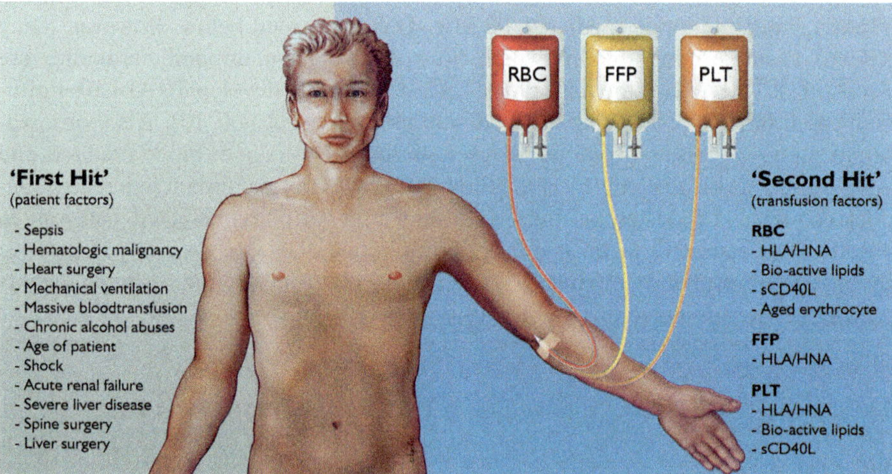

Fig. 10.1 Host and transfusion factors in the onset of transfusion-related acute lung injury (TRALI). The first hit is the underlying condition of the patient resulting in priming of the pulmonary neutrophils. Risk factors which may function as a first hit are on the left side of the panel. The second hit is the blood transfusion resulting in activation of the endothelial cells and the primed pulmonary neutrophils resulting in capillary leakage, finally resulting in pulmonary oedema (right side of the panel). Some transfusion factors are independent of the type of blood product while others are specific for a type of blood product. *HLA* human leukocyte antibodies, *HNA* human neutrophil antibodies, *RBCs* red blood cells, *FFP* fresh frozen plasma

with liver failure and massive transfusion [17, 21]. In these settings, it is not clear whether these conditions are specific risk factors or merely reflect frequent exposure to blood products.

Pathogenesis of TRALI: Antibody Mediated TRALI

HLA and HNA Antibodies

All blood products have been implicated in TRALI. Antibody mediated TRALI is caused by the passive infusion of HLA and or HNA antibodies present in the plasma of the donor product. A minority of cases are caused by antibodies of the recipient reacting with the antigens of the infused leukocytes of the donor. However, since the implementation of a universal leukoreduced blood product program this form of antibody mediated TRALI has become irrelevant. High volume plasma products such as fresh frozen plasma (FFP) and platelet concentrates are at highest risk to induce TRALI. However any plasma containing product is able to induce TRALI, even with small amounts of residual plasma in RBCs products [25]. The involved antibodies in antibody mediated TRALI are HLA class I, HLA class II, and HNA antibodies (Table 10.2). The majority of reported TRALI reactions are based on antibodies present in the transfused blood products. Observational studies report that 14–26 % of the TRALI cases are caused by HLA class I antibodies, 0–46 % by HLA class II antibodies and 16–28 % by HNA antibodies [26–29]. Studies aimed at understanding which donors are at risk for developing antibodies showed that previously exposed donors such as multiparous donors have an increased risk of developing HLA antibodies. Screening of multiparous donors showed that due to sensitization during pregnancy up to 40 % developed antibodies [30]. Based on these findings a trial was performed among critically ill patients [31] in which 100 patients in need of plasma transfusion, were randomly assigned to receive plasma from a multiparous donor or from a control donor. This study showed that transfusion of plasma from multiparous donors was associated with decreased oxygen saturation and higher TNF-alpha concentrations than transfusion of control plasma. The strong relation between the presence of antibodies and TRALI resulted in the implementation of a male-only donor policy. Two recent meta-analyses showed that

Table 10.2 Host factors involved in the onset of antibody mediated TRALI

Antibody pathway	Involved host cells	Cofactors	Alternative pathway
HLA class I	Platelet Neutrophil Monocyte	Complement	Direct on endothelium
HLA Class II	Neutrophil Monocyte		
HNA	Neutrophil		Antibody fragments

HLA human leucocyte antibody, *HNA* human neutrophil antibody the implementation of these low risk TRALI donor policies for high volume plasma products has resulted in an approximately two-thirds reduction of TRALI cases [32, 33]. A remaining discussion is whether low risk TRALI donor policies should also be implemented for low volume plasma products such as RBCs.

Downstream Host Response in Antibody Mediated TRALI

In the past decades, studies have clarified the role of host immune cells, endothelial cells, and cofactors in the onset of antibody mediated TRALI. Initially it was hypothesized that all antibodies (HLA class I, II and HNA) involved in the onset of antibody mediated TRALI induced neutrophil activation using a common pathway. Recent studies however showed that each antibody induces TRALI using separate pathways (Table 10.2). Most preclinical studies have been performed using HLA class I antibodies. The first in vivo mice model of TRALI used HLA class I antibodies [34]. Infusion of these antibodies resulted in severe pulmonary edema which made it a clinical relevant model. In this model depletion of neutrophils using vinblastine prevented the onset of TRALI. Also, depletion of platelets as well as aspirin, which prevents activation of platelets, protected mice for the onset of TRALI [35]. These studies suggest that both neutrophils and platelets are essential in the onset of TRALI. Another group, however, showed that HLA class I antibodies are able to induce TRALI in the absence of neutrophils and platelets using hydroxycarbamide and neuraminidase respectively [36]. It was suggested that complement and monocytes are key players in the onset of TRALI induced by HLA class I antibodies. Furthermore, from a TRALI case in a single lung-transplantation patient in which infusion of HLA class I antibodies resulted in TRALI only in the transplanted lung which expressed the cognate antigen and not in the native lung [37], it can be hypothesized that HLA class I antibodies are also able to directly activate and damage the endothelium.

The onset of antibody mediated TRALI through infusion of HLA class II antibodies has been studied less extensively. In vitro studies showed that HLA class II antibodies are able to activate monocytes resulting in damage to endothelial cells [38]. In an ex vivo animal model it was shown that activated monocytes are able to activate neutrophils which are hypothesized to be essential in the onset of TRALI induced by HLA class II antibodies [39].

The HNA antibodies are divided in several subtypes of which HNA-1, HNA-2, and HNA-3a are related to the most severe and even fatal TRALI reactions. HNA 3a antibodies have been shown to interact directly with the endothelial cells and cause lung injury, however neutrophils seem to be required for the onset of HNA induced lung injury [40]. Also HNA 3a antibody fragments can induce a mild form of lung injury. Of interest, HNA 3a fragments are not able to bind the Fcγ-receptor, whereas the whole antibody can. This observation suggests a neutrophil Fcγ-receptor dependent and independent pathway in the onset of HNA induced TRALI.

To summarize, antibody mediated TRALI is caused by the passive infusion of HLA class I, II and HNA antibodies reacting with the cognate antigen of the recipient.

The pathways involved in the onset of antibody mediated TRALI differ between the involved antibodies. Studies suggest that besides neutrophils, also monocytes, platelets, endothelial cells and complement are essential in the onset of antibody mediated TRALI.

Pathogenesis of TRALI: Non-antibody-mediated TRALI

Soluble Mediators

Bioactive lipids accumulating during storage of red blood cells or platelets have been implicated in TRALI. The neutral (nonpolar) lipids are only found in RBCs, whereas lysophosphatidylcholines (LysoPCs) are thought to be platelet derived. In vitro, neutrophils can be activated by LysoPCs. LysoPCs isolated from aged blood also caused lung injury in a two-hit animal TRALI model [41] and LysoPCs have been implicated in a series of ten patients with TRALI [42]. On the other hand, other study groups could not confirm a role for lipids using two-hit TRALI animal models. Clinical studies report conflicting results on the role of LysoPCs. It is hypothesized that the association between LysoPCs and TRALI merely reflects a higher total volume of products transfused and not an increased level of lysoPCs per product due to accumulation during storage [17, 43]. These differences may relate to different storage procedures. Nonpolar lipids from RBCs caused acute lung injury in a two-hit animal model [44], which could partly be prevented by filtration of donor blood before storage [4]. The role of nonpolar lipids in human TRALI has not been explored yet.

Besides lipids, soluble CD40L has been implicated in non-antibody-mediated TRALI [45]. Soluble CD40L is produced by platelets. It activates macrophages and elicits the production of pro-inflammatory cytokines. Increased levels of sCD40L in stored platelets has been associated with transfusion reactions and increased respiratory burst in granulocytes. In animals developing TRALI, the level of sCD40L was modestly increased in the supernatant of stored RBCs or platelets compared to controls [6, 46]. Also, sCD40L levels were increased in samples of platelet transfusions implicated in TRALI reactions compared to transfused patients not developing TRALI [45]. On the other hand however, blocking of CD40L expression did not modulate TRALI in an animal model [47] and in a cohort of cardiac surgery patients with TRALI, sCD40L did not differ from transfused controls [48]. Even though sCD40L is a potent mediator in inflammation, a majority of studies suggest only a minor role for sCD40L in TRALI.

Cellular Changes

Red blood cells undergo changes during storage, among others decreased deformability, depletion of 2,3 diphosphoglycerate (2,3-DPG) and reductions in concentrations of nitric oxide. During storage, human RBCs also lose Duffy antigen expression and chemokine scavenging function. In a two-hit mouse model, transfusion of stored RBCs derived from Duffy-antigen knockout resulted in increased lung injury compared to transfusion of Duffy wild-type red blood cells, implicating a key role for the Duffy-antigen in TRALI [49]. Also platelets undergo changes when stored, including shrinking and plasma membrane vesiculation. In TRALI, platelet aggregation is found in histopathologic sections of the lung [35]. Whether aging of platelets plays a role is not clear however. Aged platelets, but not the supernatant of a product treated with ultraviolet, caused acute lung injury in two-hit murine models [50]. However, a recent study did not replicate these findings [51].

Downstream Host Response in Non-antibody-mediated TRALI

In vitro, stored RBC and stored platelets can prime fMLP-induced activation of the respiratory burst in human neutrophils compared to fresh products [46, 52]. Non-antibody-mediated TRALI caused by transfusion of stored RBCs or platelets in a two-hit animal TRALI model is characterized by increased pulmonary inflammation, including elevated levels of pro-inflammatory cytokines IL-6 and chemokine CINC3, as well as increased coagulation and impaired fibrinolysis compared to animals receiving fresh products. Also there is systemic inflammation [2, 6, 7]. Clinical studies on TRALI pathogenesis cannot differentiate between the antibody and non-antibody-mediated TRALI, as no specific diagnostic test exists to distinguish the two causes. In cardiac surgery patients with possible TRALI, pulmonary neutrophil influx is present and pulmonary levels of IL-6, IL-8, IL-1, and elastase–α1-antitrypsin complexes (a marker of neutrophil activation) are elevated during a TRALI reaction. In addition, pulmonary thrombin–antithrombin complexes and plasminogen activator inhibitor-1 were increased in the bronchoalveolar lavage fluid with a concomitant decrease in plasminogen activator activity percentage, indicating enhanced coagulation with impaired thrombolysis [22]. Also, in TRALI patients, levels of biomarkers for neutrophil extracellular traps (NETs) were increased compared to healthy subjects. As implicated blood did not contain excessive NET biomarkers, NETs supposedly were formed in the recipients after transfusion, suggestive of neutrophil activation [53]. A wide range of other mediators have been implicated in TRALI, the pathogenesis of which is summarized in Fig. 10.2. Of note, a distinction between causes of TRALI is not made.

Pathogenesis of TRALI: Threshold Model

Previously, it was thought that TRALI due to antibodies did not require the presence of a priming first hit, as cases have been described in which relatively healthy recipients develop antibody mediated TRALI. However, in an experimental mouse model of TRALI, infusion of MHC-I antibodies in mice with the cognate antigen induces a TRALI reaction in the presence, but not in the absence of priming factors. A threshold model has been suggested which describes the relation between the

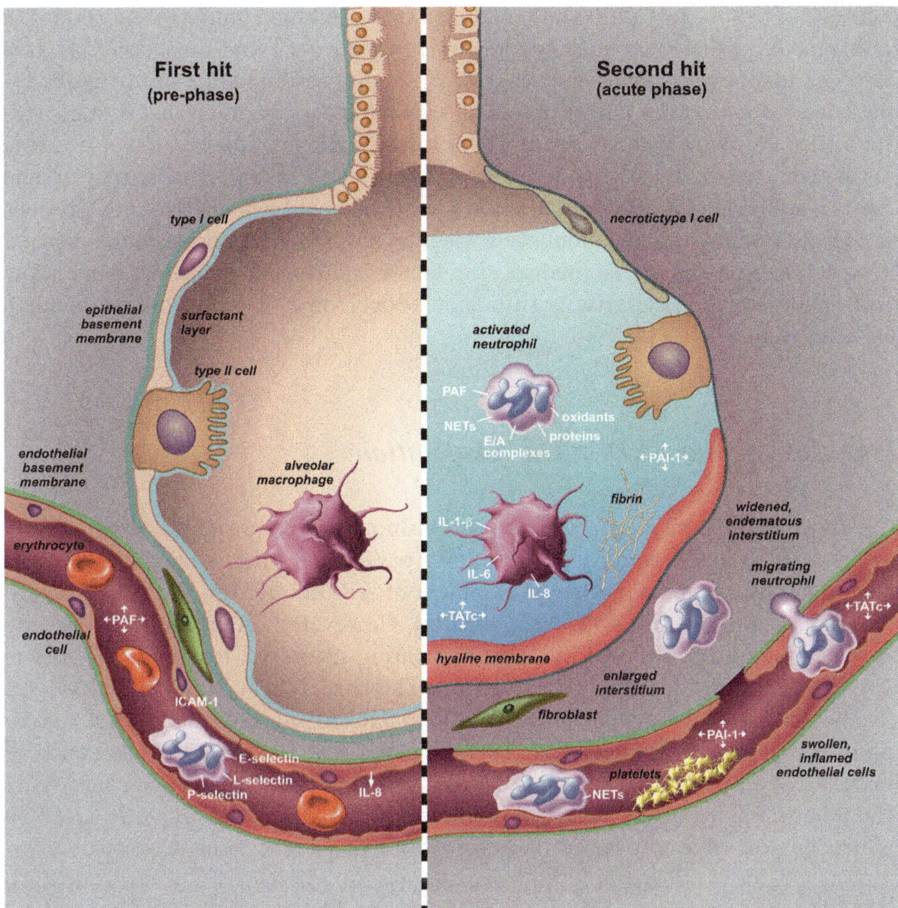

Fig. 10.2 Pathogenesis of transfusion-related acute lung injury (TRALI). In the pre-phase of the syndrome (left-hand side), there is a first hit which is mainly a systemic hit. Neutrophils are attracted to the lung by release of cytokines and chemokines from up-regulated lung endothelium. Loose binding by L-selectin takes place. Firm adhesion is realized by E-selectin and platelet-derived P-selectin and intra cellular adhesion molecules (ICAM-1). In the acute phase of the syndrome (right-hand side), there is a second hit resulting in inflammation in the pulmonary compartment. Neutrophils are shown adhering to the injured capillary endothelium and marginating through the interstitium into the air space, which is filled with protein-rich oedema fluid. In the air space, there is secretion of cytokines, interleukin-1, -6, and 8, (IL-1, IL-6, IL-8), which act locally to stimulate chemotaxis and activate neutrophils which results in elastase–α(1)-antitrypsin (EA) complex formation. Neutrophils can release oxidants, proteases, and other pro-inflammatory molecules, such as platelet-activating factor (PAF) and form neutrophil extracellular traps (NETs). Furthermore there is activation of the coagulation system illustrated by an increase in thrombin-antithrombin complexes (TATc) and decrease of the fibrinolysis system illustrated by a decrease in plasminogen activator activity (PAA%). The net result is influx of protein-rich oedema fluid into the alveolus with inactivation of surfactant

presence of host factors ("first hit") and factors in the blood product ("second hit"). In this model, a threshold must be overcome to induce a TRALI reaction [54]. It is proposed that transfusion of high titers of antibodies resulting in a strong antibody-mediated response does not "require" an inflammatory condition that primes neutrophils as a first hit, but can cause TRALI in a healthy recipient. Conversely, it is possible that activating factors in the transfusion are not strong enough to overcome the threshold when priming status is too low. This would explain why TRALI does not develop in transfused patient even when an antibody–antigen match is present. However, in a patient with a predisposing factor, transfusion of mediators with low neutrophil-activating capacity is sufficient to overcome the threshold to induce a TRALI reaction.

Transfusion and ARDS: The Association

The most striking suggestion of a relationship between transfusion and ARDS comes from a trial in critically ill and trauma patients, in which a liberal transfusion trigger was associated with the development of ARDS (OR 1.5 (CI 1.0–2.5) compared to a restrictive transfusion trigger [55]. However, a difference in pulmonary complications was not noted in a trial comparing liberal vs. restrictive triggers in patients with gastrointestinal bleeding [56]. The concept that an inflammatory predisposition may render the host susceptible to TRALI suggests that critical care or injury is a general host factor risk. Therefore, is TRALI a distinct phenomenon or the result of a synergy between transfusion and other mechanisms that cause ALI? The time frame in the conventional definition of TRALI is 6 h, which is based on expert opinion, probably based on observations of patient cases. Obviously however, a clock does not start ticking when a transfusion is started. The term "delayed TRALI" has been coined for the critically ill when ALI occurs 6–72 h after a blood transfusion [57]. Using this time frame, transfusion increases the risk for the development of the ALI 6–72 h after the transfusion in a cohort of critically ill or injured patients with an OR of 2.1 (CI 1.7–2.5). The question can be raised regarding what distinction exists, if any, between transfusion resulting in lung injury within 6 h and lung injury associated with transfusion.

Transfusion and ARDS: Is There a Two-Hit Mechanism?

The association between transfusion and ARDS is particularly clear in the critically ill, trauma, and cardiac surgery patients. In unselected critically ill populations, incidence rates of ARDS associated with transfusion are as high as 25 % [57]. In transfused trauma, incidence rates of ARDS are around 5–10 % and 4–12 % in transfused cardiac surgery. In contrast, cancer patients, who are also frequently exposed to transfusion, are not at increased risk of ARDS following transfusion as compared to other patient populations [58]. These differences in incidence suggest that an underlying inflammatory condition contributes to the risk of developing ARDS following transfusion. This is compatible with the two-hit hypothesis.

Transfusion and ARDS: Risk Factors

Patient Risk Factors

Requirement of massive transfusion has been long known as a risk factor for ARDS [59, 60]. The association between transfusion and ARDS is dose dependent. A meta analysis showed that the odds of developing ARDS following trauma or surgery are increased with each additional red blood cell unit transfused [61]. Another clear patient related risk factor is mechanical ventilation. In ventilated patients, ARDS following transfusion is reported to be as high as 30 % [62]. In a study in critically ill children, mechanical ventilation was present in all children who developed ARDS following transfusion [20]. Given that settings of the ventilator can influence the occurrence of ARDS [63], it seems clear that mechanical ventilation contributes to the risk of developing ARDS following transfusion. In trauma patients, besides massive transfusion, also shock and thoracic trauma are risk factors for ARDS following transfusion [61, 64].

Transfusion Risk Factors

As noted, red blood cells are dose dependently associated with ARDS. However, patients receiving multiple transfusions most often also receive other blood products concomitantly, rendering it difficult to determine the risk for the different types of products separately. In trauma, studies on the effect of different transfusion ratios on the outcome of severe hemorrhage following trauma. suggest that the use of high volume of plasma is an independent risk factor for the development of ARDS [61], although not all trials confirm this finding [65]. Also in critically ill patients, plasma is independently associated with ARDS, with an OR of 3.4 (CI 1.2–10.2) for each liter infused [62]. Also platelets are associated with ARDS. In a cohort of critically ill patients, the OR of developing ARDS after platelet transfusion was reported to be 3.9 (CI 1.3–11.52), which was higher than after FFP (OR 2.5 (CI 1.3–4.7) or after red blood cells (OR 1.4 (CI 0.8–2.4) [66]. This response was dose-dependent.

Transfusion and ARDS: Different Pathogenesis from TRALI?

The susceptibility of patients with the presence of a first hit, suggests that TRALI is part of the ALI/ARDS spectrum. Of note, in possible TRALI as well as in ARDS following transfusion, these patient factors are more important than transfusion factors [9]. However, a first hit is not a requirement per se for TRALI, as an antibody–antigen interaction can induce lung injury in a relatively healthy recipient. This

Table 10.3 Differences and similarities between TRALI and ARDS following transfusion

	TRALI	Post transfusion ARDS
Symptoms	Acute onset Leucopenia Thrombocytopenia Systemic inflammation Activated coagulation	Insidious onset Systemic inflammation Activated coagulation
Patient risk factors	Shock Massive transfusion Mechanical ventilation Sepsis Surgery Hematologic malignancy	Shock Massive transfusion Mechanical ventilation Trauma
Transfusion risk factors	Red blood cells Plasma Platelets	Red blood cells Plasma Platelets
Mechanisms	"Two-hit" mechanism Antileukocyte antibodies Bioactive lipids	"Two-hit" mechanism
Outcome	Mortality 5–13 %	Mortality 25 %
Post-mortem findings	Pulmonary edema Neutrophil infiltration	Diffuse alveolar damage Hyaline membranes

difference in triggering event and also in associated mortality, which is higher in transfusion and ARDS then in TRALI, suggest different pathologic mechanisms and sequelae (Table 10.3).

Causative Factors in ARDS Following Transfusion

The factor in the blood products implicated in ARDS following transfusion is unknown. After implementation of a strategy in which plasma from only males was used, thereby mitigating the risk of transfusing plasma containing HLA antibodies, the risk decreased for TRALI [32, 33], as well as for postoperative ARDS [67]. This finding suggests that cases of ARDS associated with transfusion in which TRALI was not diagnosed, may also partly be antibody mediated. Remaining cases are probably non-antibody mediated.

The impact of leukoreduction on the development of ARDS has not been studied extensively. In a trauma population comparing ARDS before and after implementation of leukoreduced blood in a 6 years time period, it was found that leukoreduction was associated with a decrease in the incidence of ARDS [68]. However, a time dependent decrease due to improved management of ARDS cannot be ruled out, as observed in other populations as well. Nowadays, leucoreduction is widely implemented.

In a study in blood components transfused to patients who developed post-transfusion pulmonary adverse reactions with dyspnea not classified as TRALI, antileukocyte antibodies and lysoPCs were measured, which are associated with

TRALI. Antibodies accounted for 0.5 % of cases, whereas the lysoPC levels and cytokine levels in blood components did not differ between patients with and without symptoms [69]. Regardless of the causative factor in the blood, patient host factors seem more important in the development of ARDS following transfusion than transfusion factors [64].

Downstream Events in ARDS Following Transfusion

In the critically ill or injured, it is extremely challenging to dissect effects from transfusion from other hits. Anti-neutrophil antibody-mediated organ injury is not a primary mechanism of action in ARDS following transfusion. The downstream pulmonary inflammatory response in TRALI resembles however the response as seen in ARDS (Table 10.3). Both entities involve interaction of activated neutrophils, platelets and pulmonary endothelium. There are some differences in platelet activation between the two syndromes. Thrombocytopenia can be observed during a TRALI reaction and during experimental TRALI [70] and development of TRALI is critically dependent on platelets [35]. In ARDS, platelets also play a role, but thrombocytopenia is not a prominent acute symptom. Platelets roll along and firmly adhere to lung endothelial cells during ARDS as well as in TRALI. This interaction is mainly mediated by platelet P-selectin [71]. However, whereas blocking of P-selectin was protective in acid-induced ALI by reducing platelet-neutrophil aggregates, a role for P-selectin has not been established so far in TRALI. Also, aspirin was shown to be protective in patients with ARDS, but not in TRALI [72].

Although less well studied in TRALI, coagulopathy seems to be an imported factor in both ARDS and TRALI. In ARDS, activated coagulation and decreased fibrinolysis in the pulmonary compartment are a hallmark of lung injury. In a cohort of transfused cardiac surgery patients with lung injury who did not comply to the diagnosis of TRALI, coagulation was also activated, as shown by increased levels of TATc in bronchoalveolar lavage fluid, whereas levels of plasminogen activator activity were decreased, indicating impaired fibrinolysis [48].

Besides some differences in host response, there are differences in pathology findings. Post mortem findings in lungs of ARDS patients classically show diffuse alveolar damage (DAD), hyaline membrane formation and neutrophil aggregation in alveoli. In contrast, autopsy findings in acute antibody-mediated TRALI, did not show DAD nor hyaline membrane formation. Instead, alveolar oedema and pleural effusion were evident [73]. However, it should be noted that the presence of hyaline membranes and DAD on autopsy may have more to do with how long the patient lived after experiencing a TRALI reaction.

A comparison of pathogenesis is given in Table 10.3. Taken together, there is considerable overlap between the two syndromes and TRALI can be considered part of the ARDS spectrum. However, clinical and pathologic differences exist.

Explanatory Model for the Occurrence of ARDS Following Transfusion

Given that patients who are more severely ill have an increased risk of having ARDS as well as being exposed to transfusion, it can be argued that transfusion is merely a confounder in the occurrence of lung injury. However, as discussed, experimental studies have clearly shown that transfusion results in pulmonary injury. Also in patients, it was shown that transfusion results in an increase in the permeability of the pulmonary vasculature, as measured by the pulmonary leakage index using Gallium-labeled transferrin [8]. Increased permeability with subsequent leakage of pulmonary edema is compatible with ARDS. Lastly, in an RCT comparing transfusion triggers, ARDS occurred less often in the restrictive arm [55]. Thereby, ARDS due to pulmonary leakage following transfusion is not merely an association but the two entities seem causally linked.

Given the dose relationship between amount of transfusion and ARDS, it could be hypothesized that at least a part of these patients have fluid overload and not permeability edema due to ARDS. However, when measuring pulmonary leakage index, increased permeability was already noted after 1 unit of red blood cells and did not increase further with multiple transfusions [8]. Also, in patients developing lung injury following transfusion, but not in those developing circulatory overload following transfusion, there is evidence of systemic inflammation [74]. Thereby, it seems that ARDS following transfusion is distinct from transfusion-associated fluid overload.

Model for the Association Between Transfusion and ARDS

We suggest the following model for the association between transfusion and ARDS. A patient who is primed by an underlying condition receives a blood transfusion and develops pulmonary inflammation and subsequent vascular leakage, the severity of which depends both on the amount of pro-inflammatory substances or antibodies in the blood product as well as on the condition of the patient.

Some patients may develop immediate symptoms compatible with TRALI. However, symptoms can also be subclinical, ranging from none to mild respiratory distress. Hemovigilance systems have occasionally received reports of cases with mild respiratory distress in timely association with transfusion, which could not be assigned to TRALI and for which the term "transfusion-associated dyspnea" was introduced (www.ehnorg.net). These symptoms are easily missed or misclassified to other causes, in particular in patients in which other ARDS risk factors are present [11]. When such a patient with subclinical pulmonary leakage is subjected to further fluid loading, this may result in increased leakage gradient with increased severity of pulmonary edema. At some point, which may take longer than 6 h, the patient complies to the definition of ARDS. The suggestion that fluid overload contributes to ARDS is underlined by the finding that a restrictive fluid balance reduces the number of ventilation days in ARDS due to other causes, suggesting that non-hydrostatic edema might contribute to the lung vascular injury [75]. Also, a positive fluid balance is a risk factor for TRALI [21].

In this scenario, ARDS can occur with subsequent transfusions but also after loading with other fluids. In line with this, in multiple transfused trauma patients, an increased ratio of crystalloids to red blood cells was also found to be associated with ARDS [76]. The clinical implication of this model is that in patients at risk for ARDS following transfusion, a restrictive fluid balance is warranted.

Further elucidation of the mechanisms involved in the onset of ARDS after transfusion is challenging, due to multiple confounding factors. Experimental studies and controlled clinical studies are a prerequisite to shed more light on this syndrome.

References

1. Marik PE, Corwin H. Efficacy of red blood cell transfusion in the critically ill: a systematic review of the literature. Crit Care Med. 2008;36(9):2667–74.
2. Hod EA, Zhang N, Sokol SA, Wojczyk BS, Francis RO, Ansaldi D, et al. Transfusion of red blood cells after prolonged storage produces harmful effects that are mediated by iron and inflammation. Blood. 2010;115(21):4284–92.
3. Silliman CC, Bjornsen AJ, Wyman TH, Kelher M, Allard J, Bieber S, et al. Plasma and lipids from stored platelets cause acute lung injury in an animal model. Transfusion. 2003;43(5):633–40.
4. Silliman CC, Kelher MR, Khan SY, Lasarre M, West FB, Land KJ, et al. Experimental prestorage filtration removes antibodies and decreases lipids in Rbc supernatants mitigating TRALI in vivo. Blood. 2014;123(22):3488–95.
5. Silliman CC, Voelkel NF, Allard JD, Elzi DJ, Tuder RM, Johnson J, et al. Plasma and lipids from stored packed red blood cells cause acute lung injury in an animal model. J Clin Invest. 1998;101(7):1458–67.
6. Vlaar AP, Hofstra JJ, Kulik W, Van LH, Nieuwland R, Schultz MJ, et al. Supernatant of stored platelets causes lung inflammation and coagulopathy in a novel in vivo transfusion model. Blood. 2010;116(8):1360–8.
7. Vlaar AP, Hofstra JJ, Levi M, Kulik W, Nieuwland R, Tool AT, et al. Supernatant of aged erythrocytes causes lung inflammation and coagulopathy in a "two-hit" in vivo syngeneic transfusion model. Anesthesiology. 2010;113(1):92–103.
8. Vlaar AP, Cornet AD, Hofstra JJ, Porcelijn L, Beishuizen A, Kulik W, et al. The effect of blood transfusion on pulmonary permeability in cardiac surgery patients: a prospective multicenter cohort study. Transfusion. 2012;52(1):82–90.
9. Toy P, Bacchetti P, Grimes B, Gajic O, Murphy E, Winters J, et al. Recipient clinical risk factors predominate in possible transfusion-related acute lung injury. Transfusion. 2015;55(5):947–52.
10. Kleinman S, Caulfield T, Chan P, Davenport R, Mcfarland J, Mcphedran S, et al. Toward an understanding of transfusion-related acute lung injury: statement of a consensus panel. Transfusion. 2004;44(12):1774–89.
11. Fadeyi EA, De Los Angeles MM, Wayne AS, Klein HG, Leitman SF, Stroncek DF. The transfusion of neutrophil-specific antibodies causes leukopenia and a broad spectrum of pulmonary reactions. Transfusion. 2007;47(3):545–50.
12. Dry SM, Bechard KM, Milford EL, Churchill WH, Benjamin RJ. The pathology of transfusion-related acute lung injury. Am J Clin Pathol. 1999;112(2):216–21.
13. Kopko PM, Popovsky MA, Mackenzie MR, Paglieroni TG, Muto KN, Holland PV. HLA class II antibodies in transfusion-related acute lung injury. Transfusion. 2001;41(10):1244–8.

14. Nicolle AL, Chapman CE, Carter V, Wallis JP. Transfusion-related acute lung injury caused by two donors with anti-human leucocyte antigen class II antibodies: a look-back investigation. Transfus Med. 2004;14(3):225–30.
15. Toy P, Hollis-Perry KM, Jun J, Nakagawa M. Recipients of blood from a donor with multiple HLA antibodies: a lookback study of transfusion-related acute lung injury. Transfusion. 2004;44(12):1683–8.
16. Silliman CC, Boshkov LK, Mehdizadehkashi Z, Elzi DJ, Dickey WO, Podlosky L, et al. Transfusion-related acute lung injury: epidemiology and a prospective analysis of etiologic factors. Blood. 2003;101(2):454–62.
17. Vlaar AP, Hofstra JJ, Determann RM, Veelo DP, Paulus F, Kulik W, et al. The incidence, risk factors, and outcome of transfusion-related acute lung injury in a cohort of cardiac surgery patients: a prospective nested case-control study. Blood. 2011;117(16):4218–25.
18. Lacroix J, Hebert PC, Fergusson DA, Tinmouth A, Cook DJ, Marshall JC, et al. Age of transfused blood in critically ill adults. N Engl J Med. 2015;372(15):1410–8.
19. Vlaar AP, Binnekade JM, Prins D, Van SD, Hofstra JJ, Schultz MJ, et al. Risk factors and outcome of transfusion-related acute lung injury in the critically ill: a nested case-control study. Crit Care Med. 2010;38(3):771–8.
20. Mulder HD, Augustijn QJ, Van Woensel JB, Bos AP, Juffermans NP, Wosten-Van Asperen RM. Incidence, risk factors, and outcome of transfusion-related acute lung injury in critically ill children: a retrospective study. J Crit Care. 2015;30(1):55–9.
21. Toy P, Gajic O, Bacchetti P, Looney MR, Gropper MA, Hubmayr R, et al. Transfusion-related acute lung injury: incidence and risk factors. Blood. 2012;119(7):1757–67.
22. Vlaar AP, Hofstra JJ, Determann RM, Veelo DP, Paulus F, Levi M, et al. Transfusion-related acute lung injury in cardiac surgery patients is characterized by pulmonary inflammation and coagulopathy: a prospective nested case-control study. Crit Care Med. 2012;40(10):2813–20.
23. Vlaar AP, Wolthuis EK, Hofstra JJ, Roelofs JJ, Boon L, Schultz MJ, et al. Mechanical ventilation aggravates transfusion-related acute lung injury induced by Mhc-I class antibodies. Intensive Care Med. 2010;36(5):879–87.
24. Kor DJ, Lingineni RK, Gajic O, Park PK, Blum JM, Hou PC, et al. Predicting risk of postoperative lung injury in high-risk surgical patients: a multicenter cohort study. Anesthesiology. 2014;120(5):1168–81.
25. Win N, Chapman CE, Bowles KM, Green A, Bradley S, Edmondson D, et al. How much residual plasma may cause TRALI? Transfus Med. 2008;18(5):276–80.
26. Fadeyi EA, Adams S, Sheldon S, Leitman SF, Wesley R, Klein HG, et al. A preliminary comparison of the prevalence of transfusion reactions in recipients of platelet components from donors with and without human leucocyte antigen antibodies. Vox Sang. 2008;94(4):324–8.
27. Kopko PM, Paglieroni TG, Popovsky MA, Muto KN, Mackenzie MR, Holland PV. TRALI: correlation of antigen-antibody and monocyte activation in donor-recipient pairs. Transfusion. 2003;43(2):177–84.
28. Porretti L, Cattaneo A, Coluccio E, Mantione E, Colombo F, Mariani M, et al. Implementation and outcomes of a transfusion-related acute lung injury surveillance programme and study of Hla/Hna alloimmunisation in blood donors. Blood Transfus. 2012;10(3):351–9.
29. Zupanska B, Uhrynowska M, Michur H, Maslanka K, Zajko M. Transfusion-related acute lung injury and leucocyte-reacting antibodies. Vox Sang. 2007;93(1):70–7.
30. Densmore TL, Goodnough LT, Ali S, Dynis M, Chaplin H. Prevalence of HLA sensitization in female apheresis donors. Transfusion. 1999;39(1):103–6.
31. Palfi M, Berg S, Ernerudh J, Berlin G. A randomized controlled trial of transfusion-related acute lung injury: is plasma from multiparous blood donors dangerous? Transfusion. 2001;41(3):317–22.
32. Muller MC, Van Stein D, Binnekade JM, Van Rhenen DJ, Vlaar AP. Low-risk transfusion-related acute lung injury donor strategies and the impact on the onset of transfusion-related acute lung injury: a meta-analysis. Transfusion. 2015;55(1):164–75.

33. Schmickl CN, Mastrobuoni S, Filippidis FT, Shah S, Radic J, Murad MH, et al. Male-predominant plasma transfusion strategy for preventing transfusion-related acute lung injury: a systematic review. Crit Care Med. 2015;43(1):205–25.
34. Looney MR, Su X, Van Ziffle JA, Lowell CA, Matthay MA. Neutrophils and their Fc gamma receptors are essential in a mouse model of transfusion-related acute lung injury. J Clin Invest. 2006;116(6):1615–23.
35. Looney MR, Nguyen JX, Hu Y, Van Ziffle JA, Lowell CA, Matthay MA. Platelet depletion and aspirin treatment protect mice in a two-event model of transfusion-related acute lung injury. J Clin Invest. 2009;119(11):3450–61.
36. Strait R, Hicks W, Barasa N, Mahler A, Khodoun M, Kohl J, et al. Mhc class I-specific antibody binding to nonhematopoietic cells drives complement activation to induce transfusion-related acute lung injury in mice. J Exp Med. 2011;208(12):2525–44.
37. Dykes A, Smallwood D, Kotsimbos T, Street A. Transfusion-related acute lung injury (TRALI) in a patient with a single lung transplant. Br J Haematol. 2000;109(3):674–6.
38. Wakamoto S, Fujihara M, Takahashi D, Niwa K, Sato S, Kato T, et al. Enhancement of endothelial permeability by coculture with peripheral blood mononuclear cells in the presence of HLA class II antibody that was associated with transfusion-related acute lung injury. Transfusion. 2011;51(5):993–1001.
39. Sachs UJ, Wasel W, Bayat B, Bohle RM, Hattar K, Berghofer H, et al. Mechanism of transfusion-related acute lung injury induced by HLA class II antibodies. Blood. 2011;117(2):669–77.
40. Seeger W, Schneider U, Kreusler B, Von WE, Walmrath D, Grimminger F, et al. Reproduction of transfusion-related acute lung injury in an ex vivo lung model. Blood. 1990;76(7):1438–44.
41. Kelher MR, Masuno T, Moore EE, Damle S, Meng X, Song Y, et al. Plasma from stored packed red blood cells and MHC class I antibodies causes acute lung injury in a 2-event in vivo rat model. Blood. 2009;113(9):2079–87.
42. Silliman CC, Paterson AJ, Dickey WO, Stroneck DF, Popovsky MA, Caldwell SA, et al. The association of biologically active lipids with the development of transfusion-related acute lung injury: a retrospective study. Transfusion. 1997;37(7):719–26.
43. Gajic O, Rana R, Winters JL, Yilmaz M, Mendez JL, Rickman OB, et al. Transfusion related acute lung injury in the critically ill: prospective nested case-control study. Am J Respir Crit Care Med. 2007;176(9):886–91.
44. Silliman CC, Moore EE, Kelher MR, Khan SY, Gellar L, Elzi DJ. Identification of lipids that accumulate during the routine storage of prestorage leukoreduced red blood cells and cause acute lung injury. Transfusion. 2011;51(12):2549–54.
45. Khan SY, Kelher MR, Heal JM, Blumberg N, Boshkov LK, Phipps R, et al. Soluble Cd40 ligand accumulates in stored blood components, primes neutrophils through Cd40, and is a potential cofactor in the development of transfusion-related acute lung injury. Blood. 2006;108(7):2455–62.
46. Tung JP, Fraser JF, Nataatmadja M, Colebourne KI, Barnett AG, Glenister KM, et al. Age of blood and recipient factors determine the severity of transfusion-related acute lung injury (TRALI). Crit Care. 2012;16(1):R19.
47. Tuinman PR, Gerards MC, Jongsma G, Vlaar AP, Boon L, Juffermans NP. Lack of evidence of Cd40 ligand involvement in transfusion-related acute lung injury. Clin Exp Immunol. 2011;165(2):278–84.
48. Tuinman PR, Vlaar AP, Cornet AD, Hofstra JJ, Levi M, Meijers JC, et al. Blood transfusion during cardiac surgery is associated with inflammation and coagulation in the lung: a case control study. Crit Care. 2011;15(1):R59.
49. Mangalmurti NS, Xiong Z, Hulver M, Ranganathan M, Liu XH, Oriss T, et al. Loss of red cell chemokine scavenging promotes transfusion-related lung inflammation. Blood. 2009;113(5):1158–66.
50. Gelderman MP, Chi X, Zhi L, Vostal JG. Ultraviolet B light-exposed human platelets mediate acute lung injury in a two-event mouse model of transfusion. Transfusion. 2011;51(11):2343–57.

51. Chi X, Zhi L, Vostal JG. Human platelets pathogen reduced with riboflavin and ultraviolet light do not cause acute lung injury in a two-event SCID mouse model. Transfusion. 2014;54(1):74–85.
52. Silliman CC, Dickey WO, Paterson AJ, Thurman GW, Clay KL, Johnson CA, et al. Analysis of the priming activity of lipids generated during routine storage of platelet concentrates. Transfusion. 1996;36(2):133–9.
53. Thomas GM, Carbo C, Curtis BR, Martinod K, Mazo IB, Schatzberg D, et al. Extracellular DNA traps are associated with the pathogenesis of TRALI in humans and mice. Blood. 2012;119(26):6335–43.
54. Bux J, Sachs UJ. The pathogenesis of transfusion-related acute lung injury (TRALI). Br J Haematol. 2007;136(6):788–99.
55. Hebert PC, Wells G, Blajchman MA, Marshall J, Martin C, Pagliarello G, et al. A Multicenter, randomized, controlled clinical trial of transfusion requirements in critical care. transfusion requirements in critical care investigators, Canadian Critical Care Trials Group. N Engl J Med. 1999;340(6):409–17.
56. Villanueva C, Colomo A, Bosch A, Concepcion M, Hernandez-Gea V, Aracil C, et al. Transfusion strategies for acute upper gastrointestinal bleeding. N Engl J Med. 2013;368(1):11–21.
57. Marik PE, Corwin H. Acute lung injury following blood transfusion: expanding the definition. Crit Care Med. 2008;36(11):3080–4.
58. Federici AB, Vanelli C, Arrigoni L. Transfusion issues in cancer patients. Thrombosis Res. 2012;129 Suppl 1:S60–5.
59. Croce MA, Tolley EA, Claridge JA, Fabian TC. Transfusions result in pulmonary morbidity and death after a moderate degree of injury. J Trauma. 2005;59(1):19–23.
60. Zilberberg MD, Carter C, Lefebvre P, Raut M, Vekeman F, Duh MS, et al. Red blood cell transfusions and the risk of acute respiratory distress syndrome among the critically ill: a cohort study. Crit Care. 2007;11(3):R63.
61. Balvers K, Wirtz MR, Van Dieren S, Goslings JC, Juffermans NP. Risk factors for trauma-induced coagulopathy- and transfusion-associated multiple organ failure in severely injured trauma patients. Front Med. 2015;2:24.
62. Rana R, Fernandez-Perez ER, Khan SA, Rana S, Winters JL, Lesnick TG, et al. Transfusion-related acute lung injury and pulmonary edema in critically ill patients: a retrospective study. Transfusion. 2006;46(9):1478–83.
63. Tards N. Ventilation with lower tidal volumes as compared with traditional tidal volumes for acute lung injury and the acute respiratory distress syndrome. N Engl J Med. 2000;342:1301–8.
64. Sadis C, Dubois MJ, Melot C, Lambermont M, Vincent JL. Are multiple blood transfusions really a cause of acute respiratory distress syndrome? Eur J Anaesthesiol. 2007;24(4):355–61.
65. Holcomb JB, Tilley BC, Baraniuk S, Fox EE, Wade CE, Podbielski JM, et al. Transfusion of plasma, platelets, and red blood cells in a 1:1:1 vs a 1:1:2 ratio and mortality in patients with severe trauma: the PROPPR randomized clinical trial. JAMA. 2015;313(5):471–82.
66. Khan H, Belsher J, Yilmaz M, Afessa B, Winters JL, Moore SB, et al. Fresh-frozen plasma and platelet transfusions are associated with development of acute lung injury in critically ill medical patients. Chest. 2007;131(5):1308–14.
67. Wright SE, Snowden CP, Athey SC, Leaver AA, Clarkson JM, Chapman CE, et al. Acute lung injury after ruptured abdominal aortic aneurysm repair: the effect of excluding donations from females from the production of fresh frozen plasma. Crit Care Med. 2008;36(6):1796–802.
68. Plurad D, Belzberg H, Schulman I, Green D, Salim A, Inaba K, et al. Leukoreduction is associated with a decreased incidence of late onset acute respiratory distress syndrome after injury. Am Surg. 2008;74(2):117–23.
69. Maslanka K, Uhrynowska M, Lopacz P, Wrobel A, Smolenska-Sym G, Guz K, et al. Analysis of leucocyte antibodies, cytokines, lysophospholipids and cell microparticles in blood components implicated in post-transfusion reactions with dyspnoea. Vox Sang. 2015;108(1):27–36.

70. Hidalgo A, Chang J, Jang JE, Peired AJ, Chiang EY, Frenette PS. Heterotypic interactions enabled by polarized neutrophil microdomains mediate thromboinflammatory injury. Nat Med. 2009;15(4):384–91.
71. Kiefmann R, Heckel K, Schenkat S, Dorger M, Goetz AE. Role of P-selectin in platelet sequestration in pulmonary capillaries during endotoxemia. J Vasc Res. 2006;43(5):473–81.
72. Tuinman PR, Vlaar AP, Binnenkade JM, Juffermans NP. The effect of aspirin in transfusion-related acute lung injury in critically ill patients. Anaesthesia. 2012;67(6):594–9.
73. Danielson C, Benjamin RJ, Mangano MM, Mills CJ, Waxman DA. Pulmonary pathology of rapidly fatal transfusion-related acute lung injury reveals minimal evidence of diffuse alveolar damage or alveolar granulocyte infiltration. Transfusion. 2008;48(11):2401–8.
74. Roubinian NH, Looney MR, Kor DJ, Lowell CA, Gajic O, Hubmayr RD, et al. Cytokines and clinical predictors in distinguishing pulmonary transfusion reactions. Transfusion. 2015;55(8):1838–46.
75. Wiedemann HP, Wheeler AP, Bernard GR, Thompson BT, Hayden D, Deboisblanc B, et al. Comparison of two fluid-management strategies in acute lung injury. N Engl J Med. 2006;354(24):2564–75.
76. Park PK, Cannon JW, Ye W, Blackbourne LH, Holcomb JB, Beninati W, et al. Transfusion strategies and development of acute respiratory distress syndrome in combat casualty care. J Trauma Acute Care Surg. 2013;75(2 Suppl 2):S238–46.

Chapter 11
Transfusion and Acute Respiratory Distress Syndrome: Clinical Epidemiology, Diagnosis, Management, and Outcomes

Hannah C. Mannem and Michael P. Donahoe

Overview

From an infectious disease standpoint, the overall safety of blood transfusion has improved over the past decade. Transmission of viral infections, including human immunodeficiency virus (HIV) and hepatitis C are as low as one per two million blood products transfused [1]. However, other transfusion related complications persist, which can be life threatening. Transfusion related acute lung injury (TRALI) is the most serious respiratory complication in transfusion medicine. Since 2003, it has been the leading cause of transfusion associated death in the USA. The Food and Drug Administration reports 43 % of transfusion related deaths due to TRALI from 2007 to 2011 [2, 3]. Due to the high morbidity and mortality, TRALI has moved to the forefront of transfusion medicine. As a consequence, a better understanding of the pathophysiology, risk factors, and mitigation strategies in TRALI prevention has developed.

Epidemiology

Definition

TRALI is defined as acute hypoxemia and respiratory distress within 6 h of a blood transfusion in the absence of hydrostatic pulmonary edema. The clinical correlation between blood transfusions and acute lung injury was first described in the 1950s [4].

H.C. Mannem, MD • M.P. Donahoe, MD (✉)
Division of Pulmonary, Allergy, and Critical Care Medicine, Department of Medicine, University of Pittsburgh School of Medicine, Pittsburgh, PA, USA
e-mail: donahoem@upmc.edu

J.S. Lee, M.P. Donahoe (eds.), *Hematologic Abnormalities and Acute Lung Syndromes*, Respiratory Medicine, DOI 10.1007/978-3-319-41912-1_11

The association was made into a distinct clinical entity with specific clinical criteria in 1983 by Popovsky and colleagues and redefined by the National Heart, Lung, and Blood Institute (NHLBI), as well as the Canadian Consensus Conference (CCC) in 2004 [5–7]. Two key points were highlighted in the revision of the definition. The first was emphasizing an *acute* and *new* presentation of respiratory distress. The second focus was to eliminate other temporally associated, alternative risk factors to explain the new lung injury (Table 11.1). Two other terms were also defined—*Possible TRALI* and *Delayed TRALI*. Possible TRALI occurs when the acute respiratory distress takes place in the setting of a blood transfusion, as well as other co-existing risk factors for development of Acute Respiratory Distress Syndrome (ARDS), including: trauma, sepsis, pancreatitis, aspiration, inhalation, drug overdose, or burns. *Delayed TRALI* is defined as TRALI which occurs after 6 h but within 72 h of a blood transfusion (Table 11.1). These distinctions between TRALI, possible TRALI, and delayed TRALI help to further elucidate incidence, pathophysiology, and treatment of this condition by clarifying the disease for future research investigations.

Mechanisms of TRALI

Two pathophysiologic mechanisms of TRALI have been recognized, *immune-mediated TRALI* and *non-antibody mediated TRALI*. Anywhere from 65 to 90 % of reported cases are found to be immune-mediated TRALI, which occurs when leuko-agglutinating antibodies from the donor blood bind to conjugate recipient antigens [8]. By definition, evidence of antibodies from the blood donor are present; most commonly anti-HLA and anti-HNA antibodies, with anti-HNA3a associated with worse clinical outcomes [9, 10]. The second mechanism for development of TRALI

Table 11.1 NHLBI/CCC definition of TRALI

TRALI	Possible TRALI*	Delayed TRALI**
•NEW, ACUTE onset of dyspnea and hypoxemia (PaO2/FiO2 < 300, SpO2 < 90% on RA, or other clinical evidence of hypoxemia) •Bilateral pulmonary infiltrates on chest x-ray •No evidence of hydrostatic pulmonary edema •No temporal relationship to an alternate risk factor for new development of ARDS* •Symptoms occurring within 6 hrs of a blood product transfusion**	•TRALI •WITH a temporal relationship to an alternate risk factor for new development of ARDS (ie-sepsis, aspiration, pneumonia, burns, inhalataion, drug overdose, drowning, trauma, cardiac bypass, acute pancreatitis)	•TRALI •Symptoms occurring > 6 hours but within 72 hours after transfusion of a blood product

is classified as non-antibody mediated TRALI and stems from an antibody independent mechanism. Approximately 15 % of TRALI falls into this category, in which no antibodies are found in the donor blood product. Silliman and colleagues have described the non-antibody mediated mechanism as a two-hit model. The first hit involves neutrophil priming and sequestration secondary to a preexisting condition in the recipient. In the second hit, biologic modifiers such as lipids in the blood product activate neutrophils and lead to capillary leak in the lung endothelium [11, 12] (see Chap. 10).

Risk Factors

Risk factors for the development of TRALI can be broken into two categories, recipient and donor related risks. The recipient of the blood product may have underlying disease states and clinical conditions, which put them at increased risk (Table 11.2). Also the donor profile and blood components being transfused may also put the recipient at higher risk for development of TRALI.

Recipient Risk Factors

Multiple recipient related risk factors are noted in the literature. Most of these studies are retrospective and small. However, it is evident from clinical data that the critically ill population is at the highest risk for the development of TRALI

Table 11.2 Recipient related risk factors for development of TRALI

Recipient related risk factors
Sepsis
Shock
Positive fluid balance
Liver disease/history of liver transplant
Chronic alcohol use
Active tobacco use
Mechanical ventilation/increased peak airway pressures
Increased IL-8 serum levels
Major surgery (i.e., cardiac, orthopedic surgery)
Hematologic malignancy
Massive transfusion
High APACHE II scores

[13]. In one multicenter, prospective trial, history of liver transplant, chronic alcohol use, active tobacco use, shock, increased IL-8 levels in serum, increased peak airway pressures of >30 cm H_2O on the ventilator, and an overall positive fluid balance were all significant risk factors for TRALI [14]. Multiple studies reveal sepsis and shock as major risk factors. Not only being critically ill, but also being on mechanical ventilation at the time of transfusion may increase risk independently. A prospective cohort study showed 33 % of patients on mechanical ventilation at the time of transfusion developed acute lung injury [15]. Multiple other studies have also shown recipient risk factors such as: major surgery within 72 h of blood transfusion, hematologic malignancy, higher APACHE II scores, and active liver disease [16]. The risk for development of TRALI also increases with the number of transfusions, as seen commonly in the trauma population where patients are receiving massive transfusions [13]. Not only critically ill patients, but cardiac and orthopedic surgery patients are also at higher risk for TRALI development [17]. The time on cardiac bypass appears to be correlated as well, with longer bypass times leading to higher risk of TRALI development [18]. Despite the multitude of recipient risk factors reported, most of which are seen in the critically ill population, TRALI is also reported in otherwise healthy individuals at the time of transfusion [19]. The development of TRALI in this healthy patient population supports the realization that the risk of TRALI is not dependent on the recipient alone.

Donor and Blood Component Risk Factors

All forms of blood products have been reported to cause TRALI, including: whole blood, packed red blood cells, apheresis platelets, fresh frozen plasma, cryoglobulin, intravenous immunoglobulin, granulocytes, and allogeneic stem cells [12]. However, blood products with higher plasma volume are at the greatest risk, specifically fresh frozen plasma, apheresis platelets, and whole blood. In the FDA reported cases of death due to TRALI, fresh frozen plasma was the most implicated [7]. In one retrospective cohort study from 2007, fresh frozen plasma and platelet transfusions led to a higher incidence of TRALI versus red blood cell transfusion in the ICU population [20]. It remains unknown the exact amount of plasma which must be transfused in order for TRALI to develop. Reports of as little as 10–20 ml of plasma transfused before TRALI development are in the literature; however, plasma volumes greater than 50–60 ml are thought to be the threshold which puts patients at a higher risk [12].

Another important risk factor is the gender of the donor, and preventive strategies in the past 15 years have focused on gender related donor deferral. Female, multiparous donors have allo-immunization from pregnancy. Blood from this particular group of donors has a much higher risk of TRALI development in the recipient secondary to the anti-HLA and anti-HNA antibodies, which bind to recipient antigens and lead to immune-mediated TRALI. The prevalence of antibodies in this population increases with parity. A 26 % approximate frequency of anti-HLA antibodies exist if a female has had more than three pregnancies [21]. Another potential risk factor where studies have shown controversial data is blood product storage time. Experts in the field hypothesize that longer storage times of red blood cells may lead to a higher incidence of TRALI. Experimental models in preclinical trials show a positive correlation between longer blood storage times and TRALI; however, there remains no overt clinical evidence to support the finding [22]. Studies done in the preemie population showed no difference in the incidence of TRALI based on blood storage time. An ongoing study in the adult intensive care unit population is underway that hopefully will help to clarify the importance of blood storage time as a potential risk factor [23].

Incidence

The true incidence of TRALI is unknown secondary to prior lack of a concise definition, the inconspicuousness of the diagnosis, and lack of a structured reporting system. It occurs in all age groups, including children and the geriatric population. It occurs at the same frequency in women and men. Reported TRALI incidence varies between 0.08 and 15 % of patients transfused and 0.01–1.12 % per product transfused, with the higher incidence in the critically ill patient population [24]. Up to 50–70 % of patients in an intensive care unit receive some form of blood product transfusion, and more independent patient risk factors exist in the critically ill population, which may account for this increase in incidence (see section "Risk Factors"). Even though the overall reported incidence of TRALI remains low, it is almost certainty an under-recognized and underdiagnosed condition. In the setting of no gold standard for diagnostic testing, a passive reporting system, and an array of mild cases which do not meet the consensus definition of the disease, TRALI remains under-reported [25]. Despite the underestimated incidence of TRALI, the overall frequency has decreased since the mid-2000s secondary to preventative strategies for plasma and platelet transfusions (see section "Prevention").

Blood Product Variation

As stated before, all blood products have been implicated in TRALI development, and the incidence of TRALI varies based on blood product components. Products with higher plasma volume have higher incidence of TRALI. Reports reveal incidences at approximately 1/432 whole blood products vs. 1/7900 fresh frozen plasma vs. 1/557,000 red blood cells [12, 22]. However, the incidence of TRALI in plasma products has decreased in the past decade secondary to risk mitigation strategies, leaving the incidence of red blood cell transfusions at a higher rate in the more recent years [26].

Diagnosis

Clinical Presentation

TRALI can present with a large variation in disease severity. By NHLBI and CCC definition 100 % of patients with TRALI have hypoxemic respiratory failure and bilateral pulmonary infiltrates on chest X-ray. Clinically, the most common complaint of patients is dyspnea. However, a large number of patients are critically ill and on mechanical ventilation at the time of blood transfusions leading symptoms to be unhelpful. Despite patients being unable to report symptoms, clinical signs of respiratory distress and failure are present, typically within one to 2 h of a blood transfusion in the majority of patients. Predominately, patients are tachypneic, and in approximately one-third of patients, fever and/or hypotension may develop. Rarely patients may develop new onset hypertension. Most notably in the vital signs, SpO2 should be decreased compared to before the transfusion. Patients on mechanical ventilation may experience a change in pulmonary compliance with an increase in peak and plateau pressures. Pink, frothy secretions from the mouth or endotracheal tube occur in roughly half of patients who develop TRALI. Physical exam should help rule out other etiologies of respiratory distress and should be thorough including a complete lung, heart, and skin exam. Lung auscultation reveals bilateral crackles. Exam findings suggestive of cardiac failure should not be present, such as jugular venous distention and an S3 on cardiac auscultation. It is important to keep in mind that very mild cases of TRALI do exist, which may not fall into the NHLBI and CCC definitions. Mild cases may go unrecognized or present with a similar presentation to the underlying disease process, albeit in a less severe form.

Diagnostic Workup

Practitioners should have a high index of suspicion for TRALI when administering blood products, especially in the critically ill population. Diagnosis can be difficult as there is no gold standard diagnostic test for TRALI. Any person who develops even the least amount of dyspnea or respiratory distress in temporal association with a blood product transfusion should have further clinical and diagnostic evaluation for TRALI. Patients who meet the 2004 NHLBI and CCC definition (Table 11.1) including, new hypoxemic respiratory failure with a PaO_2/FiO_2 ratio <300 and bilateral pulmonary infiltrates within a 6 h time frame from blood product transfusion, deserve further workup to confirm the diagnosis. One of the goals of the diagnostic workup should be to rule out other possible etiologies for the new development of ARDS, which would then classify the patient as possible TRALI. No diagnostic lab tests are available that confirm the diagnosis of TRALI. An arterial blood gas can be helpful to quantify the degree of hypoxemia. The most common laboratory finding is acute and transient leukopenia, which is thought to be secondary to neutrophil sequestration into the pulmonary vasculature and can be seen in 5–35 % of patients [27]. Thrombocytopenia has also been reported in TRALI. Other laboratory tests, although not diagnostic may also be helpful. In other etiologies of ARDS such as sepsis, a leukocytosis may be present. An elevated brain naturitic peptide can be seen in transfusion associated circulatory overload (TACO) and should not be elevated in TRALI alone. As stated before, a chest X-ray revealing bilateral pulmonary infiltrates is a ubiquitous finding in TRALI, and should be performed for any patient with suspicion of the diagnosis. Historically the pulmonary infiltrates in TRALI were described as "white out lungs." This may be the scenario in extreme cases; however, both alveolar and interstitial infiltrates have been described in a spectrum from bilateral and patchy to diffuse territories of the lung fields. Despite the findings being nonspecific, the presence of bilateral infiltrates should reach 100 % in this patient population. The chest X-ray is also helpful to eliminate other etiologies of acute respiratory failure, such as pneumothorax.

Blood Bank Reporting

For any suspected TRALI reaction, it is of vital importance the associated blood bank be contacted. Typically a transfusion reaction lab panel is sent, which is directed by the blood bank or transfusion medicine director. The panel includes a complete blood count, haptoglobin, bilirubin, direct Coombs test, and most importantly HLA and HNA antibody testing in the donor blood sample. Anti-HLA and anti-HNA antibodies strongly support the diagnosis of TRALI but are not essential for diagnosis. 15–25 % of TRALI reactions are found to be non-antibody mediated [21]. However, positive antibody results can guide future TRALI prevention if found in the donor blood product (see Section "Prevention"). Antibody testing may take days to weeks for results, and therefore no acute treatment decisions should be made based on antibody testing alone.

Differential Diagnosis

In distinguishing TRALI from other disease states it is important to consider other causes of ALI/ARDS, as well as other transfusion reactions.

Possible TRALI

In 2004, new terminology was instituted as part of the TRALI definition, termed, *possible TRALI*. This definition takes into account other etiologies of ALI/ARDS, which the patient may be at risk for at the time of blood transfusion (Table 11.1). Since no gold standard diagnostic test exist for TRALI, and it occurs most commonly in the critically ill population with multiple other comorbidities, possible

TRALI remains a very relevant diagnosis. If any of these other conditions exist or are suspected, a definitive diagnosis of TRALI cannot be made. Further diagnostic workup should be done in order to eliminate the additional etiologies. Fever can occur as part of TRALI; however, pneumonia, pancreatitis, and sepsis should be suspected as well as an etiology of the acute lung injury. CBC, blood cultures, and chest X-ray can all help to further delineate other disease states. Other conditions such as inhalation, drowning, cardiac bypass, drug overdose, and trauma may be more obvious from history alone.

Other Transfusion Reactions

Various other blood transfusion reactions exist, all of which can overlap with aspects of the clinical presentation of TRALI. Each blood transfusion reaction is managed differently, therefore it is vital to establish the correct diagnosis. The transfusion reaction that mimics TRALI the most is TACO (see Chap. 12). TACO may coexist with TRALI and distinguishing between these two diagnoses may be difficult (Table 11.3). Both conditions present acutely during or after blood product transfusion. Also, both lead to acute respiratory distress and hypoxemia with bilateral infiltrates on chest X-ray. While TRALI's clinical presentation stems from non-hydrostatic pulmonary edema with capillary leak, TACO is secondary to hydrostatic pulmonary edema. The two conditions are both transient but managed differently. Diuretics are the mainstay of treatment for TACO, but may be detrimental in the treatment of TRALI (see section "Medications"). A positive fluid balance is a risk factor for development of TRALI, and if the positive fluid balance is secondary to compromised cardiac function a higher awareness for TACO should exist. While no definitive test exists to distinguish between the two, diagnostic tools such as elevated jugular venous pressure, an S3 on cardiac auscultation, a transthoracic echo showing depressed cardiac function, and/or an elevated BNP may suggest TACO vs. TRALI. If the patient has a pulmonary artery catheter in place, an elevated pulmonary capillary wedge pressure and/or central venous pressure also

Table 11.3 Differentiating TRALI from TACO

Clinical characteristics	TRALI	TACO
SpO2	Hypoxia	Hypoxia
Blood pressure	Usually hypotensive	Usually hypertensive
Lung exam	Diffuse crackles	Diffuse crackles
Cardiac exam	+/− Tachycardia	JVD, +S3, +/− displaced PMI
CXR findings	Bilateral infiltrates	Bilateral infiltrates
PCWP/ CVP	Normal	Elevated
Arterial blood gas	Hypoxemia	Hypoxemia
CBC	Leukopenia, thrombocytopenia	Normal
BNP	Low/Normal	Elevated
Echo	Normal Cardiac function	Depressed cardiac function

favors the diagnosis of TACO. As stated before, chest X-ray is unhelpful in distinguishing between the two diagnoses.

Other transfusion reactions may also overlap in clinical presentation with TRALI; however, they are usually more obvious to diagnose. Like TRALI, an anaphylactic reaction from a blood product transfusion may also lead to hypoxia and hypotension. Conversely, the clinical presentation of patients undergoing an anaphylactic reaction may demonstrate signs of airway compromise, such as stridor, bronchospasm, laryngeal edema, and/or wheezing, as well as an associated rash, urticaria, and/or diarrhea, all of which are not seen in TRALI alone. In septicemia from blood product transfusion, which can occur in the setting of contaminated blood products, microbiology is usually positive. Patients may also have a leukocytosis, which is very uncommon in TRALI. Platelets are most commonly associated with septicemia from a transfusion. Lastly, hemolytic transfusion reactions develop acutely with blood product transfusion, but hypoxia and acute respiratory distress are not the mainstay. Fever and hypotension occur in almost all patients with hemolytic reactions and less often in TRALI. Laboratory tests will also reveal a hemolytic pattern, such as a low haptoglobin, elevated unconjugated bilirubin and an elevated lactate dehydrogenase.

Management

Similar to the diagnosis, the management of TRALI is also nonspecific. No exact therapy for TRALI exists, and supportive therapy is the mainstay for treatment. If TRALI is suspected while a blood product is actively being transfused, it should be stopped immediately. All subsequent blood product transfusions should also be held in the acute setting until the diagnosis is made and treatment ensued. As mentioned before, the blood bank or transfusion medicine physician should be notified with any suspicion of TRALI in order to potentially identify and exclude involved donors if relevant antibodies are present.

Supportive Therapy

Oxygen

Oxygen supplementation is the primary management in TRALI. Although mild cases are reported where little to no oxygen is necessary, almost all patients require some form of oxygen. Studies show up to 70–80 % of patients develop severe enough hypoxemia to require mechanical ventilation [28, 29]. There are no specific studies looking at mechanical ventilation strategies in TRALI specifically; however, it is reasonable to adopt the ventilation strategies from the ARDS Network trial [30]. The restrictive tidal volume approach with tidal volumes set at 6 ml/kg of predictive body weight vs. 12 ml/kg has been shown to improve mortality in ARDS, and therefore should be the mainstay ventilation approach in the TRALI patient population. Maintaining plateau pressures <30 cm H_2O has also been shown to improve mortality and the incidence of barotrauma in the ARDS population [30]. In severe cases where mechanical ventilation fails to support the patient's physiologic demands, the use of extracorporeal membrane oxygenation (ECMO) has been described in case reports [31, 32]. However, no randomized control studies exist to support the use of ECMO for TRALI specifically.

Hemodynamic Support

The volume status of patients who develop suspected TRALI should be examined carefully, as management decisions are dependent on this judgement. As mentioned above, in the patient who appears to be volume overloaded with depressed cardiac function the diagnosis of TACO should be strongly considered, and diuretics should be administered. Commonly patients who develop TRALI are found to be hypovolemic [33]. TRALI in the hypovolemic patient may lead to hypotension and shock. Intravenous fluids should be given in this setting, as well as pressors if needed, to support end organ perfusion during the acute episode.

Medications

Steroids

While steroids have been studied extensively in ARDS, no randomized control trials looking at the use of steroids in patients with TRALI have been completed. The use of steroids in the ARDS population remains controversial, but data suggest use after 14 days may be harmful [34]. In patients with TRALI, case reports with intravenous corticosteroids do exist [27]. However, in the setting of no true prospective clinical trials, the negative side effects, and the transient clinical course of TRALI, the use of corticosteroids is not routinely recommended in the treatment of TRALI.

Diuretics

Evidence from the FACTT trial supports the use of a conservative fluid strategy in the ARDS population [35]. However, as stated before patients who develop TRALI are at risk for hypotension and shock, especially in the setting of hypovolemia. Intravenous fluids are the mainstay of therapy for hemodynamic support early on in TRALI, especially without evidence of coexisting TACO. Diuretic therapy should be used judiciously in this patient population, as it may worsen outcomes early on. Based on evidence from the ARDS population, if patients are still requiring high levels of oxygen supplementation once they are hemodynamically stable and volume resuscitated, a role for diuretic use in TRALI may still exist [8, 36].

Prevention

With no specific management strategies for TRALI exist, prevention measures are of the utmost importance. Over the past 10 years policies have been put into place at blood product donation centers in order to guide risk mitigation. The largest risk mitigation strategies so far have focused on plasma donation. No practical risk reduction measures are established for red blood cell transfusion prevention from a donation perspective. Some experimental models suggest washing of stored red blood cell products to prevent TRALI, but it is yet to be determined if this strategy makes a difference and can be feasible in a clinical setting. However, strategies exist to assist in the prevention of all adverse transfusion reactions, most importantly being the use of conservative transfusion practices.

Restrictive Transfusion Strategy

An overall judicious approach to blood product transfusion is the simplest and most effective strategy for TRALI prevention. Evidence from a randomized, double-blinded control trial shows the incidence of ARDS is decreased with a conservative red blood cell transfusion strategy vs. a liberal one [37]. Other studies suggest FFP is still over utilized at times by physicians with no clear indications for its use [24]. With electronic medical records in the forefront of today's health care, data suggest that electronic decision support to further guide the ordering of blood product transfusions not only decreased the amount of blood transfusions given but also decreased the incidence of acute lung injury [38]. Blood utilization guidelines and blood conservation programs should be established in health care centers to help minimize unnecessary transfusions. A patient tailored approach should be taken for patients who do need non-emergent blood product transfusions. Patient related risk factors for TRALI should be considered, and an attempt to minimize these risk factors prior to transfusion is an important component of primary TRALI prevention.

Implicated Donor Deferral

As mentioned above, the reporting of any suspected or confirmed TRALI episode is vital to secondary prevention. The American Association of Blood Banks (AABB) advocates that implicated donors abstain from any type of blood product donation until leukocyte antibody testing has been complete. In the donors who are found to have leukocyte antibodies which match or are likely to match recipient leukocyte antigens, deferral from at least plasma and platelet apheresis donation is mandatory. If the donor is found to have anti-HNA3a antibodies, which have been shown to lead to an increase severity of TRALI, they are deferred from all types of blood donation [39].

Multiparous Female Donor Deferral

In the mid-2000s, risk mitigation strategies for TRALI were instilled in order to exclude "at risk" donors from certain types of blood product donation. An observational study, Leukocyte Antibody Prevalence Study (LAPS) looked at antibody levels in 8000 volunteers for blood donation using flow cytometry. Only 1–2 % of anti-HLA and anti-HNA antibodies were present in the male, never-pregnant female, and prior blood product recipient populations compared to multiparous female donors with approximately 24 % of antibodies present [40]. Other studies report higher frequency of antibodies in the multiparous, female population as well, putting patients who receive blood products from this population at an increased risk for immune-mediated TRALI [10, 41]. In 2007 the AABB published the recommendation, "…blood collecting facilities should implement interventions to minimize the preparation of high plasma-volume components from donors known to be leukocyte-allo-immunized or who are at increased risk of leukocyte allo-immunization." Based on this recommendation, the deferral of multiparous, female donors from plasma donations was implicated. The policy to use solely male donors for plasma donation led to a two-thirds decreased incidence in TRALI [24]. Data also shows since the deferral of multiparous females from plasma donation, the reported cases of deaths to the FDA from plasma associated TRALI decreased from 48 % before 2007 to 27 % from 2008 to 2011 [42]. The multiparous, female donor deferral strategy also has been used in platelet apheresis donation; however, with the shortage of donors available to meet the demanding needs of platelets, it is not completely feasible to implement complete deferral of high risk donors.

Leukocyte Reduced Blood

Another option for primary prevention of TRALI is the concept of leukocyte reduced blood. Reduction of leukocyte antibodies in high volume plasma products has been shown to reduce TRALI incidence [21]. However, patients still may be at risk for the non-immune mediated form of TRALI.

Solvent Detergent Plasma

Pooled solvent detergent plasma was approved by the FDA in 2013 as an alternative to FFP. In observational data, there was no reports of TRALI in ten million units of solvent detergent plasma [43]. Multiple studies from other countries as well have confirmed the lack of TRALI in transfusions with solvent detergent products [8, 24, 44]. The pooling and dilution of anti-HLA antibodies is thought to play a large role in this decreased incidence. Potential risks of pooling high volume plasma products also exist including, exposure to multiple donors and increased transmission of viruses.

Outcomes

The majority of patients who develop TRALI require close monitoring in an intensive care setting. The degree of hypoxemia and lung injury is variable but commonly can be very severe. However, a subset of patients who develop TRALI will only require minimal supportive care and may even go undiagnosed. No studies have shown clinical severity correlating to the type of blood product or the amount of plasma transfused. Worse clinical outcomes have been shown in patients who are positive for HNA-3a and HLA-A2 antigens [9]. Despite the potential severity of TRALI, the timeframe is short-lived. Studies show that even when patients require mechanical ventilation, the respiratory distress from TRALI resolves on average within 48 h. In the patient population who is already critically ill, the time course may extend up to 3–10 days [14, 29]. One report found that 80 % of TRALI cases resolved within 48–96 h [8, 45].

Mortality Rates

Unlike ARDS from other etiologies where mortality rates can range from 29 to 70 %, TRALI has significantly lower rates of death. Studies show that mortality rates from TRALI alone range from 5 to 10 %, with higher percentages quoted from the ICU population [24, 46]. Reports as high as 67 % mortality have been shown in TRALI patients who were critically ill at the time of TRALI diagnosis; however, the cohorts utilized in these studies included some "possible TRALI" cases as well [14, 16, 32].

Sequelae of TRALI

Despite a very similar clinical presentation as ARDS, TRALI also differs in the fact that it has minimal to no physical or pulmonary sequelae. In ARDS, patients are known to have decreased exercise capacity and decreased lung function on pulmonary function tests for up to 5 years after initial pulmonary insult [47]. In patients who recover from TRALI there are no residual pulmonary complications. This population of patients returns back to baseline pulmonary function and does not have complications of pulmonary fibrosis. Permanent lung damage is rare [48, 49]. Based on limited evidence, it also appears patients who develop TRALI are not at increased risk for recurrent episodes of blood transfusion reactions from other donors. Caution should be taken with blood transfusions from previously implicated donors; however, overall patients should not be restricted from receiving blood products in the future [27, 50, 51].

References

1. Stramer SL. Current risks of transfusion-transmitted agents: a review. Arch Pathol Lab Med. 2007;131(5):702–7. Epub 2007/05/10.
2. Holness L, Knippen MA, Simmons L, Lachenbruch PA. Fatalities caused by TRALI. Transfus Med Rev. 2004;18(3):184–8. Epub 2004/07/13.
3. Shaz BH. Giving TRALI the one-two punch. Blood. 2012;119(7):1620–1. Epub 2012/02/22.
4. Barnard RD. Indiscriminate transfusion: a critique of case reports illustrating hypersensitivity reactions. N Y State J Med. 1951;51(20):2399–402. Epub 1951/10/15.
5. Kleinman S, Caulfield T, Chan P, Davenport R, McFarland J, McPhedran S, et al. Toward an understanding of transfusion-related acute lung injury: statement of a consensus panel. Transfusion. 2004;44(12):1774–89. Epub 2004/12/09.
6. Popovsky MA, Abel MD, Moore SB. Transfusion-related acute lung injury associated with passive transfer of antileukocyte antibodies. Am Rev Respir Dis. 1983;128(1):185–9. Epub 1983/07/01.
7. Goldman M, Webert KE, Arnold DM, Freedman J, Hannon J, Blajchman MA. Proceedings of a consensus conference: towards an understanding of TRALI. Transfus Med Rev. 2005;19(1):2–31. Epub 2005/04/15.
8. Jaworski K, Maslanka K, Kosior DA. Transfusion-related acute lung injury: a dangerous and underdiagnosed noncardiogenic pulmonary edema. Cardiol J. 2013;20(4):337–44. Epub 2013/08/06.
9. Fung YL, Silliman CC. The role of neutrophils in the pathogenesis of transfusion-related acute lung injury. Transfus Med Rev. 2009;23(4):266–83. Epub 2009/09/22.
10. Triulzi DJ, Kleinman S, Kakaiya RM, Busch MP, Norris PJ, Steele WR, et al. The effect of previous pregnancy and transfusion on HLA alloimmunization in blood donors: implications for a transfusion-related acute lung injury risk reduction strategy. Transfusion. 2009;49(9):1825–35. Epub 2009/05/21.
11. Silliman CC, Curtis BR, Kopko PM, Khan SY, Kelher MR, Schuller RM, et al. Donor antibodies to HNA-3a implicated in TRALI reactions prime neutrophils and cause PMN-mediated damage to human pulmonary microvascular endothelial cells in a two-event in vitro model. Blood. 2007;109(4):1752–5. Epub 2006/10/14.
12. Triulzi DJ. Transfusion-related acute lung injury: current concepts for the clinician. Anesth Analg. 2009;108(3):770–6. Epub 2009/02/20.
13. Toy P, Gajic O, Bacchetti P, Looney MR, Gropper MA, Hubmayr R, et al. Transfusion-related acute lung injury: incidence and risk factors. Blood. 2012;119(7):1757–67. Epub 2011/11/26.
14. Gajic O, Rana R, Winters JL, Yilmaz M, Mendez JL, Rickman OB, et al. Transfusion-related acute lung injury in the critically ill: prospective nested case-control study. Am J Respir Crit Care Med. 2007;176(9):886–91. Epub 2007/07/14.
15. Rana R, Fernandez-Perez ER, Khan SA, Rana S, Winters JL, Lesnick TG, et al. Transfusion-related acute lung injury and pulmonary edema in critically ill patients: a retrospective study. Transfusion. 2006;46(9):1478–83. Epub 2006/09/13.
16. Vlaar AP, Binnekade JM, Prins D, van Stein D, Hofstra JJ, Schultz MJ, et al. Risk factors and outcome of transfusion-related acute lung injury in the critically ill: a nested case-control study. Crit Care Med. 2010;38(3):771–8. Epub 2009/12/26.
17. Sanchez R, Bacchetti P, Toy P. Transfusion-related acute lung injury: a case-control pilot study of risk factors. Am J Clin Pathol. 2007;128(1):128–34. Epub 2007/06/21.
18. Vlaar AP, Hofstra JJ, Determann RM, Veelo DP, Paulus F, Kulik W, et al. The incidence, risk factors, and outcome of transfusion-related acute lung injury in a cohort of cardiac surgery patients: a prospective nested case-control study. Blood. 2011;117(16):4218–25. Epub 2011/02/18.
19. Engelfriet CP, Reesink HW, Brand A, Palfi M, Popovsky MA, Martin-Vega C, et al. Transfusion-related acute lung injury (TRALI). Vox Sang. 2001;81(4):269–83. Epub 2002/03/21.

20. Khan H, Belsher J, Yilmaz M, Afessa B, Winters JL, Moore SB, et al. Fresh-frozen plasma and platelet transfusions are associated with development of acute lung injury in critically ill medical patients. Chest. 2007;131(5):1308–14. Epub 2007/04/03.
21. Webert KE, Blajchman MA. Transfusion-related acute lung injury. Transfus Med Rev. 2003;17(4):252–62. Epub 2003/10/23.
22. Kim J, Na S. Transfusion-related acute lung injury; clinical perspectives. Korean J Anesthesiol. 2015;68(2):101–5. Epub 2015/04/07.
23. Ho J, Sibbald WJ, Chin-Yee IH. Effects of storage on efficacy of red cell transfusion: when is it not safe? Crit Care Med. 2003;31(12 Suppl):S687–97. Epub 2004/01/16.
24. Vlaar AP, Juffermans NP. Transfusion-related acute lung injury: a clinical review. Lancet. 2013;382(9896):984–94. Epub 2013/05/07.
25. Silliman CC, Boshkov LK, Mehdizadehkashi Z, Elzi DJ, Dickey WO, Podlosky L, et al. Transfusion-related acute lung injury: epidemiology and a prospective analysis of etiologic factors. Blood. 2003;101(2):454–62. Epub 2002/10/24.
26. Sachs UJ, Kauschat D, Bein G. White blood cell-reactive antibodies are undetectable in solvent/detergent plasma. Transfusion. 2005;45(10):1628–31. Epub 2005/09/27.
27. Looney MR, Gropper MA, Matthay MA. Transfusion-related acute lung injury: a review. Chest. 2004;126(1):249–58. Epub 2004/07/14.
28. Muller MC, Juffermans NP. Transfusion-related acute lung injury: a preventable syndrome? Expert Rev Hematol. 2012;5(1):97–106. Epub 2012/01/26.
29. Popovsky MA, Moore SB. Diagnostic and pathogenetic considerations in transfusion-related acute lung injury. Transfusion. 1985;25(6):573–7. Epub 1985/11/01.
30. The Acute Respiratory Distress Syndrome Network. Ventilation with lower tidal volumes as compared with traditional tidal volumes for acute lung injury and the acute respiratory distress syndrome. N Engl J Med. 2000;342(18):1301–8. Epub 2000/05/04.
31. Nouraei SM, Wallis JP, Bolton D, Hasan A. Management of transfusion-related acute lung injury with extracorporeal cardiopulmonary support in a four-year-old child. Br J Anaesth. 2003;91(2):292–4. Epub 2003/07/25.
32. Wallis JP, Lubenko A, Wells AW, Chapman CE. Single hospital experience of TRALI. Transfusion. 2003;43(8):1053–9. Epub 2003/07/19.
33. Wallis JP. Transfusion-related acute lung injury (TRALI): presentation, epidemiology and treatment. Intensive Care Med. 2007;33 Suppl 1:S12–6. Epub 2007/11/02.
34. Peter JV, John P, Graham PL, Moran JL, George IA, Bersten A. Corticosteroids in the prevention and treatment of acute respiratory distress syndrome (ARDS) in adults: meta-analysis. BMJ. 2008;336(7651):1006–9. Epub 2008/04/25.
35. Wiedemann HP, Wheeler AP, Bernard GR, Thompson BT, Hayden D, deBoisblanc B, et al. Comparison of two fluid-management strategies in acute lung injury. N Engl J Med. 2006;354(24):2564–75. Epub 2006/05/23.
36. Swanson K, Dwyre DM, Krochmal J, Raife TJ. Transfusion-related acute lung injury (TRALI): current clinical and pathophysiologic considerations. Lung. 2006;184(3):177–85. Epub 2006/08/12.
37. Hebert PC, Wells G, Blajchman MA, Marshall J, Martin C, Pagliarello G, et al. A multicenter, randomized, controlled clinical trial of transfusion requirements in critical care. Transfusion Requirements in Critical Care Investigators, Canadian Critical Care Trials Group. N Engl J Med. 1999;340(6):409–17. Epub 1999/02/11.
38. Yilmaz M, Keegan MT, Iscimen R, Afessa B, Buck CF, Hubmayr RD, et al. Toward the prevention of acute lung injury: protocol-guided limitation of large tidal volume ventilation and inappropriate transfusion. Crit Care Med. 2007;35(7):1660–6. quiz 7. Epub 2007/05/18.
39. Sayah DM, Looney MR, Toy P. Transfusion reactions: newer concepts on the pathophysiology, incidence, treatment, and prevention of transfusion-related acute lung injury. Crit Care Clin. 2012;28(3):363–72. v. Epub 2012/06/21.
40. Kakaiya RM, Triulzi DJ, Wright DJ, Steele WR, Kleinman SH, Busch MP, et al. Prevalence of HLA antibodies in remotely transfused or alloexposed volunteer blood donors. Transfusion. 2010;50(6):1328–34. Epub 2010/01/15.

41. Reesink HW, Lee J, Keller A, Dennington P, Pink J, Holdsworth R, et al. Measures to prevent transfusion-related acute lung injury (TRALI). Vox Sang. 2012;103(3):231–59. Epub 2012/04/24.
42. On 9 June 2015. http://www.fda.gov/BiologicsBloodVaccines/SafetyAvailability/ReportaProblem/TransfusionDonationFatalities/ucm346639.htm.
43. Riedler GF, Haycox AR, Duggan AK, Dakin HA. Cost-effectiveness of solvent/detergent-treated fresh-frozen plasma. Vox Sang. 2003;85(2):88–95. Epub 2003/08/20.
44. Ozier Y, Muller JY, Mertes PM, Renaudier P, Aguilon P, Canivet N, et al. Transfusion-related acute lung injury: reports to the French Hemovigilance Network 2007 through 2008. Transfusion. 2011;51(10):2102–10. Epub 2011/03/09.
45. Aravinthan A, Sen S, Marcus N. Transfusion-related acute lung injury: a rare and life-threatening complication of a common procedure. Clin Med. 2009;9(1):87–9. Epub 2009/03/11.
46. Moore SB. Transfusion-related acute lung injury (TRALI): clinical presentation, treatment, and prognosis. Crit Care Med. 2006;34(5 Suppl):S114–7. Epub 2006/04/18.
47. Herridge MS, Tansey CM, Matte A, Tomlinson G, Diaz-Granados N, Cooper A, et al. Functional disability 5 years after acute respiratory distress syndrome. N Engl J Med. 2011;364(14):1293–304. Epub 2011/04/08.
48. Lin Y, Kanani N, Naughton F, Pendergrast J, Karkouti K. Case report: transfusion-related acute lung injury (TRALI)—a clear and present danger. Can J Anaesth. 2007;54(12):1011–6. Epub 2007/12/07.
49. Popovsky MA. Transfusion-related acute lung injury. Curr Opin Hematol. 2000;7(6):402–7. Epub 2000/10/31.
50. Silliman CC, Ambruso DR, Boshkov LK. Transfusion-related acute lung injury. Blood. 2005;105(6):2266–73. Epub 2004/12/02.
51. Win N, Montgomery J, Sage D, Street M, Duncan J, Lucas G. Recurrent transfusion-related acute lung injury. Transfusion. 2001;41(11):1421–5. Epub 2001/11/29.

Chapter 12
Transfusion Associated Circulatory Overload

Mario V. Fusaro and Giora Netzer

Introduction

In 2011, over 20.9 million blood transfusions were given in the USA [1] with an estimated one transfusion reaction per 414 transfusions given [1]. This number may be even higher, given the variations in detection and national reporting of such occurrences [2]. Among transfusion reactions, Transfusion Associated Circulatory Overload (TACO) is the most common. TACO is the second most common cause of transfusion-related death in the USA [3], and the leader in transfusion-related death in the UK [4]. In addition to morbidity and mortality, TACO is also associated with increased length of stay and increased hospital costs [5].

Definition

Although TACO has no consensus definition, it is generally described as a clinical overload state within close proximity (typically <6 h) to a blood product transfusion. The Center for Disease Control defines TACO as new onset or exacerbation of three

M.V. Fusaro, MD
Division of Telehealth, Division of Pulmonary and Critical Care Medicine, Westchester Medical Center, Valhalla, NY, USA

Division of Pulmonary and Critical Care Medicine, Department of Medicine, and Department of Epidemiology and Public Health, University of Maryland School of Medicine, Baltimore, MD, USA
e-mail: Mario.Fusaro@wmchealth.org

G. Netzer, MD, MSCE (✉)
Division of Pulmonary and Critical Care Medicine, Department of Medicine, and Department of Epidemiology and Public Health, University of Maryland School of Medicine, Baltimore, MD, USA
e-mail: gnetzer@medicine.umaryland.edu

J.S. Lee, M.P. Donahoe (eds.), *Hematologic Abnormalities and Acute Lung Syndromes*, Respiratory Medicine, DOI 10.1007/978-3-319-41912-1_12

or more of the following within 6 h post transfusion: acute respiratory distress (dyspnea, orthopnea, cough), elevated brain natriuretic peptide (BNP), elevated central venous pressure (CVP), evidence of left heart failure, evidence of positive fluid balance, or radiographic evidence of pulmonary edema [6].

Epidemiology

A review of the literature finds an incidence ranging from 2.9 to 1980 cases per 100,000 units of blood received [4, 7, 8]. Heterogeneity in definition, recognition, and reporting of TACO led to disparate case-rates [2]. Data from passive reporting, e.g., national registries, tend to estimate lower case-rates, while actively reported data find higher case-rates [11]. Additional variability is noted between patient populations. A 2015 retrospective cohort study of 4070 postoperative surgical patients found that among those receiving transfusion, 4.3 % develop TACO. Among vascular surgery patients in this study, the rate was 12.1 % [9]. In a prospective observational study from 2011, the TACO case rate among medical intensive care unit (ICU) patients was 6 % [10].

Risk Factors

While TACO may occur after any transfusion, some patient populations may be at higher risk. This includes patients greater than 70 years of age, those with renal failure, congestive heart failure, and hemorrhagic shock [7, 12]. Differences in case-rate exist according to clinical setting. Surgical patients, especially those undergoing vascular surgery, have a rate of TACO almost double that of medical ICU patients (Table 12.1) [9, 10]. Different potential mechanisms may account for these differing case rates. In the medical ICU, a larger proportion of patients may have left ventricular dysfunction or renal failure, putting them at increased risk [10].

Table 12.1 Risk factors associated with TACO

Patients specific	Iatrogenic
Age >70	Excessive transfusions
Renal failure	Infusion rate >225 mL/h
Congestive heart failure	Increased volume of transfusion
Hemorrhagic shock	Positive fluid balance
Severe liver disease	Prolonged surgical time
Cardiac surgery	
Vascular surgery	
Liver surgery	

TACO may result from intraoperative fluid resuscitation in the background of transfusion, leading to positive fluid balance. Hemodilution from fluid resuscitation may also lead to abnormally low hemoglobin levels, prompting further transfusion [12].

In addition to intrinsic patient risk, multiple iatrogenic factors contribute to the risk of developing TACO. These include a greater number of transfusions given, increased rate of transfusion, and volume of the transfusate [7, 12]. In TACO cases, the number of units transfused varies from 1.8 to 4 units but can be as few as one [2, 10, 11, 13]. In a prospective cohort study, a transfusion rate of 225 mL/h compared to 168 mL/h was associated with increased risk of TACO (Odds Ratio (OR) 1.88, 95 % confidence interval (95 % CI) of 1.06–3.33) [10], while another found that a mean positive fluid balance in patients transfused who later developed TACO was +4.7 L compared with 2.75 L in controls [OR 1.18 (95 % CI 1.08–1.28)]. The positive fluid balance per hour was +0.38 L vs. +0.26 L, respectively [OR 3.6 (95 % CI 1.52–8.5)] [12]. The amount of volume per transfusion can vary based on blood type, amount donated, and center transfusing but the approximate volume of red cells or FFP is 200–400 mL per transfusion [14, 15].

Clinical Presentation

The clinical features of TACO consist of new onset respiratory distress, hypoxemia, orthopnea, and/or cough during or after blood transfusion. Physical exam findings may include jugular venous distention, rales, and peripheral edema. Patients may exhibit abnormal vital signs such as elevated heart rate, systolic and diastolic blood pressure, respiratory rate, and lower oxygen saturation, compared to those before transfusion [7].

Pathophysiology

The driving pathophysiology in TACO is an increase in intravascular fluid, leading to elevated hydrostatic pressure in the pulmonary vasculature, and promoting fluid accumulation in the lung. Fluid dynamics and handling drive the development of pulmonary edema, contrasting with the priming, inflammation, and capillary leak occurring in Transfusion Related Acute Lung Injury (TRALI) [16].

In the lung, the main forces contributing to fluid accumulation are hydrostatic pressures, oncotic pressures, and integrity of the capillary interface, otherwise known as Starling Forces [17]. As hydrostatic pressures in the lung increase relative to oncotic forces, more fluid is forced into the interstitium. Normal or marginally elevated hydrostatic pressures in the setting of low oncotic pressure may cause the same effect such has in hypoalbuminemia. It is unclear whether the hypervolemic effect of blood products may be amplified by their increased extrapulmonary oncotic pressure compared to that of isotonic fluid [18].

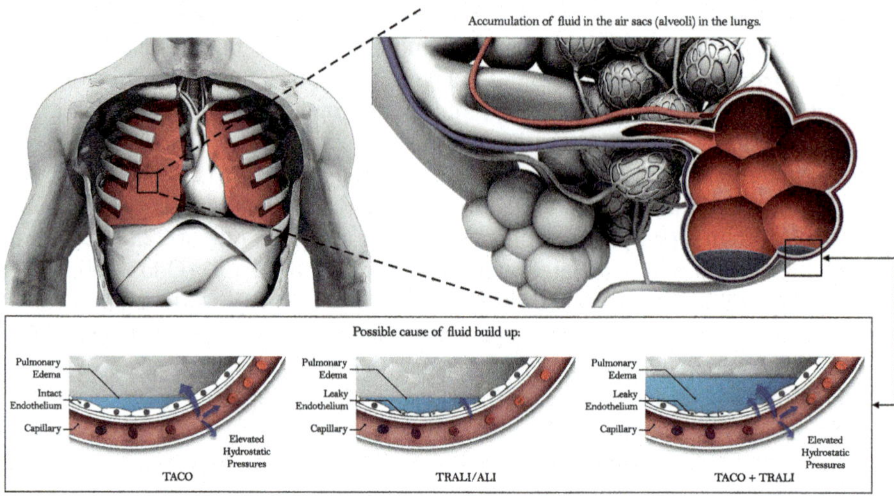

Fig. 12.1 Transfusion associated circulatory overload (TACO) represents movement of fluid into alveoli secondary to hydrostatic pressure. Transfusion related acute lung injury/acute lung injury (TRALI/ALI) occurs when the integrity of the endothelial interface is compromised. TACO and TRALI/ALI may occur concurrently with pulmonary edema occurring from both leaky endothelium and elevated hydrostatic pressures. Courtesy of Peter L. Gibfried

In critically ill patients, an overlap syndrome may exist between TRALI and TACO [19]. In these critically ill patients, disruption of the capillary interface is thought to magnify the effect of elevated hydrostatic pressures (Fig. 12.1). A study evaluating the differences between pulmonary edema secondary to cardiogenic and noncardiogenic etiologies noted a more positive relationship between elevated PAOP and amount of "lung water" in Acute Respiratory Distress Syndrome (ARDS) compared with cardiogenic etiologies [20]. This relationship was again noted in The Fluid and Catheter Treatment Trial (FACTT) which investigated two different fluid strategies in ARDS patients [21].

Diagnostic Evaluation

While no single test can defines the diagnosis of TACO, several are highly suggestive (Fig. 12.2). As the mechanism driving TACO is elevated cardiac filling pressures secondary to excess volume, diagnostic techniques can be used for its identification. The pulmonary artery catheter is one of the most direct modalities to measure elevated cardiac filling pressures. In the setting of transfusion related pulmonary edema, the finding of a pulmonary artery occlusion pressure (PAOP) greater than 18 mmHg can suggest TACO versus TRALI which would be below 18 mmHg [22]. While once a mainstay guiding ICU therapy, for a variety of reasons, the pulmonary artery catheter has fallen out of favor in recent practice [23].

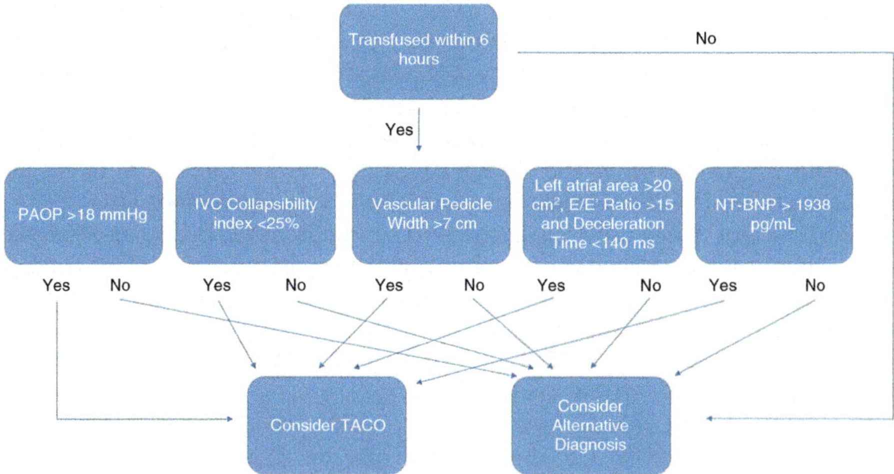

Fig. 12.2 Diagnostic algorithm for TACO

One of the simplest and most informative studies performed for the investigation of TACO is the chest roentgenogram (X-ray). Pulmonary edema can be visualized in the lung fields and is characterized by perihilar opacities and bibasilar effusions. Additionally, elevated cardiac pressures may be inferred from findings of cephalization, pleural effusions, and the increased vascular pedicle width on chest X-ray. The measurement of vascular pedicle width has been studied and correlated to elevated PA catheter wedge pressures [24]. The technique is performed by making a perpendicular line from left subclavian artery exit of the aortic arch and measuring across to the point at which the superior vena cava crosses the right main stem bronchus [25]. A vascular pedicle width >7 cm has a 56 % sensitivity and 74 % specificity for a PAOP >18 mmHg. In situations in which echo is unavailable and PA catheter is not being considered, this may be a simple and useful strategy to suggest fluid overload in a patient receiving blood transfusion.

Bedside ultrasound and echocardiography are increasingly common in ICU practice. Evaluation of the thorax can be rapidly performed in a patient with acute respiratory distress using ultrasound. Multiple anterior diffuse B-lines may be suggestive of pulmonary edema with sensitivity of 97 % and specificity of 95 % [26]. Identification of pleural effusions can be made by sitting the patient upright and directing the ultrasound superior to the costovertebral angle. Simple anechoic fluid may be suggestive of pleural effusion and fluid overload. Although these findings are seen in pulmonary edema of any etiology, left heart failure or elevated central venous pressures are prerequisite for the diagnosis TACO.

In recent years, interest in the noninvasive evaluation of intravascular fluid status using ultrasound and echocardiography has grown. Many iterations of the ultrasound exam have been devised for this purpose, with respirophasic inferior vena cava (IVC) variation being the most widely studied. While this technique has not been evaluated in its diagnostic accuracy for TACO, it may be extrapolated that the determination of intravascular fluid balance in a recently transfused patient with pulmonary edema can be helpful in determining the potential etiology of respiratory distress. Respirophasic IVC variation is measured by directing a phased array ultrasound probe just inferior to the xiphoid process 1–2 cm to the right with marker dot position toward the operator. The probe can then be angled perpendicularly to the patient and then adjusted to angle cephalad. The operator can then sweep the probe until the IVC is visualized longitudinally. The ultrasound can then be switched to M-mode and evaluation of the IVC diameter during respirophasic variation can be made.

This modality has been investigated in both intubated [27] and non-intubated [28] patients for the purpose of determining fluid responsiveness. The IVC collapsibility index (IVC-CI) defined as the percent change between IVC diameter at end expiration and end inspiration has been inversely correlated. 90 % of patients with IVC-CI of <25 % will have a CVP of >7 mmHg while 85 % of patients with IVC-CI >75 % will have a CVP of 0–6 mmHg [29].

In addition to IVC parameters, echocardiographic parameters have also been associated with elevated PAOP. These include: mitral *E*/*E*′ ratio, left atrial area, and deceleration time. The mitral *E*/*E*′ ratio is the ratio of early diastolic mitral inflow velocity to early diastolic mitral annulus velocity which is a marker of end diastolic filling pressures [30]. Deceleration time is the time from peak flow to stasis across the mitral valve. These parameters are associated with PAOP of >15 mmHg for a left atrial area of ≥20 cm^2, a mitral *E*/*E*′ ratio of ≥15, and a deceleration time <140 ms. The sensitivity and specificity for each was 66 and 89 % for mitral *E*/*E*′ ratio, 55 and 96 % for left atrial area and 51 and 93 % for deceleration time, respectively. If all three tests were used, the sensitivity and specificity was 92 and 85 %, respectively. Lastly, if all were positive, the odds ratio for PAOP >15 mmHg was 48 (CI 10–289, $p < 0.001$) [31].

Laboratory tests may also suggest the diagnosis. One of the most studied biomarkers in the determination of TACO is N-terminal Brain Natriuretic Peptide (NT-BNP). NT-BNP was initially isolated from porcine neural tissue. It is released in humans in response to myocardial stretch and counteracts the renin-angiotensin system to reduce excess salt and water retention as well as inhibit vasoconstriction, promote vascular relaxation, and reduce sympathetic outflow [32].

In non-ICU populations, the marker had sensitivity and specificity of 87.5 and 95.8 %, respectively, for a level of >1923 pg/mL [33]. In patients with TACO, pre- and post-N-terminal BNP (NT-BNP) levels are elevated compared to controls who received transfusion and did not have TRALI or TACO [33]. A prospective cohort study evaluating the utility of BNP and NT-BNP in differentiating between TRALI and TACO in ICU patients found that levels differed significantly between entities. The area under the curve was 0.63 (95 % confidence interval [CI] 0.51–0.74) and 0.70 (95 % CI 0.59–0.80) for BNP and NT-BNP, respectively [34]. As such, the use of this biomarker may be limited in differentiating TRALI from TACO in an ICU population [35].

Several additional biomarkers have been investigated including pulmonary fluid protein concentration, radiolabeled albumin and interleukins (IL) 6, 8 and 10 with variable success. Previous studies have revealed that TRALI patients will have elevated IL-6 and 8 levels prior to the event relative to controls. A recent nested case–control study evaluating the use of IL-6, 8, 10, tumor necrosis factor-α (TNF-α), and granulocyte-macrophage colony stimulating factor (GM-CSF) were used to distinguish TACO versus TRALI [36]. While in multivariate analysis a good correlation existed between these levels might distinguish TRALI from TACO, but in univariate analysis specificity was only 59 % compared with 90 % in multivariate analysis. At this time, insufficient data exist to recommend routine clinical use of these assays [37–39].

Prevention

Recognition of populations at higher risk as well as modifiable risk can guide not only early identification of TACO, but also in its prevention. As always, the decision to transfuse should be given proper deliberation. An ever-growing body of data indicates the need for judicious use of blood transfusion at lower transfusion thresholds [40–42]. The best way to prevent any transfusion reaction is to not transfuse at all. Like all clinical interventions, the decision to transfuse should occur only after assessing that the benefits of transfusion outweigh the risks.

Older patients, those with heart failure, renal failure, and hemorrhagic shock should be carefully monitored when receiving blood products. Clinical suspicion for TACO should remain high. Careful monitoring of intake and outtake recording is important. Attention should also be paid to the patient's fluid balance, both for the day of transfusion and cumulatively. Physical examination should be recorded both before and after transfusion as initial signs might be subtle. These include increased respiratory distress, elevated blood pressure, tachypnea, hypoxemia, elevated JVD, third heart sounds, crackles, decreased breath sounds, or edema. Transfusion of single units should be considered for high risk patients. While The American Association of Blood Banks (AABB) Technical Manual 17th edition recommends a transfusion rate of 240 mL/h, a rate of 168 mL/h (as discussed above) has been associated with reduced risk of TACO [10] and should be considered for high risk patients.

While definitive data for prophylactic diuretic use are lacking, these may be of benefit. A recent Cochrane Review, including four randomized controlled studies, found a decrease in PAOP and improvement in fraction of inspired oxygen with diuretics prior to transfusion. However, no differences were noted in clinically meaningful endpoints defined as acute respiratory distress, tachycardia, increased blood pressure or acute/worsening pulmonary edema on chest X-ray [43].

Treatment

Acute Support

Goals of acute management are consistent with the general support of the patient with volume overload of any type. Airway, breathing, and circulation should be addressed first. The transfusion should be stopped immediately. Supplemental oxygen,

Table 12.2 Treatment modalities

Supportive care	Volume removal
Transfusion cessation	Loop diuretic
Endotracheal intubation	Hemodialysis
Oxygen therapy	Ultrafiltration
Nitroglycerine	Inotropes
ACE inhibitor	
Morphine	
Noninvasive positive pressure ventilation	

noninvasive or invasive ventilation should be considered. While high flow oxygen is an option [44], given the pathophysiology of TACO, noninvasive positive pressure ventilation may be more appropriate [45]. In patients with systolic dysfunction, preload and afterload reduction should be initiated. This can be performed using nitroglycerine, angiotensin converting enzyme inhibitors. Morphine might also be used to reduce dyspnea and provide further preload reductions, similar to its use in patients with acute heart failure [46] (Table 12.2).

Volume Removal

Aggressive therapy with diuretics should be the initial therapy [11]. If diuresis cannot be achieved in this fashion, then dialysis or ultrafiltration may need to be utilized [11]. TACO in patients with cardio-renal syndromes may present a particularly challenging scenario. In these patients, diuresis and preload/afterload reduction should be attempted. Ultrafiltration or step-up inotropic therapy using dobutamine may need to be considered [47].

Reporting

If TACO is suspected, the blood bank should be notified immediately to being investigation of the blood product. This is to evaluate for possible TRALI, including antibody testing. This may reduce the risk of harm to other potential recipients of the same donor. AABB leaves investigation of TACO to the provider's discretion but recommends white blood cell antibody screening as well as Human Leukocyte Antigen (HLA) typing of the recipient if any question of TRALI exists [48].

Outcomes

The clinical sequelae of TACO vary from mild shortness of breath to ICU transfer and death. Patients may undergo excess radiologic testing and diuretic administration. The ICU transfer rate is between 18 and 35 % [7] with case-fatality rate ranging from 5.1 to 16.9 % [7, 12]. Li et al. performed a nested case–control study evaluating outcomes in TACO patients with regard to long-term survival, ICU length of stay, and quality of life. Compared to those with TRALI, TACO patients did not have a worsened 1 and 2 year mortality compared to matched controls but did have a significantly longer ICU length of stay [13]. In both groups, no differences were noted in quality of life afterward.

Conclusion

In summary, TACO is a common cause of transfusion-related mortality. TACO has significant associated morbidity, and is likely underreported and under-recognized. The patients most at risk are the elderly, those with heart or renal failure, and those receiving excessive transfusion volumes at faster infusion rates. The diagnosis is made when a patient suffers cardiogenic pulmonary edema in the setting of a recent blood transfusion. Prevention with concurrent diuretics, slower transfusion speed, and smaller transfusion volumes should be pursued. In patients with TACO, treatments consist of volume reduction and/or usual heart failure therapy.

References

1. Whitaker BI, Hinkins S. The 2011 national blood collection and utilization survey report. 2011;0990–0313.
2. Narick C, Triulzi DJ, Yazer MH. Transfusion-associated circulatory overload after plasma transfusion. Transfusion. 2012;52(1):160–5. doi:10.1111/j.1537-2995.2011.03247.x.
3. FDA. Fatalities reported to FDA following blood collection and transfusion annual summary for fiscal year 2013. 2013.
4. Bolton-Maggs P, et al. Annual SHOT report 2012. 2012.
5. Magee G, Zbrozek A. Fluid overload is associated with increases in length of stay and hospital costs: pooled analysis of data from more than 600 US hospitals. Clinicoecon Outcomes Res. 2013;5:289–96. doi:10.2147/CEOR.S45873.
6. Division of Healthcare Quality Promotion, National Center for Emerging and Zoonotic Infectious Diseases, Centers for Disease Control and Prevention (CDC). The national healthcare safety network (NHSN) manual, biovigilance component. Atlanta, GA.
7. Lieberman L, Maskens C, Cserti-Gazdewich C, et al. A retrospective review of patient factors, transfusion practices, and outcomes in patients with transfusion-associated circulatory overload. Transfus Med Rev. 2013;27(4):206–12. doi:10.1016/j.tmrv.2013.07.002.
8. Bierbaum BE, Callaghan JJ, Galante JO, Rubash HE, Tooms RE, Welch RB. An analysis of blood management in patients having a total hip or knee arthroplasty. J Bone Joint Surg Am. 1999;81(1):2–10.

9. Clifford L, Jia Q, Yadav H, et al. Characterizing the epidemiology of perioperative transfusion-associated circulatory overload. Anesthesiology. 2015;122(1):21–8. doi:10.1097/ALN.0000000000000513.
10. Li G, Rachmale S, Kojicic M, et al. Incidence and transfusion risk factors for transfusion-associated circulatory overload among medical intensive care unit patients. Transfusion. 2011;51(2):338–43. doi:10.1111/j.1537-2995.2010.02816.x.
11. Andrzejewski Jr C, Casey MA, Popovsky MA. How we view and approach transfusion-associated circulatory overload: pathogenesis, diagnosis, management, mitigation, and prevention. Transfusion. 2013;53(12):3037–47. doi:10.1111/trf.12454.
12. Murphy EL, Kwaan N, Looney MR, et al. Risk factors and outcomes in transfusion-associated circulatory overload. Am J Med. 2013;126(4):357.e29–38. doi:10.1016/j.amjmed.2012.08.019.
13. Li G, Kojicic M, Reriani MK, et al. Long-term survival and quality of life after transfusion-associated pulmonary edema in critically ill medical patients. Chest. 2010;137(4):783–9. doi:10.1378/chest.09-0841.
14. Elzik ME, Dirschl DR, Dahners LE. Correlation of transfusion volume to change in hematocrit. Am J Hematol. 2006;81(2):145–6. doi:10.1002/ajh.20517.
15. AABB, the American Red Cross, America's Blood Centers, and the Armed Services Blood Program. Circular of Information for the Use of Human Blood and Blood Components. 2013.
16. Marik PE, Corwin HL. Acute lung injury following blood transfusion: expanding the definition. Crit Care Med. 2008;36(11):3080–4. doi:10.1097/CCM.0b013e31818c3801.
17. Starling EH. On the absorption of fluids from the connective tissue spaces. J Physiol. 1896;19(4):312–26.
18. Weaver DW, Ledgerwood AM, Lucas CE, Higgins R, Bouwman DL, Johnson SD. Pulmonary effects of albumin resuscitation for severe hypovolemic shock. Arch Surg. 1978;113(4):387–92.
19. Gajic O, Gropper MA, Hubmayr RD. Pulmonary edema after transfusion: how to differentiate transfusion-associated circulatory overload from transfusion-related acute lung injury. Crit Care Med. 2006;34(5 Suppl):S109–13. doi:10.1097/01.CCM.0000214311.56231.23.
20. Sibbald WJ, Short AK, Warshawski FJ, Cunningham DG, Cheung H. Thermal dye measurements of extravascular lung water in critically ill patients. Intravascular starling forces and extravascular lung water in the adult respiratory distress syndrome. Chest. 1985;87(5):585–92.
21. National Heart Lung, and Blood Institute Acute Respiratory Distress Syndrome (ARDS) Clinical Trials Network, Wiedemann HP, Wheeler AP, et al. Comparison of two fluid-management strategies in acute lung injury. N Engl J Med. 2006;354(24):2564–75. doi: NEJMoa062200 [pii].
22. Skeate RC, Eastlund T. Distinguishing between transfusion related acute lung injury and transfusion associated circulatory overload. Curr Opin Hematol. 2007;14(6):682–7. doi:10.1097/MOH.0b013e3282ef195a.
23. Connors Jr AF, Speroff T, Dawson NV, et al. The effectiveness of right heart catheterization in the initial care of critically ill patients. SUPPORT investigators. JAMA. 1996;276(11):889–97.
24. Rice TW, Ware LB, Haponik EF, et al. Vascular pedicle width in acute lung injury: correlation with intravascular pressures and ability to discriminate fluid status. Crit Care. 2011;15(2):R86. doi:10.1186/cc10084.
25. Milne EN, Pistolesi M, Miniati M, Giuntini C. The vascular pedicle of the heart and the vena azygos. Part I: the normal subject. Radiology. 1984;152(1):1–8. doi:10.1148/radiology.152.1.6729098.
26. Lichtenstein DA, Meziere GA. Relevance of lung ultrasound in the diagnosis of acute respiratory failure: the BLUE protocol. Chest. 2008;134(1):117–25. doi:10.1378/chest.07-2800.
27. Feissel M, Michard F, Faller JP, Teboul JL. The respiratory variation in inferior vena cava diameter as a guide to fluid therapy. Intensive Care Med. 2004;30(9):1834–7. doi:10.1007/s00134-004-2233-5.
28. Yildirimturk O, Tayyareci Y, Erdim R, et al. Assessment of right atrial pressure using echocardiography and correlation with catheterization. J Clin Ultrasound. 2011;39(6):337–43. doi:10.1002/jcu.20837.
29. Stawicki SP, Adkins EJ, Eiferman DS, et al. Prospective evaluation of intravascular volume status in critically ill patients: does inferior vena cava collapsibility correlate with central venous

pressure? J Trauma Acute Care Surg. 2014;76(4):956–63. doi:10.1097/TA.0000000000000152. discussion 963–4.

30. Burgess MI, Jenkins C, Sharman JE, Marwick TH. Diastolic stress echocardiography: hemodynamic validation and clinical significance of estimation of ventricular filling pressure with exercise. J Am Coll Cardiol. 2006;47(9):1891–900. doi: S0735-1097(06)00637-1 [pii].
31. Rafique AM, Phan A, Tehrani F, Biner S, Siegel RJ. Transthoracic echocardiographic parameters in the estimation of pulmonary capillary wedge pressure in patients with present or previous heart failure. Am J Cardiol. 2012;110(5):689–94. doi:10.1016/j.amjcard.2012.04.055.
32. Levin ER, Gardner DG, Samson WK. Natriuretic peptides. N Engl J Med. 1998;339(5):321–8. doi:10.1056/NEJM199807303390507.
33. Tobian AA, Sokoll LJ, Tisch DJ, Ness PM, Shan H. N-terminal pro-brain natriuretic peptide is a useful diagnostic marker for transfusion-associated circulatory overload. Transfusion. 2008;48(6):1143–50. doi:10.1111/j.1537-2995.2008.01656.x.
34. Li G, Daniels CE, Kojicic M, et al. The accuracy of natriuretic peptides (brain natriuretic peptide and N-terminal pro-brain natriuretic) in the differentiation between transfusion-related acute lung injury and transfusion-related circulatory overload in the critically ill. Transfusion. 2009;49(1):13–20. doi:10.1111/j.1537-2995.2008.01941.x.
35. Forfia PR, Watkins SP, Rame JE, Stewart KJ, Shapiro EP. Relationship between B-type natriuretic peptides and pulmonary capillary wedge pressure in the intensive care unit. J Am Coll Cardiol. 2005;45(10):1667–71. doi: S0735-1097(05)00468-7 [pii].
36. Roubinian NH, Looney MR, Kor DJ, et al. Cytokines and clinical predictors in distinguishing pulmonary transfusion reactions. Transfusion. 2015. doi: 10.1111/trf.13021.
37. Fein A, Grossman RF, Jones JG, et al. The value of edema fluid protein measurement in patients with pulmonary edema. Am J Med. 1979;67(1):32–8.
38. Schuster DP, Stark T, Stephenson J, Royal H. Detecting lung injury in patients with pulmonary edema. Intensive Care Med. 2002;28(9):1246–53. doi:10.1007/s00134-002-1414-3.
39. Roubinian NH, Looney MR, Toy P, et al. Distinguishing pulmonary transfusion reactions using cytokines and cardiopulmonary biomarkers. Am J Respir Crit Care Med. 2014;189:A6639.
40. Carson JL, Terrin ML, Noveck H, et al. Liberal or restrictive transfusion in high-risk patients after hip surgery. N Engl J Med. 2011;365(26):2453–62. doi:10.1056/NEJMoa1012452.
41. Hebert PC, Wells G, Blajchman MA, et al. A multicenter, randomized, controlled clinical trial of transfusion requirements in critical care. transfusion requirements in critical care investigators, Canadian critical care trials group. N Engl J Med. 1999;340(6):409–17. doi:10.1056/NEJM199902113400601.
42. Holst LB, Haase N, Wetterslev J, et al. Lower versus higher hemoglobin threshold for transfusion in septic shock. N Engl J Med. 2014;371(15):1381–91. doi:10.1056/NEJMoa1406617.
43. Sarai M, Tejani AM. Loop diuretics for patients receiving blood transfusions. Cochrane Database Syst Rev. 2015;2:CD010138. doi:10.1002/14651858.CD010138.pub2.
44. Frat JP, Thille AW, Mercat A, et al. High-flow oxygen through nasal cannula in acute hypoxemic respiratory failure. N Engl J Med. 2015;372(23):2185–96. doi:10.1056/NEJMoa1503326.
45. Peter JV, Moran JL, Phillips-Hughes J, Graham P, Bersten AD. Effect of non-invasive positive pressure ventilation (NIPPV) on mortality in patients with acute cardiogenic pulmonary oedema: a meta-analysis. Lancet. 2006;367(9517):1155–63. doi: S0140-6736(06)68506-1 [pii].
46. Braunwald E, Bonow RO. Braunwald's heart disease: a textbook of cardiovascular medicine. 9th ed. Philadelphia: Saunders; 2012. p. 1961.
47. Bart BA, Goldsmith SR, Lee KL, et al. Ultrafiltration in decompensated heart failure with cardiorenal syndrome. N Engl J Med. 2012;367(24):2296–304. doi:10.1056/NEJMoa1210357.
48. American Association of Blood Banks. Standards Program Committee. Blood Bank/ Transfusion Service Standards Program Unit. Standards for blood banks and transfusion services. 25th ed. Bethesda, MD: American Association of Blood Banks; 2008. p. 134.

Chapter 13
Transfusion-Related Immunomodulation (TRIM): From Renal Allograft Survival to Postoperative Mortality in Cardiac Surgery

Eleftherios C. Vamvakas

Transfusion-related immunomodulation (TRIM) encompasses the documented laboratory immune alterations that follow allogeneic blood transfusion (ABT), as well as any established or purported, beneficial or deleterious, clinical effects that may be ascribed to immunosuppression resulting from ABT, including enhanced survival of renal allografts, increased risk of recurrence of resected malignancies and of postoperative bacterial infections, increased short-term (up to 3-month post-transfusion) mortality from all causes, and activation of endogenous Cytomegalovirus (CMV) or human immunodeficiency virus (HIV) infection in transfused compared with untransfused patients [1]. Any ABT-related increase in short-term post-transfusion mortality (perhaps secondary to an increased risk of multiple-organ failure [MOF]) would likely be mediated by "pro-inflammatory"' rather than "immunomodulatory" mechanisms; however, the term TRIM has been used more broadly, to encompass transfusion complications mediated via either immunomodulatory or pro-inflammatory pathways [1].

The only *established* clinical TRIM effect is beneficial; not deleterious. It is the enhanced survival of renal allografts after pretransplant ABT [2]. The existence of deleterious clinically relevant TRIM effects has not yet been established; neither do we know the mechanism(s) of TRIM or the specific blood constituent(s) that mediate(s) TRIM. TRIM may be mediated by one (or more) of the following: allogeneic mononuclear cells (AMCs) present in red-blood-cell (RBC) units stored for less than 2 weeks; pro-inflammatory soluble mediators released from WBC granules or membranes and accumulating progressively in the supernatant of RBCs during storage; and/or soluble, class I HLA molecules circulating in allogeneic plasma [3–5].

E.C. Vamvakas, MD, PhD, MPH (✉)
Formerly, Rita and Taft Schreiber Chair in Transfusion Medicine,
Cedars-Sinai Medical Center, Los Angeles, CA, USA
e-mail: vamvakas@post.harvard.edu

J.S. Lee, M.P. Donahoe (eds.), *Hematologic Abnormalities and Acute Lung Syndromes*, Respiratory Medicine, DOI 10.1007/978-3-319-41912-1_13

Enhanced Survival of Renal Allografts

In both observational studies and randomized controlled trials (RCTs), patients transfused with allogeneic blood have been shown to have a significantly better renal-allograft survival than untransfused patients, regardless of the number of HLA-A, HLA-B, and HLA-DR locus mismatches between recipient and donor [6]. This is true also when there is a common HLA haplotype, or shared HLA-B and HLA-DR antigens between donor and recipient [7]. The TRIM effect has further been reported to be associated with allografts between HLA-identical siblings [8].

The ABT-related enhancement of renal-allograft survival has been confirmed by animal data and clinical experience worldwide [6]. In the past it was a standard policy in many renal-transplant units to deliberately expose patients on transplant waiting lists to one or more allogeneic RBC transfusions. Subsequently, the beneficial effect of pretransplant ABT was thought to be less important with the advent of cyclosporine and other potent immunosuppressive drugs and, as a consequence, many centers discontinued its use.

However, a multicenter observational study, reporting on 58,036 renal allografts from cadaveric donors after the advent of cyclosporine, indicated that patients who had received ABT were still more likely to have a successful renal allograft than those who had not [9]. This study reported that the 1-year renal-allograft survival of patients receiving pretransplant ABT was 3–5 % better than that of those who did not receive ABT. Similar results were also reported for patients who received renal allografts from living-related donors [10]. The beneficial effect of pretransplant ABT in the outcome of cadaveric renal allografts was confirmed by a RCT conducted at 14 transplant centers [11]. Patients were randomly assigned to receive either three pretransplant, *non-WBC-reduced* RBC transfusions or no ABT. The renal-allograft survival was significantly higher in the 205 transfused patients than in the 218 untransfused subjects (90 % versus 82 % at 1-year, $p=0.02$; 79 % versus 70 % at 5-years, $p=0.025$). The beneficial effect of ABT was found to be independent of age, gender, underlying disease, prophylaxis with lymphocyte antibodies, or the presence of pre-formed lymphocytotoxins [11].

There have been two more RCTs [12, 13] that compared types of pretransplant ABTs given to prolong graft survival. Both studies were small, enrolling 52 and 144 patients, respectively. The first RCT [12] compared non-WBC-reduced and WBC-reduced RBCs and found no difference in graft survival. However, the WBC-reduced RBCs administered in this 1985 RCT did not meet the current European WBC reduction standard ($<10^6$ WBCs/unit) and all transfused RBC components may have been equally effective in mediating the ABT effect. The other RCT [13] compared recipients of one HLA-DR-mismatched ABT, one HLA-DR-matched ABT, and no ABT. There was no difference in graft survival at 1 year or at 5 years. The risk of acute rejection in patients who had received a HLA-DR-shared ABT was lower than that observed in the other two groups (19 % versus 33 %), but this difference did not attain statistical significance in this small RCT. The three available RCTs [11–13] have employed different study designs and have addressed different clinical questions, so that the integration of their results in a meta-analysis is not possible owing to the clinical heterogeneity of the studies.

In observational studies, recipients of non-WBC-reduced whole blood or RBCs have had better 1-year cadaveric-allograft survival than patients given WBC-reduced blood components such as frozen-thawed-deglycerolized RBCs. Such data indicate that allogeneic WBCs are involved in eliciting this beneficial TRIM effect [14]. However, the mechanism(s) involved in the ABT-related enhancement of renal allograft survival remain(s) to be elucidated. An experimental-animal model has suggested that the beneficial effect of donor-specific ABT might be related to the type of transplanted organ. Whereas ABT appears to lead to permanent acceptance of all renal allografts, this benefit was not observed with pancreas, skin, or heart allografts [15]. ABT administered during the actual operation for renal transplantation has not been shown to affect subsequent allograft survival [16]. In observational studies, patients who receive more than 10 RBCs have a better 1-year allograft survival than patients who receive only 1 or 2 RBC units. However, patients who receive more than 10 RBCs appear to have a poorer overall allograft survival than those who receive fewer than 10 RBC units [17].

Such data suggest that multi-transfused patients often develop cytotoxic antibodies and are thus at greater risk for earlier and more severe allograft-rejection episodes [10]. Along these lines, another potential benefit from pretransplant ABTs has been advanced [18], which is especially relevant in settings where there is a shortage of organs for transplantation. When several prospective recipients on a renal-transplant list produce crossmatch-negative results with an available organ, pretransplant ABTs could help identify high-responder patients (i.e., patients most likely to form cytotoxic antibodies in response to pretransplant ABTs, and also most likely to reject a transplanted kidney because of formation of cytotoxic antibodies after a negative crossmatch). Transplant surgeons could thus channel the scarce organ away from such patients, and give it to a patient in whom the allograft is most likely to survive [18].

A recent Agency for Healthcare Research and Quality (AHRQ) review of all available clinical evidence [19] suggested that pretransplant ABT has a neutral to beneficial effect on graft rejection, graft survival, and patient survival compared with no ABT. However, such benefits were reported mostly in studies conducted before the introduction of modern immunosuppressive drugs and solid-phase technology to detect formation of cytotoxic antibodies. In addition, the strength of the evidence was low.

Three other recent reviews of the clinical literature concluded that pretransplant ABTs place patients at increased risk of forming cytotoxic antibodies, and that the ensuing HLA alloimmunization reduces renal allograft survival and increases wait time for transplantation [20–22]. By searching the MEDLINE, Embase, and Cochrane Library datasets for English-language publications between January 1984 and March 2011, the latest analysis [22] captured 180 studies and data from publically available registries. The authors noted that implementation of universal WBC reduction had not decreased HLA alloimmunization in patients receiving renal allografts to any significant extent [23]. While a recent study again reported a beneficial effect of pretransplant ABT with current immunosuppression protocols such as cyclosporine [24], most current evidence appears to indicate that improvements in graft survival comparable to those previously ascribed to the beneficial "ABT effect" are now attainable without pretransplant ABTs. For this reason, the graft outcome risk/benefit ratio has now become too high to justify consideration of pretransplant ABTs when these can be avoided [20–22].

In summary, the beneficial ABT effect in renal transplantation is established, and it used to be clinically relevant before the advent of cyclosporine and similar immunosuppression regimens. Before 1984, the demonstration of this beneficial ABT effect had led to the consideration of pretransplant ABT(s) as a strategy to improve renal allograft survival in transplant recipients. However, with the rapid improvement in peri-transplant immunosuppression therapy, the additional effect of ABT became marginal. For this reason, the relevance of such pretransplant ABT protocols in clinical practice diminished because of the improvements in HLA technology and the remarkable advances in targeted and safe immunosuppression. Alloimmunization to HLA antigens can occur despite the use of WBC-reduced blood components. Therefore, in the modern era, use of pretransplant ABTs should be avoided whenever possible. When ABT is necessary in patients awaiting renal transplantation, WBC-reduced blood components must be given to reduce the risks of HLA alloimmunization and CMV transmission.

Clinical Studies of Adverse TRIM Effects

Some 200 observational studies and 21 RCTs reported before 2005 examined the purported adverse TRIM effects in humans [25–30]. The reasons for the disagreements between the reported studies have been extensively and acrimoniously debated [25–30]. The RBC components transfused in these studies reflected the RBC components used in Europe and North America between the mid-1980s and the first few years of the twenty-first century. Fifteen RCTs assumed that the TRIM effect is mediated by allogeneic WBCs and compared recipients of non-WBC-reduced versus WBC-reduced allogeneic RBCs or whole blood (Fig. 13.1) [31–45]. Five RCTs assumed that the TRIM effect is mediated by either allogeneic WBCs or allogeneic plasma and compared recipients of non-WBC-reduced allogeneic versus autologous blood (Fig. 13.2) [46–51]. Thus, the reported RCTs differed in ways that determined the conclusions to be drawn about mechanisms of TRIM. Patients randomized to receive non-WBC-reduced allogeneic RBCs received units that were either buffy-coat-reduced (in Europe) or buffy-coat-rich (in the US) [30]. Buffy-coat-reduced RBCs are units from which approximately two-thirds of WBCs are removed, without filtration, by the method used to separate blood into components. If WBCs mediate TRIM, buffy-coat-rich (non-WBC-reduced) RBCs should have more of a TRIM effect than buffy-coat-reduced (non-WBC-reduced) RBCs.

Patients randomized to receive autologous or WBC-reduced allogeneic RBCs received units that were either replete with or devoid of WBC-derived soluble

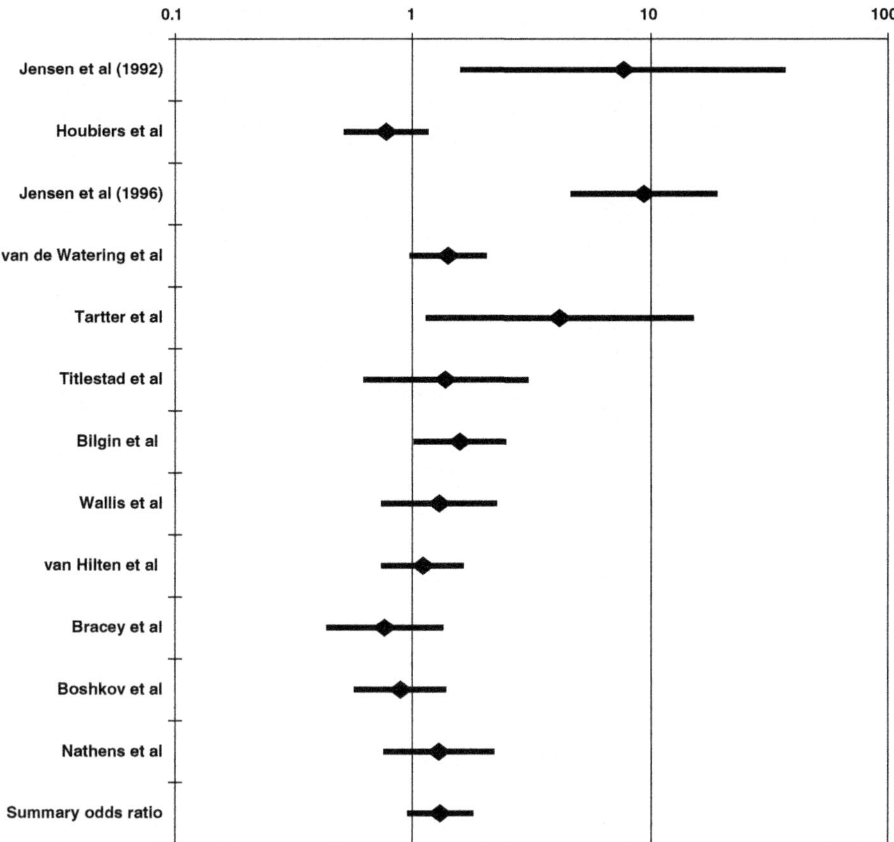

Fig. 13.1 Risk of postoperative infection after transfusion of non-WBC-reduced allogeneic RBCs or whole blood, as compared with transfusion of WBC-reduced allogeneic RBCs or whole blood. Randomized controlled trials (RCTs) of ABT and postoperative infection, depicted on a logarithmic scale and in the order of their publication or presentation, and administering either buffy-coat-rich or buffy-coat-reduced allogeneic RBCs or whole blood to the non-WBC-reduced arm, and either pre-storage or post-storage-filtered allogeneic RBCs or whole blood to the WBC-reduced arm [31–42]. The figure shows the odds ratio (OR) of postoperative infection in recipients of non-WBC-reduced versus WBC-reduced allogeneic RBCs or whole blood, as calculated from an intention-to-treat analysis of each study. Although the heterogeneity among the 12 available RCTs precludes any integration of their findings by the methods of meta-analysis, the figure shows a summary OR calculated by the random-effects method of DerSimonian–Laird *solely* for the purpose of illustration. A deleterious ABT effect (and thus a benefit from WBC reduction) across the 12 RCTs would be demonstrated by an OR > 1, provided that the effect were statistically significant ($p < 0.05$; i.e., provided that the associated 95 % confidence interval [CI] of the summary OR did not include the null value of 1). No such effect is detected here because the 95 % CI of the summary odds ratio includes the null value of 1. More specifically, with the caveat that this exercise reflects no real biologic effect owing to the medical heterogeneity of the studies, when all 6290 patients randomized in the 12 available RCTs are included in intention-to-treat analyses of the 12 studies, no TRIM effect is detected (summary OR = 1.24; 95 % CI, 0.98–1.56; see figure). Similarly, when only the 4460 actually transfused patients are retained in "as-treated" analyses of the 12 studies, again no TRIM effect is detected (summary OR = 1.31; 95 % CI, 0.98–1.75; data not shown) [1, 30]

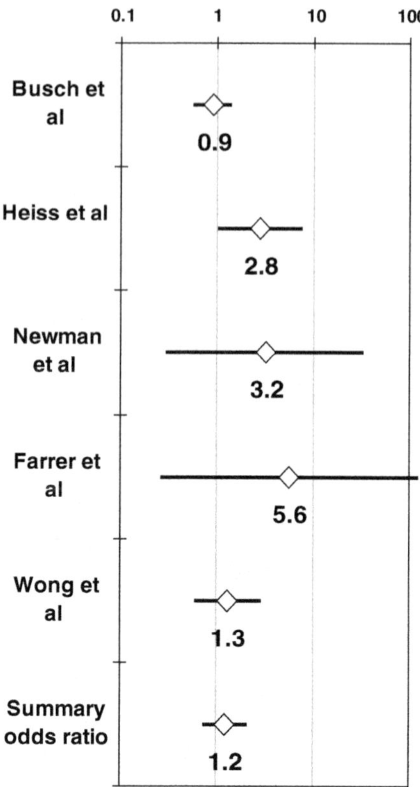

Fig. 13.2 Risk of postoperative infection after transfusion of allogeneic RBCs, as compared with transfusion of autologous RBCs or whole blood. Randomized controlled trials (RCTs) of ABT and postoperative infection, depicted on a logarithmic scale and administering either buffy-coat-rich or buffy-coat-reduced allogeneic RBCs or whole blood to the allogeneic arm, and either autologous RBCs or whole blood obtained by preoperative blood donation [46, 47] or blood procured by ANH, IBR, or PBR to the autologous arm [48–50]. The figure shows the odds ratio (OR) of postoperative infection in recipients of allogeneic versus autologous RBCs or whole blood, as calculated from an intention-to-treat analysis of each study; as well as a summary OR across the 5 RCTs, as calculated from a meta-analysis [51]. There is no deleterious ABT effect (and thus no benefit from autologous transfusion), because the 95 % CI of the summary odds ratio includes the null value of 1 [51]

mediators. During storage of a non-WBC-reduced RBC unit, WBCs deteriorate over 2 weeks, progressively releasing soluble mediators. RBC units that are WBC-reduced by filtration following storage are still replete with WBC-derived mediators because these mediators (in addition to apoptotic or necrotic WBCs) are not removed by WBC reduction filters. RBCs that are WBC-reduced by filtration prior to storage are free of WBC-derived mediators, because their WBCs are removed before they can release mediators into the supernatant fluid [30]. WBCs in stored autologous blood, obtained by preoperative donation, also deteriorate during storage and release mediators. Fresh autologous blood, obtained by acute normovolemic hemodilution

(ANH), intraoperative blood recovery (IBR), or postoperative blood recovery (PBR), and transfused within hours of collection and processing, is free of WBC-derived soluble mediators [51].

WBC reduction, performed either before or after storage, can prevent TRIM effects mediated by allogeneic mononuclear cells (AMCs), but it cannot prevent TRIM effects mediated by soluble molecules circulating in allogeneic plasma. Only pre-storage, as opposed to post-storage, WBC reduction can prevent TRIM effects mediated by WBC-derived, soluble mediators. Autologous transfusion can prevent TRIM effects mediated by AMCs as well as by soluble molecules circulating in allogeneic plasma. Only fresh, as opposed to stored, autologous blood can prevent TRIM effects mediated by WBC-derived, soluble mediators [30, 51].

TRIM Effects Mediated by Allogeneic Mononuclear Cells

The only established TRIM effect (i.e., the beneficial effect of pretransplant ABT on renal allograft survival) appears to require viable WBCs. Patients awaiting renal transplantation derived less immunologic benefit from pretransplant RBC transfusions that are WBC-reduced, washed, or frozen-thawed. Mincheff et al. [52] implicated the dendritic antigen-presenting cells (APCs) of the allogeneic donor in the induction of a state of anergy in the recipient, proposing that during refrigeration APCs lose their ability to deliver co-stimulation. These investigators hypothesized that, following ABT, the recipient's T cells are stimulated by allogeneic donor APCs in the absence of co-stimulation, and this interaction induces a state of anergy in the recipient's T cells.

Animal data suggest that TRIM effects are most likely mediated by transfused allogeneic mononuclear cells [53]. Kao [54] induced immune suppression in mice receiving donor WBCs free of plasma and platelets. A recent theory [55] proposes that donor dendritic cells expressing both alloantigen and the OX-2 (CD200) co-stimulatory molecule are required for the production of the TRIM effect.

Clark et al. [55] demonstrated ABT-induced tumor growth in a murine model that employed BALB/c mice as allogeneic donors and C57B1/6 mice as blood recipients. The recipient mice received a tail vein injection of syngeneic FSL10 fibrosarcoma cells, followed by transfusion of 50–200 μL of allogeneic blood. Pulmonary tumor nodules were counted 3 weeks after the FSL10 cell infusion. There was a dose-response relationship between the volume of transfused allogeneic blood and the number of pulmonary tumor nodules, along with proliferation of TGF-β-positive suppressor T-cells in the spleen.

Donor myeloid dendritic cells that expressed both CD11c and CD200 on their surface appeared to mediate the tumor-growth-promoting effect of ABT, as the effect could be blocked by monoclonal antibodies to either CD11c or CD200. However, the effect could not be blocked by antibodies to CD200R, an observation that implicated a subset of donor myeloid dendritic cells expressing both CD11c and CD200 in the pathogenesis of TRIM. The interaction between the donor CD200 and presumably the cognate receptor on the recipient's T cells induced proliferation of γδ-suppressor T cells that released cytokines, especially TGF-β. Physiological concentrations of TGF-β stimulated proliferation of FSL10 fibrosarcoma cells in vitro. As TGF-β can also suppress host defenses against infectious agents, it could be the basis of the TRIM effect with regard to both postoperative infections and tumor growth, at least with regards to sarcomas.

Bordin and Blajchman [56] reviewed the findings of animal models of ABT and cancer recurrence and reported that 17 published models had found stimulation of tumor growth by ABT, as compared with three models that had reported inhibition of tumor growth and 4 models that had found no effect. Data from both inbred and outbred animal models have indicated that ABT accelerates tumor growth and enhances formation of metastatic nodules [57–60]. Allogeneically transfused mice inoculated intramuscularly with either syngeneic malignant melanoma (B16) or mastocytoma (P815) cells developed larger tumors than did syngeneically transfused mice [58]. Similar results were obtained when syngeneic B16 tumor cells were infused intravenously and the numbers of pulmonary nodules enumerated [58, 59]. Experiments performed to investigate the effect of the tumor-cell dose showed that the ABT effect was only evident when small numbers ($1.25–2.5 \times 10^5$) of tumor cells were inoculated into the host animal. The effect was not evident when larger numbers of tumor cells were inoculated, suggesting that the tumor burden had a strong bearing on whether the ABT effect became manifest.

Studies in both inbred (mice) and outbred (rabbits) animals have shown that ABT has a tumor-growth-promoting effect when administered prior to the infusion of syngeneic tumor cells [57, 60]. In the murine model, male C57Bl/6J mice (MHC type H-2b) were blood recipients; Balb/c mice (MHC type H-2d) were allogeneic donors; and the tumor cells were syngeneic (H-2b) methylcholanthrene-induced fibrosarcoma cells [60]. To better replicate the situation seen clinically, the enhancement of tumor growth by ABT was investigated in animals (mice and rabbits) that received such syngeneic and allogeneic transfusions subsequent to the inoculation of the tumor cells, and the data indicated that ABT-enhanced tumor growth also occurs in animals with established tumors [57]. Is was also shown that animals with either non-established or established tumors receiving non-WBC-reduced ABT developed significantly larger numbers of pulmonary nodules than did animals given WBC-reduced ABT [57, 60].

Finally, the tumor-growth-promoting effect of ABT can be adoptively transferred to naive animals by spleen cells harvested from allogeneically transfused animals [60]. In these experiments, the number of pulmonary nodules observed in animals that had received spleen cells from allogeneically transfused animals was significantly higher than that observed in animals that had received spleen cells from animals transfused with syngeneic blood. Importantly, the ABT effect could not be adoptively transferred to naive animals that received spleen cells derived from animals transfused with pre-storage-WBC-reduced allogeneic blood. Despite convincing results from animal models regarding tumor-promoting effects of non-WBC-reduced ABT [53–60], the findings of RCTs investigating the association between non-WBC-reduced ABT and cancer recurrence in humans [32, 46, 47] have been negative.

The only RCT to study the effect of AMCs has been the Viral Activation Transfusion Study, which studied transfusion-induced activation of endogenous CMV or HIV infection [45]. All RBCs transfused in this study had been stored for less than 2 weeks and could thus be presumed to contain immunologically competent AMCs. There was no difference between the arms of the RCT in HIV-RNA level, the number of CD4-positive T cells, or any other end-point studied. Median survival was 13.0 months in recipients of pre-storage filtered, WBC-reduced allogeneic RBCs, as compared with 20.5 months in recipients of buffy-coat-rich, non-WBC-reduced allogeneic RBCs. This difference was not siginificant in the intention-to-treat analysis ($p=0.12$) but, after adjustment for various prognostic factors, transfusion of non-WBC-reduced RBCs was associated with a better outcome.

TRIM Effects Mediated by White-Cell-Derived Soluble Mediators

Soluble immune response modifiers accumulating during storage of blood components include elastase, histamine, soluble HLA, soluble Fas ligand, transforming growth factor (TGF)-β1 and proinflammatory cytokines IL-1β, IL-6, and IL-8. In vitro, soluble WBC-derived factors from stored RBCs induce immediate up-regulation of expression of inflammatory genes in third-party WBCs. Apoptosis of WBCs begins immediately after the collection of donor blood. Gradual apoptosis and necrosis begins with granulocytes and continues with monocytes, while lymphocytes can remain viable for >25 days at 2–6 °C. Apoptotic cells engage the phosphatidylserine/annexin-V receptor on macrophages, inducing release of prostaglandin E-2 and TGF-β—factors that suppress macrophages and natural-killer cells and impair antigen-presenting capacity.

However, the 12 RCTs that compared the risk of postoperative infection between patients randomized to receive non-WBC-reduced versus WBC-reduced ABT (in the event that they needed perioperative transfusion) have not supported the theory that attributes TRIM to WBC-derived soluble mediators. These RCTs are medically heterogeneous, having been conducted at various settings, having transfused various blood products, and having diagnosed infection based on varying criteria. Thus, not all 12 RCTs targeted a TRIM effect that was *biologically* similar in all cases, making it inappropriate to combine the results of all 12 RCTs in a meta-analysis [1, 30]. However, if we were to integrate these findings despite the extreme heterogeneity of the studies, we would find no association between non-WBC-reduced ABT and an increased risk of infection across all the available RCTs, whether we relied on "intention-to-treat" analyses (that retain all randomized subjects, whether transfused or not) or on "as-treated" analyses (that remove the untransfused subjects—Fig. 13.1).

What has medical relevance, however, is the integration of medically homogeneous studies. Integration of such subsets of homogeneous studies produced results antithetical from those expected from theory. Across 9 RCTs transfusing allogeneic RBCs filtered before storage to the WBC-reduced arm, and enrolling approximately 5000 subjects, no TRIM effect was detected. If WBC-derived, soluble mediators did cause TRIM, pre-storage filtration should abrogate any increased infection risk associated with non-WBC-reduced ABT. Thus, a deleterious TRIM effect would be expected in this analysis, but no such effect was found (summary odds ratio [OR] = 1.06; 95 % confidence interval [CI], 0.91–1.24; $p > 0.05$) [30].

In contrast, across the 4 RCTs transfusing allogeneic RBCs or whole blood filtered after storage to the non-WBC-reduced arm, there was a 2.25-fold increase in the risk of infection in association with non-WBC-reduced ABT (summary OR = 2.25; 95 % CI, 1.12–4.25; $p < 0.05$) [30]. Thus, the TRIM effect appeared to be prevented by post-storage filtration, contradicting the theory that attributes TRIM to WBC-derived, soluble mediators. Such mediators would have been present equally in both the non-WBC-reduced and WBC-reduced RBCs, because they would not have been removed by post-storage filtration.

TRIM Effects Mediated by Soluble Molecules Circulating in Allogeneic Plasma

Only 1 RCT has been specifically designed to study the effects of soluble HLA molecules circulating in allogeneic plasma as mediators of TRIM. Wallis et al. [38] randomized patients undergoing open-heart surgery to receive plasma-reduced, buffy-coat-reduced, or WBC-reduced RBCs. The highest risk of infection was observed in the plasma-reduced arm, although the difference between the three arms was not significant. This finding suggested that plasma removal does not prevent TRIM; or, by extension, that allogeneic plasma does not mediate TRIM. Similarly, integration of the 5 RCTs [46–50] that compared recipients of allogeneic versus autologous blood demonstrated no increased risk of infection in association with ABT [51], whether the analysis included all studies (Fig. 13.2) or was limited to RCTs transfusing blood obtained through ANH, IBR, or PBR to the autologous arm of the studies [48–50].

Association of Non-white-cell-reduced Allogeneic Blood Transfusion with Postoperative Mortality

The association of non-WBC-reduced ABT with short-term mortality from all causes started out as a data-derived hypothesis to account for an unexpected transfusion effect. The RCT of van de Watering et al. [34] had been designed to investigate differences in postoperative infection between recipients of non-WBC-reduced versus WBC-reduced allogeneic RBCs. However, it detected, instead, differences in 60-day mortality between the arms (Fig. 13.3). The authors suggested that non-WBC-reduced ABT may predispose to MOF, which, in turn, may predispose to mortality.

If 11 medically heterogeneous RCTs reported before 2005 and comparing recipients of non-WBC-reduced versus WBC-reduced ABT and reporting on short-term mortality [33, 34, 36–44] were to be combined, there would be no increase in mortality in association with non-WBC-reduced ABT (Fig. 13.3) [1]. These studies transfused to the non-WBC-reduced arm either buffy-coat-rich or buffy-coat-reduced allogeneic RBCs; as already discussed, the former should have more of an effect than the latter. However, this theoretical prediction is the opposite of what the analysis actually showed. Across 6 RCTs transfusing buffy-coat-reduced RBCs to the non-WBC-reduced arm, and pre-storage filtered RBCs to the WBC-reduced arm, there was a 60 % increase in mortality in association with non-WBC-reduced ABT (summary OR = 1.60; 95 % CI, 1.14–2.24; $p<0.05$) [1]. In this analysis, pre-storage filtration appeared to abrogate an increased mortality risk, but the benefit from pre-storage filtration was not seen where more of an ABT effect would have been expected. Across the RCTs that transfused buffy-coat-rich RBCs to the non-WBC-reduced arm, no ABT effect was detected, although some 4500 subjects had been enrolled in these studies.

Perhaps, the benefit observed in the analysis of studies transfusing buffy-coat-reduced versus pre-storage filtered RBCs was due to overrepresentation in that analysis of the cardiac surgery studies: three of the six RCTs included in that analysis (i.e., the studies by van de Watering et al. [34], Bilgin et al. [37], and Wallis et al. [38]) had been conducted in open-heart surgery. Across all 5 RCTs conducted in cardiac surgery [34, 37, 38, 40, 41] (Fig. 13.3), there was a 72 % increase in mortality in association with non-WBC-reduced ABT (summary OR = 1.72; 95 % CI, 1.05–2.81; $p<0.05$). In contrast, across the remaining 6 RCTs conducted in other surgical settings (Fig. 13.3), there was no ABT effect (summary OR = 0.99; 95 % CI, 0.73–1.33; $p>0.05$) [1].

Thus, the ABT-related mortality risk, which is not seen in any other setting, may relate to another effect present in patients undergoing cardiac surgery. During open-heart surgery, blood is exposed to the extracorporeal circuit, as well as to hypothermia and to ischemic and reperfusion injury. These insults are potent inducers of a stress response, triggering a systemic inflammatory response syndrome (SIRS), which is immediately counteracted by a compensatory anti-inflammatory response syndrome (CARS) [61]. SIRS manifests with leukocytosis, capillary leakage, and organ dysfunction; overwhelming SIRS causes a dormant state of metabolism referred to as multiple-organ-dysfunction syndrome (MODS). CARS has an immune-paralyzing effect characterized by anti-inflammatory cytokines, such as TGF-β1, IL-4, and IL-10. Through the intervention of CARS, the post-perfusion SIRS of cardiac surgery generally resolves. However, any intervention by biologic response modifiers during an already-existing inflammatory cascade can push the SIRS/CARS equilibrium toward SIRS, thereby leading to MODS, MOF, and death. WBC-

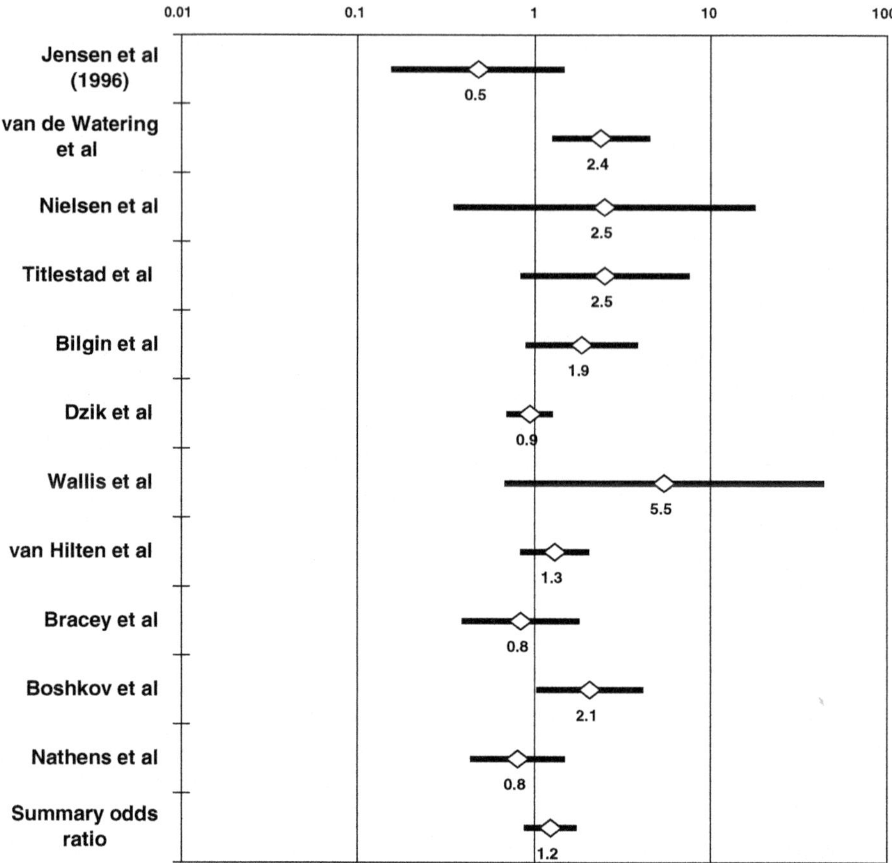

Fig. 13.3 Postoperative mortality after transfusion of non-WBC-reduced allogeneic RBCs, as compared with transfusion of WBC-reduced allogeneic RBCs. Randomized controlled trials (RCTs) investigating the association of non-WBC-reduced allogeneic blood transfusion (ABT) with short-term (up to 3-months post-transfusion) mortality from all causes, depicted on a logarithmic scale and in the order of their publication or presentation, and administering either buffy-coat-rich or buffy-coat-reduced allogeneic RBCs to the non-WBC-reduced arm, and either pre-storage or post-storage-filtered allogeneic RBCs to the WBC-reduced arm [33, 34, 36–44]. For each RCT, the figure shows the odds ratio (OR) of short-term mortality in recipients of non-WBC-reduced versus WBC-reduced allogeneic RBCs, as calculated from an intention-to-treat analysis of each study. Although the heterogeneity among the 11 available RCTs precludes their integration by the methods of meta-analysis, the figure shows a summary OR calculated by the random-effects method of DerSimonian–Laird *solely* for the purpose of illustration. There is no deleterious ABT effect (and thus no benefit from WBC reduction), because the 95 % CI of the summary odds ratio includes the null value of 1 [1]

containing ABT administered during cardiac surgery may provide this "second hit," exacerbating the SIRS and potentially causing the patient's death [61]. However, this explanation is speculative as, hitherto, no cardiac-surgery RCT has reported an association between non-WBC-reduced (versus WBC-reduced) ABT and MOF. In the completed cardiac-surgery RCTs, non-WBC-reduced ABT was not associated with any particular cause of death, yet the aggregate mortality was higher in the non-WBC-reduced arm than in the WBC-reduced arm [1].

Bilgin et al. [62] investigated the pro- and anti-inflammatory cytokine profiles in patients participating in their cardiac-surgery RCT that compared recipients of buffy-coat-reduced versus WBC-reduced allogeneic RBCs [37]. Patients who developed postoperative infection had higher IL-6, and patients who developed MODS had higher IL-12 concentrations, in the subgroup of subjects who received more than three non-WBC-reduced RBC units. These findings supported the authors' thesis that non-WBC-reduced ABT amplifies an inflammatory response which is a "second hit" superimposed upon the on-going SIRS induced by cardiac surgery. Such a "second-hit" inflammatory response may subsequently lead to a more profound CARS which amounts to transfusion-induced immunosuppression predisposing to enhanced susceptibility to postoperative infection.

Bilgin et al. [63] also presented a combined observational analysis of the data from the 2 Dutch RCTs [34, 37] conducted in cardiac surgery. After adjusting for confounding factors in the combined data set, it was the *plasma* (rather than the RBC) transfusions that were associated with higher mortality in patients undergoing open-heart surgery. Non-WBC-reduced RBC transfusion was also significantly associated with postoperative infection [63]. The authors concluded that, although it is difficult to separate the effects of the concomitantly administered allogeneic blood components (non-WBC-reduced or WBC-reduced RBCs, platelets, and plasma), future ABT studies in cardiac surgery should consider the possible adverse effects of all these various transfused blood components.

More recently there have been challenges [64, 65] to the two-hit SIRS/CARS model postulated by Bilgin et al. [61] to account for the mechanism of the TRIM effect(s) in cardiac surgery. Jackman et al. [64] studied immunomodulation in transfused trauma patients and delineated distinct roles of trauma and ABT in inducing immune modulation post-injury. They demonstrated broad shifts in the expression of soluble immune mediators following traumatic injury and ABT, including *early* anti-inflammatory responses in contrast with the *later* anti-inflammatory (hence immunomodulatory) responses envisioned by the SIRS/CARS model. Xiao et al. [65] found that, of the 20,720 genes investigated, expression of 16,820 (>80 %) was significantly altered in blood WBCs after blunt trauma, appropriately naming this response a "genomic storm." Early responses involved an increase in the expression of genes regulating innate immunity, microbial recognition, and inflammation; but also in anti-inflammatory mediators such as those involved with the IL-10 signaling pathway.

Observational Studies "Before-and-After" White-Cell Reduction

As initially conceived, adverse TRIM effects such as cancer recurrence and postoperative infection pertained to *all* patients, as opposed to immunocompromised patients or patients from specific clinical settings (such as open-heart surgery). Accordingly, if such adverse TRIM effects were confirmed by RCTs, and if allogeneic WBCs were shown to mediate the TRIM effects, implementation of *universal* WBC reduction (of *all* transfused cellular blood components) would be indicated for the prevention of the adverse TRIM effects. Although the European debate focused on the appropriateness of implementing universal WBC reduction for the prevention of transmission of variant Creutzfeldt-Jakob disease prions by transfusion, the North-American debate concentrated on the appropriateness of introducing universal WBC reduction for the prevention of the adverse TRIM effects. The outcome of this policy debate in the early twenty-first century was that Canada implemented universal WBC reduction, but the US did not [66, 67].

After Canada and many western European countries implemented universal WBC reduction by means of pre-storage filtration of the cellular blood components, it became possible to compare the risk of infection or mortality in recipients of non-WBC-reduced RBCs before implementation of WBC reduction with the risk of infection or mortality in recipients of WBC-reduced RBCs after implementation of WBC reduction. Such observational studies cannot establish causal relationships. Five studies have reported data on the risk of infection and/or short-term mortality [68].

A large Canadian study included 9525 patients undergoing cardiac surgery, 1731 patients undergoing orthopedic surgery, and 3530 patients admitted to the ICU. A statistically significant ($p=0.04$) decrease in short-term mortality (from 7.0 to 6.2 %) after WBC reduction was found but without a concomitant reduction in the risk of postoperative infection [69]. The data-derived hypothesis offered was that the observed decrease in the number of deaths was not mediated through suppression of the recipient's immune function, but through a pro-inflammatory microvascular effect of transfused WBCs that affects several organ systems. This hypothesis was buttressed by the findings of a companion before-and-after study in premature infants [70]. In that setting, the implementation of universal WBC reduction coincided with a reduction in several secondary morbidity outcomes from several organ systems (i.e., bronchopulmonary dysplasia, retinopathy of prematurity, necrotizing enterocolitis)—an observation consistent with a diffuse pro-inflammatory microvascular effect of allogeneic WBCs.

However, when all before-and-after studies were considered together in a meta-analysis [68], and the findings of the unadjusted analyses from five studies were integrated, there was an unadjusted association of WBC reduction with a decreased risk of postoperative infection. This association did not persist when findings from the multivariate analyses of the three observational studies that had adjusted for the effects of prognostic factors were integrated. There was neither an unadjusted nor an adjusted association of WBC reduction with decreased short-term mortality [68].

Conclusions

TRIM appears to be a real biologic phenomenon resulting in at least one established beneficial clinical effect in humans, the enhanced survival of renal allografts in patients receiving pretransplant ABT, but the existence of deleterious clinical TRIM effects manifest across other clinical settings has not been demonstrated in RCTs. Except for cardiac surgery, there is no setting where the results of the RCTs of deleterious TRIM effects have been consistent. In cardiac-surgery patients, the use of non-WBC-reduced ABT has been consistently associated with increased mortality, but, even in this setting, the reasons for the excess deaths remain elusive. Until further studies are conducted to pinpoint the mechanisms for these excess deaths (or to refute this association), all cellular blood components transfused in cardiac surgery should be WBC-reduced. However, at this time, the totality of the evidence from RCTs does not support a policy of universal WBC reduction of *all* transfused cellular blood components introduced specifically to prevent TRIM [66, 67].

The evidence for implementing universal WBC reduction for the prevention of the TRIM effects may not be available, because the requisite studies have not been conducted. The design of the available RCTs has not been based on specific hypotheses about the mechanisms of TRIM formulated in the preclinical studies. For example, animal models of ABT and tumor growth have convincingly documented that allogeneic blood containing functional dendritic cells can facilitate the growth of selected tumors. However, none of the available RCTs of ABT and cancer recurrence has transfused fresh, non-WBC-reduced RBCs to test this theory. Indeed, in many cases, the preclinical studies were conducted and the hypotheses about mechanisms formulated after clinical studies (including RCTs) had already presented data-derived hypotheses to account for unexpected ABT effects. Because it has not been possible to conduct further RCTs after the hypotheses about TRIM mediators were crystallized, we may never know whether some adverse TRIM effects exist (or not) in humans, since we have been unable to test for them in RCTs. Moreover, it is possible that the available RCTs have targeted outcomes that did not capture the true nature of the ABT effect. If this effect were "pro-inflammatory" rather than "immunomodulatory," it would have been expected to result not in clinical impairment of the recipient's immunity, but in multiple-organ dysfunction. MOF and related outcomes were not studied in most completed RCTs.

Following a great interest in TRIM in the 1990s and the early years of the twenty-first century, remarkably few clinical studies on the adverse TRIM effects (and even the mechanisms of these effects) appeared in the last decade. This is partly due to the fact that each country's policy decisions vis-à-vis implementing universal WBC reduction had already been made in the early years of the twenty-first century [66, 67]; it is partly also due to the fact that funding of research was redirected from research into *bona fide* TRIM effects to the investigation of the deleterious effects of RBCs stored for prolonged periods. After RCTs from 1993 to 2004 of non-WBC-reduced versus WBC-reduced ABT reported no adverse TRIM effect(s) vis-à-vis cancer recurrence and postoperative infection (with the exception of cardiac surgery), funding for further investigation was directed instead to the possible deleterious effects of the transfusion of "old" (versus "fresh") RBCs (Chap. 9).

References

1. Vamvakas EC, Blajchman MA. Transfusion-related immunomodulation (TRIM): an update. Blood Rev. 2007;21:327–48.
2. Opelz G, Sengar DP, Mickey MR, et al. Effect of blood transfusions on subsequent kidney transplants. Transplant Proc. 1973;5:253–9.
3. Brunson ME, Alexander JW. Mechanisms of transfusion-induced immunosuppression. Transfusion. 1990;30:651–8.
4. Blajchman MA, Bordin JO. Mechanisms of transfusion-associated immunosuppression. Curr Opin Hematol. 1994;1:457–61.
5. Vamvakas EC. Possible mechanisms of allogeneic blood transfusion-associated postoperative infection. Transf Med Rev. 2002;16:144–60.
6. Blajchman MA, Singal DP. The role of red blood cell antigens, histocompatibility antigens, and blood transfusions on renal allograft survival. Transfus Med Rev. 1989;3:171–9.
7. van Twuyver E, Mooijaart RJD, Tem Berge IJM, et al. Pretransplantation blood transfusion revisited. N Engl J Med. 1991;325:1210–3.
8. Norman DJ, Wetzsteon P, Barry JM, Fisher S. Blood transfusion are beneficial in HLA-identical sibling kidney transplants. Transplant Proc. 1985;17:23–6.
9. Ross WB, Yap PL. Blood transfusion and organ transplantation. Blood Rev. 1990;4:252–8.
10. Sells RA, Scott MH, Prieto M, Bone JM, Evans GM, Millar R, et al. Early rejection following donor-specific transfusion prior an HLA-mismatched living related renal transplantation. Transplant Proc. 1989;21:1173–4.
11. Opelz G, Vanrenterghem Y, Kirste G, et al. Prospective evaluation of pretransplant blood transfusions in cadaver kidney recipients. Transplantation. 1997;63:964–7.
12. Sanfilippo FP, Bollinger RR, Macquin JM, Brooks BJ, Koepke JA. A randomized study comparing leukocyte-depleted versus packed red cell transfusions in prospective cadaver renal allograft recipients. Transfusion. 1985;25:116–9.
13. Hiesse C, Busson M, Buisson C, et al. Multicenter trial of one HLA-DR matched or mismatched blood transfusion prior to cadaveric renal transplantation. Kidney Int. 2001;60:341–9.
14. Horimi T, Terasaki PI, Chia D, Sasaki B. Factors influencing the paradoxical effect of transfusions on kidney transplants. Transplantation. 1983;35:320–3.
15. Bektas H, Jörns A, Klempnauer J. Differential effect of donor-specific blood transfusions after kidney, heart, pancreas, and skin transplantation in major histocompatibility complex-incompatible rats. Transfusion. 1997;37:226–30.
16. Opelz G, Terasaki PI. Improvement of kidney-graft survival with increased numbers of blood transfusions. N Engl J Med. 1978;299:799–803.
17. Opelz G. Current relevance of the transfusion effect in renal transplantation. Transplant Proc. 1985;17:1015–21.
18. Solheim BG. The role of pre-transplant blood transfusions. Transplant Proc. 1979;11:140–4.
19. Chen W, Lee S, Colby J, et al. The impact of pre-transplant red blood cell transfusions in renal allograft rejection. Rockville, MD: Agency for Healthcare Research and Quality Technology Assessment Report (Project ID# RENT0610); 2012.
20. Macdougall IC, Obrador GT. How important is transfusion avoidance in 2013? Nephrol Dial Transplant. 2013;28:1092–9.
21. Obrador GT, Macdougall IC. Effect of red cell transfusions on future kidney transplantation. Clin J Am Soc Nephrol. 2013;8:852–60.

22. Scornik JC, Bromberg JS, Norman D, Bhanderi M, Gitlin M, Petersen J. An update on the impact of pre-transplant transfusions and allosensitization on time to renal transplant and on allograft survival. BMC Nephrol. 2013;14:217.
23. Scornik JC, Meier-Kriesche HU. Blood transfusions in organ transplant patients: mechanisms of sensitization and implications for prevention. Am J Transplant. 2011;11:1785–91.
24. Marti HP, Henschkowski J, Laux G, et al. Effect of donor-specific transfusions on the outcome of renal allografts in the cyclosporine era. Transpl Int. 2006;19:19–26.
25. Vamvakas EC, Blajchman MA, editors. Immunomodulatory effects of blood transfusion. Bethesda, MD: AABB Press; 1999. 295 pp.
26. Blumberg N, Heal JM. Effects of transfusion on immune function: cancer recurrence and infection. Arch Pathol Lab Med. 1994;118:371–9.
27. Vamvakas E. Perioperative blood transfusion and cancer recurrence: meta-analysis for explanation. Transfusion. 1995;35:760–8.
28. Vamvakas E, Moore SB. Blood transfusions and postoperative septic complication. Transfusion. 1994;34:714–27.
29. Blumberg N, Zhao H, Wang H, Messing S, Heal JM, Lyman OH. The intention-to-treat principle in clinical trials and meta-analyses of leukoreduced blood transfusions in surgical patients. Transfusion. 2007;47:573–81.
30. Vamvakas E. Why have meta-analyses of the randomized controlled trials of the association between non-white-blood-cell-reduced allogeneic blood transfusions and postoperative infection produced discordant results? Vox Sang. 2007;93:196–207.
31. Jensen LS, Andersen AJ, Christiansen PM, et al. Postoperative infection and natural killer cell function following blood transfusion in patients undergoing elective colorectal surgery. Br J Surg. 1992;79:513–6.
32. Houbiers JGA, Brand A, van de Watering LMG, et al. Randomized controlled trial comparing transfusion of leucocyte-depleted or buffy-coat-depleted blood in surgery for colorectal cancer. Lancet. 1994;344:573–8.
33. Jensen LS, Kissmeyer-Nielsen P, Wolff B, et al. Randomized comparison of leucocyte-depleted versus buffy-coat-poor blood transfusion and complications after colorectal surgery. Lancet. 1996;348:841–5.
34. van de Watering LMG, Hermans J, Houbiers JGA, et al. Beneficial effect of leukocyte depletion of transfused blood on post-operative complications in patients undergoing cardiac surgery: a randomized clinical trial. Circulation. 1998;97:562–8.
35. Tartter PI, Mohandas K, Azar P, et al. Randomized trial comparing packed red cell blood transfusion with and without leukocyte depletion for gastrointestinal surgery. Am J Surg. 1998;176:462–6.
36. Titlestad IL, Ebbesen LS, Ainsworth AP, et al. Leukocyte-depletion of blood components does not significantly reduce the risk of infectious complications: results of a double-blind, randomized study. Int J Colorectal Dis. 2001;16:147–53.
37. Bilgin YM, van de Watering LMG, Eijsman L, et al. Double-blind, randomized controlled trial on the effect of leukocyte-depleted erythrocyte transfusions in cardiac valve surgery. Circulation. 2004;109:2755–60.
38. Wallis JP, Chapman CE, Orr KE, et al. Effect of WBC reduction of transfused RBCs on postoperative infection rates in cardiac surgery. Transfusion. 2002;42:1127–34.
39. van Hilten JA, van de Watering LMG, van Bockel JH, et al. Effects of transfusion with red cells filtered to remove leukocytes: randomized controlled trial in patients undergoing major surgery. BMJ. 2004;328:1281–4.
40. Bracey AW, Radovancevick R, Nussimeier NA, et al. Leukocyte-reduced blood in open-heart surgery patients: effects on outcome. Transfusion. 2002;42(Suppl):5S.
41. Boshkov LK, Furnary A, Morris C, Chien G, van Winkle D, Reik R. Pre-storage leukoreduction of red cells in elective cardiac surgery: results of a double-blind randomized controlled trial. Blood. 2004;104:112a.
42. Nathens AB, Nester TA, Rubenfeld GD, Nirula R, Gernsheimer TB. The effects of leukoreduced blood transfusion on infection risk following injury: a randomized controlled trial. Shock. 2006;26:342–7.

43. Nielsen HJ, Hammer JH, Kraup AL, et al. Pre-storage leukocyte filtration may reduce leukocyte-derived bioactive substance accumulation in patients operated for burn trauma. Burns. 1999;25:162–70.
44. Dzik WH, Anderson JK, O'Neill EM, et al. A prospective, randomized clinical trial of universal WBC reduction. Transfusion. 2002;42:1114–22.
45. Collier A, Kalish L, Busch M, et al. Leukocyte-reduced red blood cell transfusions in patients with anemia and human immunodeficiency virus infection. JAMA. 2001;285:1592–601.
46. Busch ORC, Hop WCJ, van Papendrecht MAWH, et al. Blood transfusion and prognosis in colorectal cancer. N Engl J Med. 1993;328:1372–6.
47. Heiss MM, Mempel W, Jausch K-W, et al. Beneficial effect of autologous blood transfusion on infectious complications after colorectal cancer surgery. Lancet. 1993;342:1328–33.
48. Newman JH, Bowers M, Murphy J. The clinical advantages of autologous transfusion: a randomized, controlled study after knee replacement. J Bone Joint Surg Br. 1997;79:630–2.
49. Farrer A, Spark JI, Scott DJ. Autologous blood transfusion: the benefits for the patient undergoing abdominal aortic aneurysm repair. J Vasc Nurs. 1997;15:111–5.
50. Wong JCL, Torella F, Haynes SL, et al. Autologous versus allogeneic transfusion in aortic surgery: a multicenter randomized clinical trial. Ann Surg. 2002;235:145–51.
51. Vamvakas E. Meta-analysis of randomized controlled trials comparing the risk of postoperative infection between recipients of allogeneic and autologous blood transfusion. Vox Sang. 2002;83:339–46.
52. Mincheff MS, Meryman HT, Kapoor V, et al. Blood transfusion and immunomodulation: a possible mechanism. Vox Sang. 1993;65:18–24.
53. Bordin JO, Heddle NM, Blajchman MA. Biologic effects of leukocytes present in transfused cellular blood products. Blood. 1994;84:1705–21.
54. Kao KJ. Induction of humoral immune tolerance to major histocompatibility complex antigens by transfusions of UV-B irradiated leukocytes. Blood. 1996;88:4375–82.
55. Clark DA, Gorczynski RM, Blajchman MA. Transfusion-related immunomodulation due to peripheral blood dendritic cells expressing the CD200 tolerance-signaling molecule and alloantigen. Transfusion. 2008;48(5):814–21.
56. Bordin JO, Blajchman MA. Blood transfusion and tumor growth in animal models. In: Vamvakas EC, Blajchman MA, editors. Immunomodulatory effects of allogeneic blood transfusion. Bethesda, MD: AABB Press; 1999. p. 29–42.
57. Bordin JO, Bardossy L, Blajchman MA. Growth enhancement of established tumors by allogeneic blood transfusion in experimental animals and its amelioration by leukodepletion: the importance of timing of the leukodepletion. Blood. 1994;84:344–8.
58. Shirwadkar S, Blajchman MA, Frame B, Singal DP. Effect of allogeneic blood transfusion on solid tumor growth and pulmonary metastases in mice. J Cancer Res Clin Oncol. 1992;118:76–180.
59. Shirwadkar S, Blajchman MA, Frame B, Orr FW, Singal DP. Effect of blood transfusions on experimental pulmonary metastases in mice. Transfusion. 1990;30:188–90.
60. Blajchman MA, Bardossy I, Carmen R, Sastry A, Singal DP. Allogeneic blood transfusion-induced enhancement of tumor growth: two animal models showing amelioration by leukodepletion and passive transfer using spleen cells. Blood. 1993;81:1880–2.
61. Bilgin YM, Brand A. Transfusion-related immunomodulation (TRIM): a second hit in an inflammatory cascade? Vox Sang. 2008;95:261–71.
62. Bilgin YM, van de Watering LMG, Versteegh MIM, van Oers MHJ, Brand A. The effects of allogeneic blood transfusions during cardiac surgery on inflammatory mediators and postoperative complications. Crit Care Med. 2010;38:546–52.
63. Bilgin YM, van de Watering LMG, Versteegh MIM, van Oers MHJ, Brand A. Postoperative complications associated with transfusions of platelets and plasma in cardiac surgery. Transfusion. 2011;51:2603–10.
64. Jackman RP, Utter GH, Muench MO, et al. Distinct roles of trauma and transfusion in induction of immune modulation post-injury. Transfusion. 2012;52:2533–50.

65. Xiao W, Mindrinos MN, Seok J, et al. A genomic storm in critically-ill injured humans. J Exp Med. 2011;208:2581–90.
66. Thurer RL, Luban NLC, AuBuchon JP, et al. Universal WBC reduction. Transfusion. 2000;40:751–2.
67. Vamvakas EC, Blajchman MA. Universal WBC reduction: the case for and against. Transfusion. 2001;41:691–712.
68. Vamvakas EC. White-blood-cell containing allogeneic blood transfusion, postoperative infection, and mortality: a meta-analysis of observational, "before-and-after" studies. Vox Sang. 2004;86:111–9.
69. Hébert PC, Fergusson D, Blajchman MA, et al. Clinical outcomes following institution of the Canadian universal leukoreduction program for red blood cell transfusions. JAMA. 2003;289:1941–9.
70. Fergusson D, Hébert PC, Lee SK, et al. Clinical outcomes following institution of universal leukoreduction of blood transfusions for premature infants. JAMA. 2003;289:1950–6.

Index

J.S. Lee, M.P. Donahoe (eds.), *Hematologic Abnormalities and Acute Lung Syndromes*, Respiratory Medicine, DOI 10.1007/978-3-319-41912-1

CPSIA information can be obtained
at www.ICGtesting.com
Printed in the USA
LVOW02*2305031116
R11553600001B/R115536PG511374LVX3B/1/P